AMERICA FOOLED

FOOLED

The Truth About Antidepressants, Antipsychotics and How We've Been Deceived

DR. TIMOTHY SCOTT

Argo Publishing, LLC
Victoria, Texas

NOTE TO READERS CURRENTLY
ON ANTIDEPRESSANTS OR ANTIPSYCHOTICS
Stopping antidepressants or antipsychotics abruptly commonly results in mild withdrawal symptoms, but for some individuals the withdrawal reaction is severe. Appendix 1 should be read before stopping these drugs.

Printed and bound by Maple–Vail Book Manufacturing Group

Library of Congress Cataloging–in–Publication Data
Scott, Timothy, 1954–
America fooled : the truth about antidepressants, antipsychotics, and how we've been deceived / Timothy Scott.
    p. ; cm.
Includes bibliographical references and index.
ISBN–13: 978–0–9773075–0–0 (hardcover : alk. paper)
ISBN–10: 0–9773075–0–6 (hardcover : alk. paper)
1. Medical misconceptions. 2. Depression, Mental—Chemotherapy—Side effects. 3. Schizophrenia—Chemotherapy—Side effects. 4. Psychoses—Chemotherapy. 5. Drugs—Side effects. 6. Medical ethics. 7. Consumer education.
[DNLM: 1. Psychotropic Drugs—adverse effects. 2. Biological Psychiatry—ethics. 3. Clinical Trials—ethics. 4. Psychopharmacology—ethics. 5. Research Design. QV 77.2 S429a 2006] I. Title.

RM333.5.S36 2006
338.4'76157882—dc22
                                        2005034904

ISBN   0–9773075–0–6

To my wife Nita —

*For more than three decades
my best friend, greatest encourager,
constant helper and faithful partner
in all things truly important*

Acknowledgments

As this work comes to a conclusion, I feel a great sense of appreciation for so many who have assisted me in writing a better book than I could have written on my own. Many have graciously contributed their knowledge, their expertise or their experiences from their own lives. Every personal story is factual (though names have been changed), and I appreciate the friends and former clients who consented to be interviewed (some two or three times). Ronald Wilson, whose father's work is described in Chapter 1, courageously revealed facts that are painful and very personal in order to contribute to the greater good—facts I would never have learned without his openness during our conversations. Numerous researchers (unfortunately, too many to name) graciously responded to inquiries concerning their research, and often shared insights which I would have otherwise missed. Shirley Parkan has for many years been the ideal library assistant, cheerfully gathering research materials from libraries near and far. She and her helpers Susan, JoAnn and Lou Ellen are greatly appreciated. Ray McGlothlin, Sara Sawey, Lula Jackson and Leanna Paul carefully examined every word and made numerous helpful comments and suggestions. Glenn Hand, Bernie Fulks, Beverly Bruns and Jean Gisler also helped with editing. My wife Nita, to whom this book is dedicated, has given beyond measure to what—like every project throughout our lives together——has been a joint effort. Redletter Digital's Christopher Rampey provided much assistance with the design and development of both the dust jacket and the americafooled.com website. My students have also made this a better book. The personal experiences they have shared put flesh on the dry bones of research. The questions they asked clarified issues I most needed to address. I will greatly miss our experiences together during my retirement from the classroom. To those dedicated men and women who are now building a new body of evidence–based medicine I am very grateful. There is a battle being waged between those who are profiting from antidepressants and antipsychotics and those thousands of dedicated researchers contributing to an honest search for truth. Marcia Angell, Jerry Avorn, Fred Baughman, Peter Breggin, David Graham, Joseph Glenmullen, David Healy, Eliot Spitzer, Elliot Valenstein and Sidney Wolfe have been leaders in the effort to see truth prevail. All Americans should be grateful to these individuals. Lastly I must express gratitude to my own parents and my parents by marriage, both of whom are examples of service to others and, thus, an inspiration to me.

Table of Contents

"All truth passes through three stages:
First, it is ridiculed;
Second, it is violently opposed;
Third, it is accepted as being self–evident."[1]
— *Arthur Schopenhauer*
German philosopher

PREFACE

Tom Cruise's appearance on the "Today" show with Matt Lauer in 2005 became the topic of water cooler conversation all across America.[2] Though he was supposed to be promoting his newest movie, "War of the Worlds," the conversation turned to antidepressants and whether or not depression and other mental problems are caused by a chemical imbalance in the brain. Cruise asserted,

> I'm saying that drugs aren't the answer. These drugs are very dangerous. They're mind–altering. . . . There is no such thing as a chemical imbalance.[3]

The American Psychiatric Association's president responded that Cruise's comments were irresponsible.[4] St. Louis psychiatrist Charles Conway declared, "I was shaking my head in disbelief. . . . It's safe to say that we know that metabolic changes in the brain are present for all major mental illnesses."[5]

Harvard psychiatrist Joseph Coyle responded by defending the role of genes, an essential component of the chemical imbalance view. "Scientists have identified some genes that clearly play a role in causing mental illnesses such as depression."[6] A psychiatrist at Washington University in St. Louis defended the traditional view as well while pointing to the influence of both genes and two environmental factors—influenza and oxygen deprivation.

> Babies who suffer low oxygen to the brain during birth are more likely to develop schizophrenia. Children of mothers who got the flu in the second trimester of pregnancy also have a greater risk of getting schizophrenia.[7]

Few psychiatrists came to Cruise's defense. Perhaps his association with the Church of Scientology caused psychiatrists to be standoffish, but the reality is that most psychiatrists are fully convinced that mental problems are caused by chemical imbalances and that there is a strong genetic influence behind these disorders. Put the views of a Hollywood actor next to the declarations of the American Psychiatric Association as well as several psychiatrists involved in scientific research, and deciding which side is right would seem to be easy. The psychiatrists appear to win hands down. But they don't. Cruise was right.

I have been a psychology professor for most of my adult life. What I have long believed is that the single most important skill college students should receive from their education is the ability to read and critique research. Unfortunately, most college graduates have never taken a single research design course. They do not know how to evaluate the research they read. They cannot accurately assess whether a study is of high quality and its findings and conclusions are valid or whether the study's findings and conclusions are completely invalid distortions of truth. They are not aware of how much research is funded by those with a financial interest in a positive outcome. Neither are most physicians aware. They may have been highly trained and be very knowledgeable about a host of issues, but few know how to evaluate research studies. Thus we have a nation where even our college–educated populace can be easily fooled. And they have been.

What Is True?

Truth should never be decided by a vote, by massive multi–million dollar advertising campaigns or by antidepressant drug studies designed and paid for by drug manufacturers. Truth should be decided by an honest, objective assessment of the evidence and by logic. It is not enough to say "I'm right" or "I'm right, and peer–reviewed research found in medical journals proves it." You need to have exact references to the facts which are used to support arguments and conclusions. This book contains over 1,800 references to some of the best of the scientific research. I have sought to present this research using plain and simple language so that it can be clearly understood by those without a research background. But to be convinced, you will have to possess good logical thinking skills as well. For example, see if the following facts and associated questions related to the chemical imbalance theory of depression and the use of antidepressants cause you at least to suspect that something might be wrong with psychiatry's approach to treating depression today.

(1) A study by the National Institute of Mental Health of 18,244 Americans found that among those born before 1905, only 1% had a major depression by age 75. However, younger generations who have had the "benefits" of antidepressants are much more likely to experience a major depression—6% of those born since 1955 having at least one episode by age 25.[8] These facts are not intended to suggest that antidepressants are responsible for the huge increases in depression. But ask yourself this question: Is it reasonable to believe that we would have such dramatic increases if depression is primarily due to a chemical imbalance?

(2) Women, who are much more likely to be given antidepressant prescriptions than men, experience approximately twice as much major depression as men.[9] Are we to believe that women's minds are weaker than men's minds—that is, more prone to develop a chemical imbalance—or that if it were not for antidepressants the disparity between women and men would be even greater? Consider the next related fact before giving an answer.

11

(3) There is huge variation in the amount of depression among the world's countries. Adults in Taiwan and Korea, where antidepressants are rarely used, have very low rates of major depression. Adults in America, Canada and France, where antidepressants are commonly prescribed, have much higher rates.[10] Are western people born inherently inferior to Asian people mentally; that is, more prone to develop a mental disease?

(4) In 1950, when no antidepressants existed,[11] the suicide rates for children and young people were less than half the rates for those same age groups in 2000 despite dramatic growth in antidepressant use among America's youth.[12] In 1950 suicide among the elderly, the age group which is the least likely to use antidepressants, was double today's rate.[13] Someone might argue that the reduction in suicide among the aged can be credited to antidepressants, but are we then to assume that if antidepressants had not been developed and prescribed to children, their increase in suicide would have been even greater?

These facts do not prove that antidepressants cause depression or suicide since correlational studies can never prove antidepressants cause these problems (see Box #P–1, It's So Easy To Be Fooled). However, the fact that growing antidepressant use and increases in depression so often go together should make us at least wonder whether or not antidepressants are really capable of improving mental health.

(5) In 1987 the German equivalent of America's Food and Drug Administration refused to allow Prozac (the only antidepressant drug approved for use by children in America) to be marketed in Germany when studies revealed three times as many suicides among study participants as among those on a placebo.[14] Their studies were particularly disconcerting because, unlike correlational studies which can lead to false conclusions, the Germans used an experimental design. If antidepressants correct the chemical imbalance, why would there be more suicide among those on these drugs?

BOX #P-1

It's So Easy To Be Fooled

How certain can you be? See how many items you can honestly answer with either a "1" or a "5."

Fact 1: Those who were given Flintstones Vitamins as children are more likely to divorce as adults than those not given Flintstones Vitamins.

　　Certain It's True　　1　2　3　4　5　　Certain It's Not True

Fact 2: Foot size is related to knowledge.

　　Certain It's True　　1　2　3　4　5　　Certain It's Not True

Fact 3: Those who grew up eating oatmeal are more likely to develop cancer this year than those who grew up eating Sugar Frosted Flakes.

　　Certain It's True　　1　2　3　4　5　　Certain It's Not True

Fact 4: Those who grew up eating broccoli, asparagus, and cauliflower are less likely to commit violent crimes than those who did not eat those vegetables when they were young.

　　Certain It's True　　1　2　3　4　5　　Certain It's Not True

Do not be insulted even if you are wrong on every item. These are tricky. I will tell you which are true and even explain why in the box on the next page, but, before you turn there, I would challenge you to examine that list again, use your best thinking skills and seek to be certain about which items are true and which are false.

The Bigger Issue

In 2004, following several published studies which found that antidepressants might be increasing suicide among America's children, Congress initiated hearings. I was pleased Congress chose to begin investigating. However, the suicide link is but a small part of a problem which has damaged or destroyed lives beyond number in America and elsewhere. Today Americans have generally become convinced that antidepressants, even if

BOX #P–2

"It's So Easy To Be Fooled" Answers

Here are the answers for Box #P–1: Fact 1 is true as are Facts 2–4. Really! The "why" can be very difficult to see until you hear the explanation (at which point each will likely seem obvious).

Explanation for Fact 1: Flintstones Vitamins did not exist prior to the 1960s. (The Flintstones television show debuted in 1960.[1*]) Earlier generations who did not take Flintstones Vitamins (because they did not exist when they were young) have lower divorce rates than more recent generations.

Explanation for Fact 2: One–year–olds have very small feet and very little knowledge. Two–year–olds have larger feet and more knowledge. Ten–year–olds know much more and have much larger feet than babies. Get it? Even if all adults are considered, there are enough babies and children in the world to make the fact true.

Explanation for Fact 3: The number one predictor of cancer is age.[2] Those in their 80s and 90s who commonly get cancer grew up eating oatmeal, not Sugar Frosted Flakes. That cereal was not marketed until 1952.[3]

Explanation for Fact 4: Poor children are less likely to receive a diet that includes fresh vegetables. Poor children are also more likely to commit violent crime as they grow older.[4]

The point? Even "obvious" answers are often wrong. I keep a file labeled "Research Errors" which is filled with scientific research studies that we later came to realize were erroneous. What do all these studies have in common? Nearly all are correlational studies. Most of the research that has ever been published is correlational research—a research design that fools the public and the researcher, oh, so easily. The far better design which will be discussed in Chapter 1 is what is called a randomized, placebo–controlled trial or RCT. Before you finish this book you will have a great appreciation for the importance of using an RCT research design.

*Endnotes for references inside boxes begin on p. 407.

they do not prove to be effective for children, are clearly effective for adults. And today these mind drugs are taken by adults and children for every imaginable mental problem—anxiety, compulsive behavior, anger, fear, PMS, shyness and even lying.

When a concerned mother wrote "Dear Abby" about her son's habitual lying, her questions clearly indicated that she had been successfully indoctrinated. She wondered if lying was not simply just lying but was perhaps a psychological "condition" caused by a chemical imbalance that could be fixed with a pill.

> Please check with your resources and tell me if there is such a condition as habitual lying. Can it be cured? Is it hereditary? Can it be overcome with age and maturity? I have heard there is such a condition and that medication is available. Is this true?[15]

Unfortunately, "Dear Abby" has also been indoctrinated. Instead of saying "Of course, it is not hereditary," she responded that "the trait is not necessarily inherited." She then suggested psychotherapy (an unfortunate bit of advice) and added, "I have been told that anti–depressants are somewhat effective, but the cure is psychotherapy."[16] If "Dear Abby" is right, then most young boys in America could be helped by antidepressants (and fully cured with psychotherapy) since most young boys are not always truthful.

Because it is increasingly believed that mental and even behavioral problems originate in chemical imbalances in the brain and drugs can improve this chemical imbalance, receiving a prescription for these problems seems reasonable. Questions such as "How helpful are these drugs?", "Are there any long–term health consequences?" and "Do these drugs ever make things worse?" are seldom asked. Those who do ask are nearly always given answers that are wrong. I am convinced most of those answering the questions (physicians) are not purposefully intent on deceiving anyone. It is instead a matter of a nation having come to believe ideas which simply are not true. That is a bold statement, but, using some simple logic again, consider this next set of facts concerning antipsychotics and see if you find them surprising.

(1) Those who develop schizophrenia (that is, lose touch with reality) in many third world countries (India, Nigeria and Columbia) which have

---

BOX #P–3
Schizophrenia Defined

In the past a person with what we term "schizophrenia" today was said to have "gone mad," "lost his mind" or become crazy, demented, disturbed, unbalanced, unhinged or brainsick. In simple terms, those words and phrases described someone who was not thinking clearly, had illogical ideas (false delusions), was seeing or hearing things that were not actually there, was acting in bizarre ways, had very flat or extreme emotions, was speaking in ways that did not make sense or was just mumbling—someone who, in a nutshell, had lost touch with reality.

The condition has always existed though the term "schizophrenia" was not coined until 1911[1] and, unfortunately, the word's literal meaning implies a "multiple personality" condition, not the word's definition. Of course, terms can have both practical common usage meanings and technical definitions. The technical definition comes from the American Psychiatric Association's *Diagnostic and Statistical Manual of Mental Disorders,* 4th ed., and reads as follows:

> Schizophrenia is a disorder that lasts for at least 6 months and includes at least 1 month of active–phase symptoms (i.e. two [or more] of the following: delusions, hallucinations, disorganized speech, grossly disorganized or catatonic behavior, negative symptoms.)[2]

---

less access to antipsychotic drugs have much higher recovery rates than do those in the United States and other wealthy nations who are prescribed these drugs.[17]

(2)   Schizophrenics in America and in other developed countries (high antipsychotic drug–use nations) are nearly twice as likely to receive a "worst possible outcome" diagnosis upon follow–up, compared with those who are diagnosed with schizophrenia in less developed nations.[18]

(3)   Those given antipsychotics have much higher, not lower, relapse rates than those never given these drugs.[19]

(4)   Those on antipsychotics put themselves at risk for numerous health problems, permanent brain damage and early death.[20]

(5)   Two hundred years ago, long before antipsychotics were invented, when someone lost his or her mind and was sent to a moral treatment center

or state hospital practicing moral treatment, he or she was much more like-ly to recover than are Americans who lose their minds today.[21]

If you are a person possessing even an average measure of critical think-ing skills or even an average ability to think logically, then these facts will likely surprise you and should concern you. After all, the primary treatment strategy for dealing with mental disorders today is to prescribe medication.

We as a nation have come to believe mind drugs, whether antidepressants or antipsychotics, are highly effective in treating the chemical imbalances which nearly everyone now believes are the cause of mental problems. And it has been our faith in drugs that has taken our eyes off what does work. That may be the greatest danger of all for mind drugs. This is what *America Fooled* is all about.

A Brief Overview

This book is divided into three parts. Part 1 is focused primarily on anti-depressants, their effectiveness, their side effects and how America has come to believe that chemical imbalances are responsible for depression and other mental problems. Part 2 deals with the various approaches used throughout our history to treat more serious mental problems including the use of antipsychotics, the side effects of antipsychotics and the real reasons people sometimes lose their minds. This is an important part of the book as the story of antidepressants cannot be fully understood without knowing the story of antipsychotics. Part 3 discusses what I call the Continuum Model of mental health and how good mental health can be achieved.

The book also contains 59 boxes which provide additional information to increase your insight and understanding. I do not want you to "just read" this book any more than I have ever wanted my students to "just listen" to my lectures. I want you to make applications and have experiences related to our topic that, hopefully, you will long remember. Thus, some of the boxes require your involvement. If you actually sought to determine with some degree of certainty which of the four "It's So Easy To Be Fooled" facts were true, it was a more profitable experience for you than if you had only read over the facts, the answers and the explanations quickly. Sometimes I will ask you to discover a truth on your own. If you have access to a computer, you can discover for yourself that many of the published antidepressant drug studies are conducted by the very pharmaceutical companies who own the drugs (see Box #7–2, Investigation: How Much Research *Is* Published by the Drug Companies?) or you can experience how drug studies are "authored" by researchers who likely never even saw their article before it was published (see Box #6–1, Guess How Many Authors Wrote This Article). These experiences are enriching, and I hope you will take advantage of them. Please notice that these boxes have their own endnote section beginning on p. 407.

It was the realization that the kind of information I have been sharing in this preface is unknown to most physicians and to most of the public that led me to write this book. I am delighted you are reading it. As I have told my students, I need helpers. I need helpers willing to learn and then willing to share their discoveries with others. I have no doubt that, in today's America, your having this information can help you keep yourself, your family and your friends from being fooled.

A Personal Note to Physicians

Each semester I discover I have several students who have been prescribed antidepressants. I occasionally have students who are on antipsychotics. Typically I learn these facts after one of my lectures on depression, mind drugs or the drug approval process. The students who approach me often express anger that their physician would put them on Zoloft, Paxil or another mind drug in view of the research. I want you to know what I routinely say to these students. The following dialogue is reflective of those conversations and includes my standard response.

My response: I don't think you should get angry at your physician. She is probably very conscientious and works very hard to provide you good medical care. The blame lies not so much with individual physicians as with the drug approval system and the drug companies which today are very knowledgeable about how to design a study that is fraudulent yet capable of getting their drug approved and still be used in marketing and advertising.

Student: But my physician should never have prescribed that drug to me unless she knows it's safe!

My response: You have to remember three facts. First, the information they were taught in college and medical school, the information they receive at medical conferences and the information they are given by drug reps all say that these drugs work. Second, they are seeing patients all day long. I finish teaching my classes by 10:00 a.m. most days. I can spend hours every day reading and critiquing mind drug studies—one issue among the hundreds of issues they have to know about. And third, though physicians in private practice know a lot more than I know about hundreds of health issues, very few have a strong research design background. Most academic physicians could look at many of the studies used to promote these drugs and know very quickly they are worthless, but this is not a skill that many private practice physicians have.

This is a conversation I have every semester—over and over. I have always believed that the only reason you have routinely prescribed mind drugs is because you have genuinely believed that they help your patients. I do not believe you would have done so, any more than you would have routinely prescribed estrogen for all post–menopausal women if you had known the facts we know today. I have written this book to help educate both physicians and the public, not simply to criticize or to make money. (All profits from this first edition will be contributed to Habitat for Humanity.) I appreciate your taking the time to learn more about mind drugs.

Part One

The Antidepressant Story

1

"When I began at FDA, I had no idea of the costs that would be demanded of my family or of me personally. Had I known the cost, and the extreme difficulty of working in an environment that routinely dismisses or twists the truth about drug safety, and punishes you severely for speaking the truth, I'm certain that I would have chosen a different path." [1]

— *David Graham, MD*
FDA Drug Scientist

INTRODUCTION

Every semester I surprise many students (perhaps shock or anger are even more accurate terms) as I share facts related to the FDA's drug approval process. Most students, like most Americans, assume that if a drug has been approved by the FDA, it is both safe and effective. That was an assumption I also presumed to be true at one time. However, the research on many FDA–approved drugs led me to realize that I, too, had been fooled.

Every semester I have students on mind drugs who react with skepticism when I make my initial comments about antidepressants and other mind drugs. I am always impressed with the fact that by the time I conclude the related lectures and have the students do some additional reading, the skepticism is gone. But for the average American, it is hard to believe that the research studies used to get these drugs approved were purposely designed to get the desired results, that the FDA drug approval process relies on the studies provided to them by the drug companies, not by independent or government–sponsored research, or that some FDA employees involved in approving these drugs have been paid huge sums by the very drug companies they are supposed to be regulating.

Add to this the fact that hundreds of millions of dollars (literally) are spent by the drug companies each year convincing the public and physicians that these drugs are the answer to mental problems, and we should not be surprised that my students and many who come to learn the facts feel like they have been fooled. These hundreds of millions are spent promoting mind drugs, but who is willing to spend millions to inform the public of the research on the increase in diabetes, endometrial cancer, breast cancer, permanent brain damage, sexual dysfunction and abnormal bone growth associated with mind drug use? (See Chapters 10, 11 and 13.) There are no deep pockets on this side.

On the other side are pharmaceutical companies which have supported thousands of studies by university professors and other medical researchers with research grants—and have cut off funding to professors who have published papers with a negative view that might hurt drug sales. These are by no means the only ways to control what people come to believe. But, generally, when America gets fooled, there is money involved. The antidepressant and antipsychotic story is still being played out. Huge amounts are still being spent to convince all of us these drugs work. We are still in a kind of battle. My task is to lay out the research so that

(1) you will be less willing to take a pill if you are stressed or depressed;

(2) you will have the information you need to discourage your family members and friends from being harmed; and

(3) you will understand what does work in maintaining and improving good mental health.

In recent years I "prepared" my students for the mind drug saga by first sharing another story. That story also involved a battle for truth. As in the case of the mind drug story, the drug companies controlled what Americans believed, and the harm was immense. But it is now a story we can examine with hindsight as truth has finally prevailed—as it eventually will with mind drugs. The story involves my mother and her experience with hormone replacement therapy (HRT). No one now argues that what has been called "the greatest experiment ever performed on women" was the right course. But it took many years before we were certain that it was a huge mistake, and some continued the experiment years after it should have ended. Those familiar with the research on antipsychotics and antidepressants cannot keep from seeing the parallels with HRT.

My Mother's Life Threatened

My mother's physician recommended she begin taking estrogen following her hysterectomy in 1961. However, my father had concerns about her taking hormone supplements, so she avoided those pills for years—until she began experiencing "hot flashes" shortly before she turned 60. Her friends were also on estrogen, and one declared, "Well, I sure don't want to get osteoporosis in old age. I'm going to keep taking my estrogen." That concern, combined with the discomfort of hot flashes, was enough for Mom to decide it was time to take it herself.[2] For nearly 12 years she faithfully took her Premarin brand of estrogen.[3] (Premarin is derived from **preg**nant **mar**es' **urine**; hence, the name.)

At that time it was not universally agreed that estrogen was linked to breast cancer and endometrial (uterine) cancer, although those concerns had been discussed for decades.[4] Yet even after these cancer risks became widely acknowledged, because estrogen was believed to lower the risk of developing heart disease (and more women died of heart disease than endometrial cancer), the overall benefits were believed to outweigh the possible costs.[5] Other benefits were also observed among long–time estrogen users. In addition to reducing the symptoms of menopause, they reportedly experienced less diabetes, less depression, less Alzheimer's disease and increased longevity. Receiving all those benefits while accepting only a slight endometrial cancer risk seemed so reasonable to so many American women (or to so many American physicians) that Premarin became the nation's top–selling drug.[6]

Although some women underwent elective hysterectomies to eliminate the risk of endometrial (uterine) cancer, the drug researchers at Wyeth soon came up with a better option. Knowing that progesterone actually blocked the effect of estrogen, the Wyeth researchers found that they could reduce the risk of endometrial cancer by simply adding progesterone to some of the estrogen pills.[7] This new and improved pill, Prempro, was perfect for all those women who had never had a hysterectomy. The women like my mother who had already had that surgery could stay on Premarin since there was no uterus in which cancer could develop.

At the time progesterone was added, no one realized that, although the added progesterone did decrease endometrial cancer, it also significantly increased the rate of breast cancer.[8] We will never know how many women have or will get breast cancer as a result of taking Prempro or the higher dosage of Premarin that used to be the standard, but my mother must be added to that total, whatever it is. Despite having no sisters, cousins, aunts or nieces who ever experienced breast cancer and despite having breastfed her children, having a healthy diet, having the healthy, trim body of a daily walker and never having smoked, in September of 1994 my mother was diagnosed with breast cancer and was faced with either full breast removal (mastectomy) or doing a partial breast removal (lumpectomy). Her oncologist would not recommend one or the other. She had to decide on her own.

My initial response was clear. "Why take any chances, Mom? You're 70 years old. There's no reason to save breast tissue. However, let me investigate what the risks are, and I'll let you know what I find." My work as a college professor involved reading medical literature on an almost daily basis. Becoming familiar with the breast cancer research was now far more than simply a research interest. I went to the library and began gathering and ordering research on the type of cancer my mother had. I was soon surprised to learn that survival rates were actually higher for those who did the lumpectomy rather than the full mastectomy—information her oncologist undoubtedly knew but would not share.[9]

The Truth is Discovered

In 1998 a large, well–designed study of hormone replacement therapy[10] appeared in the *Journal of the American Medical Association.*[11] The results made the evening news and surprised and concerned millions of women. Not only did estrogen not protect against heart disease, those taking estrogen had an increased chance of having a heart attack. In 2002 another well–designed study appeared in *JAMA* which essentially quieted most of those who continued to advocate HRT for menopause after the 1998 report. That 2002 study found HRT increased heart attacks, strokes and cancer.[12]

Subsequent research has found that long–term use of hormones results in more breast cancer,[13] ovarian and endometrial cancers,[14] heart attacks, strokes (including TIAs), asthma, cognitive declines and twice the chance of developing Alzheimer's disease—though there is less osteoporosis and less colon cancer.[15]

What Went Wrong

How could a drug which we now know causes heart attacks, strokes, endometrial cancer, breast cancer and so many other physical dangers become the most prescribed pill in the nation? The most fundamental answer is that the drug approval and prescription process in America is faulty. It allowed a drug to be prescribed which could kill and allowed it to be prescribed for far more than the originally approved limited use. But it is not just the drug approval process which was at fault.

Poorly designed studies which fool not just the public but also the researcher responsible for the study are published daily. This happened hundreds and hundreds of times with the HRT research. And of course, the books, journal articles, continuing education conferences, literature provided by drug representatives and advertising all led the American public and physicians to assume HRT was the best medical practice. We were all fooled. Today we are being fooled about mind drugs. The mind drug story remarkably parallels the estrogen (HRT) story, though there are at least three significant differences:

(1)   The degree to which mind drug studies are manipulated and even fraudulent is far greater than what occurred with HRT studies.

(2)   The degree to which FDA standards need to be raised is greater in the area of mind drug research since "depression," "anxiety" and "confusion" are more difficult to measure than heart attacks, strokes and cancer.

(3)   The amount of money being made with mind drugs is greater than was made with hormone pills, and thus their promotion is greater.

A Closer Look

In many of the lectures I give, I provide an example of a poorly designed study which fooled the researchers and the public. And yes, I have often been fooled also. In the early 1980s, I lectured to communities in Nebraska concerning family and health issues, including the results of a discredited 1976 study by Klaus and Kennel. Klaus and Kennel had studied babies born prematurely who, because of their special needs, were not given directly to their parents after birth. They reported that these premies were at greater risk of being returned to the hospital as a result of being physically abused by their own parents than were babies not born prematurely.

It was not the first report of this phenomenon. It had actually been reported often, and mother–offspring contact was long known to be important among various animals. In the 1930s Konrad Lorenz won a Nobel prize for his research and documentation of this "imprinting" effect. Using goslings he showed that these newborn geese will bond to whatever is present and moving when they are born.[16] Newborn kids given five minutes with the mother goat, removed for 1–3 hours, and then returned to the mother goat are always accepted by their mothers. Newborn kids removed immediately upon birth for 1–3 hours and then given to their mothers are nearly always rejected.[17]

Klaus and Kennel knew the threats to the accuracy of their research and tried to control for those variables but were still innocently fooled by their own study. I, in turn, fooled the people of Nebraska. Observational studies, where we simply observe what is, are always dangerous. It is simply impossible not to have error creep into observational studies. The erroneous results of Klaus and Kennel were related to what we know to be fact today—that premies are more likely to be born to those who did not receive good prenatal care, who have an abusive marriage, who abuse alcohol or other drugs, and who are living with an abundance of stress.

Far better than observational studies are randomized, placebo–controlled trials (RCTs). In time large RCTs will be required for any new drug which manufacturers want to market, and then frequent blunders will become a thing of the past.[18] RCT studies randomly assign subjects to experimental groups (one group getting the real drug and one group getting a sugar pill "placebo," for example) and randomly assign some subjects to a "control group." Dramatically different results can emerge by using these two almost diametrically opposed designs. (Hundreds of observational studies had found that women taking estrogen or estrogen and progesterone hormones had *fewer* heart attacks. RCT studies found women on these hormones had far *more* heart attacks.) Suffice it to say that, if an observational design is used, it is just not always possible to keep the variables which can distort the search for truth from doing so, no matter how much education, ability or money the researchers may possess.

And now the bombshell: There had never been even one large RCT study examining the benefits and risks of HRT by the time my mother got breast cancer in 1994![19] Every one of the hundreds of studies was an observational study. Those studies are easier and cheaper to conduct, but what a price we have paid and will continue to pay for not doing RCTs. Today we realize, finally, why we had so many erroneous study results. Just as Klaus and Kennel's sample of women who gave birth to premies had unique characteristics, the women who were on hormones were fundamentally different than a group would be which was randomly selected.

How They Differed

The women receiving hormones during the last several decades were not typical in that they

(1) visited their doctors more often (gaining an opportunity to be prescribed hormones with each visit)

(2) were more health conscious and more aware of medical research findings

(3) were more inclined actually to take their prescription daily (The number of prescriptions that are never filled or that are filled but are never taken is surprisingly high.[20] But women in the observational studies, being very health conscious, were quite compliant.)

(4) were more likely to be white

(5) were less likely to smoke

(6) were more physically active

(7) were less likely to be obese

(8) were more likely to have Type A personalities

(9) were more likely to see gynecologists (who are more likely to prescribe hormones than are internists and general practitioners) and

(10) were more likely to be wealthier and better educated.[21]

This last fact by itself could explain all the perceived benefits the women on estrogen appeared to receive as could the fact which preceded it. And even now that list is not comprehensive. Consider one more difference that, again, taken all by itself could explain why it seemed women on estrogen enjoyed better health when in fact it was putting their health at risk. Women who had high blood pressure, heart disease or diabetes were less likely to be put on hormones.[22] The women on hormones in the observational studies were less likely to have serious health problems, but it was not because the hormones were protecting them.

The "Chemical Imbalance" Theory is Adopted

In 1964 the newsweekly *Time* reported on a presentation made at a conference of the American College of Surgeons. Gynecologist Robert W. Kistner declared,

> Women are the only mammalian females to live beyond their reproductive usefulness. So it is by that evolutionary standard that they live too long. But since we do keep them around we should recognize that during the menopause they are living in a state of hormonal imbalance, and we should treat it.[23]

There you have it, women. You are valuable only until you are about 40 or 50. After that age you suffer from a chemical imbalance (a hormonal imbalance in this case) which does far more than just prevent you from bearing children. Dr. Kistner argued that women who lived to and beyond menopause suffered excessive wrinkles, osteoporosis and humped backs because of these hormonal deficiencies.

And his proof? He had none. There is no standard against which humans can be compared unless we simply look at other healthy humans. But if we do that, we find all of us experience chemical changes throughout life. We will never have catecholamine levels that are as high as they are at birth.[24] We have more melatonin as teens than we do later in life.[25] For men and women, testosterone peaks when we are about 20 years old.[26] But should we assume all 30–year–olds have a chemical imbalance? Or should we assume that because we produce more melatonin at night than during the day (whether we are children or centenarians)[27] that we have a chemical imbalance during the daytime? Or should we assume that our greater melatonin production from April to September[28] means we need extra in October through March?

Many times during the 20th century someone decided that we lacked enough catecholamines, melatonin, testosterone or some other chemical, and yet supplements of these body chemicals have often proved surprisingly dangerous. For example, men given extra testosterone (to maintain the levels of a 20–year–old) are more likely to develop prostate cancer.[29] No, the evidence actually indicates we are made just right for every stage of life. God knew what He was doing.

Now, considering again how America became convinced that women had a chemical imbalance after menopause, we need to return once more to the 1960s. Eighteen months after Dr. Kistner's declaration that women had not properly evolved beyond their role as childbearing factories, *Time* again reported on the miracles of estrogen.[30] Under the title "Pills to Keep Women Young" the article began,

> All over the U.S. women in their 40s and 50s are going to doctors and demanding "the pills that will keep me from growing old." Women in their 60s and over are asking for "pills to make me young again." In each case what they are really asking for are doses of hormones to slow down or reduce the ravages of age.[31]

The *Time* article also noted that the clamor of 1966 was "stimulated by recent magazine articles and especially by a book."[32] Major medical blunders do not start and end in the medical literature. No one, especially a busy private practice physician, has the time to scour the hundreds (literally) of medical articles that are published daily. No, to really impact America, the research has to make it to the popular media.

The popular media report on the most interesting or important studies from the leading medical journals each week—*Journal of the American*

Medical Association (on Tuesdays), the *New England Journal of Medicine* (on Wednesdays), the *British Medical Journal* (on Saturdays) and the *Lancet* (on various days).[33] Research found in other medical journals makes it to popular media outlets less frequently. But there are other ways to get medical information into the mass media. Being sensational and being willing to spend lots of money on marketing can work wonders.

Promotion by Drug Companies

New York gynecologist Dr. Robert A. Wilson believed that spreading the hormone replacement message was so important that he quit his private practice, established the Wilson Research Foundation and began working on a book which he hoped would widely educate the public. That book, *Feminine Forever*, came out in 1966 and became a national bestseller. *Look* magazine, which had a circulation of nearly 8 million at that time,[34] excerpted portions, announcing this fact on its cover with the words "A Famous Doctor's Key to Staying Young."[35] The first paragraph described the estimated 6,000 to 12,000 women then on estrogen. "Instead of being condemned to witness the death of their womanhood during what should be their best years, they will remain fully feminine—physically and emotionally—for as long as they live."[36] What woman would not read the rest of the article?

Wilson's book, articles, and interviews had tremendous impact on what Americans came to believe about menopause and aging. He had four purposes:

(1) To convince women that the decrease in estrogen which occurred during menopause was not just part of a new stage of life but was a medical disease similar to diabetes.

> In the course of my work, spanning four decades and involving hundreds of carefully documented clinical cases, it became evident that menopause is in fact a deficiency

33

disease. By way of rough analogy, you might think of menopause as a condition similar to diabetes. Both are caused by lack of a certain substance. To control diabetes we supply the lacking substance in the form of insulin. To prevent menopause, we replace the deficient or missing hormones.[37]

(2) To convince women that, without estrogen, mental and emotional stability would be harmed. Dr. Wilson reported that women with estrogen deficiencies tended to cry more easily, think less clearly and be more nervous, anxious, irritable and depressed. These were the typical symptoms. But for some women, the result of the low–estrogen chemical imbalance caused the development of "a neurosis so severe as to make personal adjustments impossible. A disturbing number take refuge in alcohol, sleeping pills and, sometimes, even in suicide."[38]

(3) To convince women that those not taking estrogen would lose their youthful attractiveness and would suffer more aging effects.

The breasts become flabby and shrink . . . . The tissues dry out, the muscles weaken, the skin sags. The bones . . . become brittle and porous, easily fractured. The weakening of the bones leads to an increasingly hunchbacked condition known as 'dowager's hump' . . . . Arms and legs lose their suppleness and strength, becoming gaunt and stringy. The neck grows scrawny; grace and rhythm soon depart, along with proper muscular coordination.[39]

(4) To convince women that estrogen was completely safe and even protected against heart disease and cancer. Wilson, of course, was well aware of concerns about the estrogen–cancer link. He tackled that matter head on, calling it a "misconception" and then reported the results of his own study which appeared in *JAMA* four years earlier. He shared that among the 304 women in the study, some treated up to 27 years, 18 cases of either breast cancer or cancer of the uterus should have been expected, but "instead, not a single case of cancer occurred!"[40] But estrogen did more than prevent cancer. "It tends to prevent the development of high blood pressure, heart disease and strokes, diabetes and diseases of the urinary bladder."[41]

Wilson's book and countless articles in the popular media led to the conclusion that menopause did indeed bring on a chemical imbalance that needed to be corrected. The number of women on estrogen or estrogen and progesterone skyrocketed. By the end of 1966, Premarin was America's most prescribed drug, and the estrogen pills of other pharmaceutical companies were also bringing them millions of dollars.

BOX #1-1

The Man Who Knew Too Much

The year 1966 saw the release of Dr. Robert A. Wilson's *Feminine Forever*. It was in 1966 that *Look* excerpted parts of that book. Discussions of hormones and their ability to keep one forever young appeared in *Time*, *Reader's Digest*, *Science Digest* and newspapers across the country during that same year. It was also in 1966 that Alfred Hitchcock's film "The Man Who Knew Too Much" starring Jimmy Stewart and Doris Day came to America's theaters.

Pay close attention to the dialogue, and you will see Dr. Wilson's influence in a light–hearted comment about Jimmy Stewart's youthful appearance. Stewart (playing the role of a doctor) is told, "You haven't changed a bit" to which another admirer declares, "Why should he? He's a doctor—probably gets free hormones."

That one line likely resulted in thousands of new estrogen prescriptions. But that free commercial for HRT cannot compare to the relentless barrage of testimonials coming from Hollywood stars today who are regularly heard sharing how life–changing and even life–saving antidepressants have been for them.

Dr. Wilson's Secret Ties with the Drug Companies

Dr. Wilson's 1962 *JAMA* article[42] caught the attention of the drug companies that marketed estrogen. They approached him shortly after its publication with a series of proposals—all of which were to be withheld from the public. No one knew when Robert Wilson established his foundation and published his book what some of the financial arrangements were behind these endeavors. Two *New Republic* journalists were, however, suspicious and obtained the 1965 tax–exempt filings of Wilson's foundation. What they found confirmed their suspicions. Financial support came from Searle & Company, Ayerst Laboratories (today's Wyeth) and The Upjohn Company—all manufacturers of estrogen.[43]

No one knew that the Wilson Research Foundation's employees were members of Wilson's family—including his wife and his son—or that the informational brochures they provided free of charge were paid for by a manufacturer of estrogen.[44] No one suspected that the public speeches Wilson's wife presented all over the nation for several years were paid for by Wyeth.[45] And no one knew that Wyeth supported Wilson during the writing of his book, paid for its publication and purchased so many books for free distribution by drug "reps" (representatives) to physicians that it actually helped push *Feminine Forever* onto the best seller list. No one knew that G. D. Searle and Company which manufactured the estrogen–progestin drug Enovid made Wilson a paid research consultant. (Progesterone is the only naturally produced hormone of its kind, supporting the menstrual cycle, conception and pregnancy. Progestins are synthetic forms of progesterone.) Other financial arrangements may still be unknown.

It is impossible to prove that the financial ties that developed between the drug manufacturers and Dr. Wilson influenced his words or his writing. However, without substantial ties, it is difficult to believe that he would have left the temperate language of science for the dramatic (sometimes even frightening) and consistently promotional language we read in his book, articles and interviews.[46] He even made up new medical terms and renamed others for the obvious purpose of promotion. The normal reduction in estrogen became "estrogen–deficiency disease," a disease which resulted in the "defeminization" of a woman. He even renamed the vaginal cytology test which measured estrogen levels, calling it instead the "femininity test."[47] Such promotional efforts with only a minimal amount of research on the effects of hormones (and, again, animal studies had consistently pointed to the dangers of cancer) clearly angered the newly appointed and reform–minded head of the FDA, Dr. James L. Goddard. Dr. Goddard contacted Searle and Company and informed them that "test data submitted by Dr. Wilson will no longer be considered acceptable."[48]

Dr. Wilson's Demise

By his assessment, Dr. Wilson had treated more women with estrogen than any other physician "by a wide margin."[49] By the time *Feminine Forever* was published, he personally had prescribed estrogen for approximately 5,000 women, most beginning treatments by their mid–30s but many starting in their late teens. It was a treatment that he wanted them to continue the rest of their lives. His own wife was one of those who followed his advice, and a year after *Feminine Forever* was published, she developed breast cancer. That fact was not even made known to family members. If word got out, it would have made the papers and news magazines. Even the medical records were falsified. It was years later that Mrs. Wilson told her son Ronald the truth—after she was diagnosed with breast cancer again, the disease which took her life.

Eventually the pharmaceutical companies no longer needed Dr. Wilson's services. The nation had been convinced. Financial support came to an end. The Wilson Research Foundation was closed. As the research of the mid-1970s removed any doubt about the estrogen–endometrial cancer link, Robert Wilson was no longer a forerunner and hero but, in the eyes of many former patients, something of a villain. He took his own life in 1981.[50]

More Marketing Strategies

As noted earlier, Premarin became the nation's top–selling drug in 1966. Profits for Wyeth were huge. By 1975, 28 million prescriptions were being written per week just in the United States, and sales in other nations were also rising.[51] But when the *New England Journal of Medicine* published two independent studies in 1975 showing that women on estrogen supplements had a 4.5 times increased risk of endometrial cancer, sales of Premarin began plummeting.[52] The fear of cancer trumped the desire to be feminine forever. It is not hard to imagine that lawsuits could have brought on bankruptcy for Wyeth. That didn't happen. In fact, by 1995 over 44 million Premarin prescriptions were being filled each year in the U.S., making it once again the nation's top–selling drug. But how? How could a drug that causes cancer become the nation's #1 drug—again? The answer can be summed up with one word: marketing.

Premarin had been a cash cow and, with a multifaceted marketing effort (to the tune of over $16 million dollars each week), it would be again. But how? It involved one fortunate research discovery. Between 1975 and 1979 no major marketing efforts were possible for Premarin. That would have brought nothing but problems. But in 1979 when the *Lancet* reported that adding progestin made the risk of endometrial cancer disappear,[53] Wyeth decided that it was time once again to promote their estrogen pills. They chose a New York public relations and marketing firm, Burson–Marsteller, to conduct the hormone promotion campaign. Burson–Marsteller focused on the studies which found that women taking estrogen experienced less osteoporosis in old age. Ads in medical journals from those years can still be seen in any large library, and they are convincing. Older women with disfiguring humps, X–rays of weak bones and other creative ads all proclaimed, "Avoid osteoporosis."

Of course, ads from drug companies are seen in a very different light than information coming from non–profits. When we know that a group has been organized for the sole purpose of benefitting the rest of us, we are more open to their message. So when the National Osteoporosis Foundation began encouraging estrogen use, its recommendation had great influence. The National Osteoporosis Foundation was started in 1984, the same year the National Institutes of Health reported that estrogen could help prevent osteoporosis.[54] Wyeth, which was the leading estrogen manufacturer, saw an opportunity and helped organize and fund the new group—a fact no one publicized at the time.[55]

Another Burston–Marsteller strategy involved publishing articles on the benefits of estrogen in women's magazines as well as medical journals. Articles by medical doctors would have the most influence on women and other medical doctors, but it wasn't possible to gather enough MDs to write as many pro–estrogen articles as the campaign called for. Solution? Both types of articles would utilize professional medical writers who would write the articles but then send them to physicians who would read over the articles and agree to allow their names (and MD initials) to appear as authors. The physicians who participated with the "ghostwriters" would receive checks for thousands of dollars for this service.[56] Articles were then identified that were very positive about estrogen use, and tens of thousands of these were reproduced for distribution by drug reps to physicians. Articles that voiced concerns were not mass produced and distributed. On and on the marketing strategies continued.

When the result of the observational study of postmenopausal women and heart disease erroneously found that hormones actually reduced the risk of heart disease,[57] Wyeth and the other drug manufacturers had the medical research they needed to restore sales of Premarin to its top position. Ads appeared in the journals, literature was given to physicians, and dinners and conferences were held on the benefits of HRT (paid for by drug companies). Sales soared. That is how, despite the reality that Premarin was killing more and more women each year, it once again rose to the very top of the best–selling drugs list.

Ignoring, Discounting or Fighting Research Results

Were there no early warnings? There were lots of them. But put yourself in the position of a physician who has for years not just been willing to prescribe hormones but has been actively encouraging patients to take hormones in the honest belief that it will really benefit their health. You now hear that it may be very dangerous to be on hormones. Do you immediately call all these patients and tell them you were wrong and it now seems that the hormones may actually increase their cancer, heart disease and Alzheimer's risk? I wouldn't want to do so. I would hope that the newest findings were simply wrong. I would likely look at the fact that the bulk of the studies found that HRT resulted in health benefits. I might even dig in my heels.

I cannot be certain what I would do since I have never been in that situation. But several years ago I recognized there is a tendency to stubbornly ignore the truth when an Ob/Gyn whom I had invited to speak on HRT came to one of my classes. I did not learn until he began speaking that he put every female patient on estrogen from puberty on. He believed estrogen levels should not be allowed to fluctuate throughout the month. Since I followed the topic closely, I knew to tell my students during the next class session that there was no research on such a practice, and it would likely prove to cause cancer in time. When I later discussed this practice with him and pointed out that his own professional association, the American College of Obstetricians and Gynecologists (ACOG), did not recommend the practice, he insisted that he was certain his practice was best and the ACOG would support it in time.

The FDA never did approve such indiscriminate use of Premarin or any other estrogen, but unknown to most Americans, once the FDA approves a drug for any use, a physician has a legal right to prescribe it to any patient for any reason. My Ob/Gyn colleague could prescribe Premarin to every 12- or 13- or 14-year-old girl that ever came to his office quite legally, though the FDA approved it for menopause symptoms only. That is the law and, practically speaking, it means that in America there are millions of "off-label" prescriptions written each week for uses that have never been properly researched.

Nowhere is this more true than it is with antidepressants. The HRT story has finally been exposed. But this did not occur immediately after the research was published indicating health risks attributable to HRT. Despite the *JAMA* articles of 1998[58] and 2000,[59] both of which made clear that hormone supplements were killing women, supplemental hormone sales of Premarin in 2001 were robust, generating Wyeth $2 billion in sales.[60] It was not until after the widespread media attention given *JAMA*'s 2002[61] article that dramatic change came.

It is time the same errors, marketing strategies and resistance to change that applied to HRT be more fully exposed with regards to antidepressants and antipsychotics. Parts 1 and 2 of this book do just that. If carefully read, they will give you the knowledge you need not to be fooled yourself as well as information I hope you will actively share so fewer and fewer Americans will stay fooled.

2

*"Falsehood flies and the truth comes limping after;
so that when men come to be undeceived it is too late:
the jest is over and the tale has had its effect."*[1]
— *Jonathan Swift, 1710*

ARE MENTAL PROBLEMS MENTAL DISEASES?

Good mental health is no accident. Yet most psychiatrists, if asked "Why is my brother's thinking so crazy?" or "Why is my child so depressed?", will respond with an answer that implies it is indeed an accident. "These problems occur in the best of families. We are getting closer to understanding how they develop, but ultimately it is just like some cancers. They sometimes strike young children or healthy athletes and miss the person who has never taken care of his health. That is why we call these mental diseases."

If that view is correct, the implication must be that there is little, if anything, you can do to be sure you avoid insanity or severe depression or any other mental health problem. That is the view which dominates psychiatry today, a view generally termed "biological psychiatry." It has been so dominant that even dictionary definitions sometimes disparage the *other* view (sometimes called the functional view). Consider the following definition of "functional psychosis" from the On–line Medical Dictionary:

43

An obsolete term once used to denote schizophrenia and other severe mental disorders before modern science discovered a biological component to some aspects of each of the disorders.[2]

Obsolete? Hardly. Yet even suggesting that biological psychiatry has it all wrong will really upset most psychiatrists. No issue is more important to how they practice. For many, their view determines the future of their careers and their annual income. That sounds hard to believe, I know. But before you finish this book you will understand how very true it is.

Biological psychiatry is wrong, and more and more psychiatrists and mental health researchers are now saying so. The movement away from biological psychiatry was inevitable since truth does ultimately triumph. Unfortunately, truth is often slow to conquer. For example, one might assume that within 15 years of the first lobotomies the procedure would be outlawed. But in reality, Egas Moniz won the Nobel prize for developing the lobotomy 15 years after he began severing the frontal lobes from the rest of the brain. (And even today a small number of psychosurgeries continue to be performed though they are generally limited to cases of "obsessive compulsive disorder, chronic anxiety states and major depression."[3]) Lobotomies are but one example of how we have been fooled. In this and in subsequent chapters you will learn that the American public has been led to believe many ideas that simply are not true. All I will ask of you is that you keep your mind open as you read. You may be surprised by what you are about to learn.

Objective Medicine Comes to the Rescue

In 2002 I spent part of my summer teaching in Kampala in the east African nation of Uganda. Five days after my return, my wife and I were sitting with my parents in their home in southern California. As the evening came to a close, I headed toward my room when I suddenly began shaking violently. I made it to the bathroom and was determined to brush my teeth before crawling into bed. However, my mouth and hands were shaking so uncontrollably that brushing was almost impossible. Then the chills began. I quickly called out to my wife and then got to bed. When she entered our room I told her I thought I had malaria.

Little did I know that I had falciperum malaria or I would have headed to the hospital immediately. (There are four types of malaria. Only falciperum can kill within 24 hours.) It was a miserable night marked by shaking, fever, chills and sweats. When I got to the emergency room the next morning, I told the admitting nurse that I was sure I had malaria. She found it hard to believe. "I've worked here for 16 years, and I've never seen a case of malaria." (Southern California is malaria free and almost mosquito free so cases of malaria are rare—seen only in those who have recently arrived, like myself, from a malaria–infested part of the world.) I was not going to argue. As soon as they could take some of my blood and have it analyzed, the question would be settled, and I could begin taking the parasite--killing medication I knew I needed. The point to be made is that there is a definite, objective means of determining whether or not I had malaria. Once the blood sample was examined, all debate would come to an end. Such is the case for all true diseases.

My wife has Type 1 diabetes. One simple blood glucose test can confirm diabetes in only moments. If we needed to confirm that she has Type 1 diabetes (insulin dependent diabetes) and not Type 2 diabetes, we could do a C–peptide test. If we find a patient with an enlarged prostate, we run a PSA test. If symptoms indicate a thyroid problem, we request a thyroid stimulating hormone test. If someone appears jaundiced, we do a bilirubin test. On and on it goes. There are hundreds of tests which can be ordered, most of which involve an analysis of a patient's blood or urine which is compared against universally accepted norms. The point is we have objective measures. Many people believe the same is true for depression or other mental problems. The truth? The truth is that there is no objective test for determining depression, schizophrenia or any purely mental disorder—no blood test, urine test or brain scan.

The Chemical Imbalance Theory

Many of those familiar with the research in this area speak of the "chemical imbalance myth." My concern with this phrase is that it implies that there is no evidence that brain chemistry is related to mental problems. The evidence is obvious and overwhelming (and no one actually questions the fact) that the mind can be harmed by disease. Late stage syphilis can cause paranoia, delusions, disorientation and eventually complete insanity and death. But we understand it is caused by a spiral–shaped bacterium, the treponema pallidum spirochete. We know we can determine if the mental changes are caused by this bacteria through a cerebrospinal fluid test.[4]

Viral encephalitis can also infect and damage the brain, causing confusion, disorientation and hallucinations. But, again, we can identify the specific microorganism responsible. General mental declines or irrational thinking can emerge out of a whole host of physical challenges. These include severe anemia, vitamin B_{12} deficiency, pellagra, alcohol abuse, chronic meningitis, and consumption of arsenic or mercury.[5] However, this is in no way parallel to what the drug companies would have us believe and what the public has come to believe about mental "diseases" and brain chemistry. Their chemical imbalance theory cannot be supported by the research. That theory can be summarized in three major points:

(1) Depression, anxiety, schizophrenia and other mental disorders are diseases just like asthma, diabetes or cancer. They result from flaws in brain chemistry, not from flaws in character, and consequently these mental disorders can attack anyone—regardless of age, race, gender, educational level, financial status or other personal characteristics.

(2) Depression, anxiety, schizophrenia and other mental disorders may arise from many sources, but the genetic contribution to the development of a chemical imbalance is beyond question.

(3) Taking the appropriate drugs can restore normal brain chemistry and normal mental function.

Each of these three major tenets is widely believed, but each is false. Depression, schizophrenia and other mental problems are not due to a "flaw in chemistry" despite all the ads that say they are. Consider the following statements from others who have researched and published on this issue:

- "As a practicing psychiatrist, I have watched with growing dismay and outrage the rise and triumph of . . . biologic psychiatry [which] now completely dominates the discourse on the causes and treatment of mental illness. . . . I am constantly amazed by how many patients who come to see me believe or want to believe that their difficulties are biologic and can be relieved by a pill. This is despite the fact that modern psychiatry has yet to convincingly prove the genetic/biologic cause of any single mental illness . . . . Patients [have] been diagnosed with chemical imbalances despite the fact that no test exists to support such a claim."[6]
  —David Kaiser, MD, psychiatrist

- "In reality, science does not have the ability to measure the levels of any biochemical in the tiny spaces between the nerve cells (the synapses) in the brain of a human being. All the talk about biochemical imbalances is sheer speculation aimed at promoting psychiatric drugs."[7]
  —Peter Breggin, MD, psychiatrist

- "Many physicians tell their patients that they are suffering from a chemical imbalance, despite the reality that there are no tests available for assessing the chemical status of a living person's brain. . . . The evidence does not support any of the biochemical theories of mental illness."[8]
  —Elliott Valenstein, PhD, neuropsychologist

- "In recent decades, we have had no shortage of alleged biochemical imbalances for psychiatric conditions. Diligent though these attempts have been, not one has been proven. Quite the contrary. In every instance where such an imbalance was thought to have been found, it was later proven to

be false."[9]
—Joseph Glenmullen, MD, psychiatrist

- "The day will come when people will look back at our current medicines for schizophrenia and the stories we tell to patients about their abnormal brain chemistry, and they will shake their heads in utter disbelief."[10]
—Robert Whitaker, award–winning medical journalist

- "The values and ideology of biological psychiatry are transmitted in our clinical language and educational institutions. Largely unquestioned, these ideas form the basis on which our field trains future psychiatrists."[11]
—Susan Kemker, MD, psychiatrist

- "The ascendant belief that 'mental illnesses are brain diseases' is due far more to the cultural belief that only biologically based illnesses are 'real' illnesses than to any empirical findings that the causes of mental disorder are brain based. The view that real illnesses must have biological causes is, paradoxically, a cultural construction. Advocacy groups lobby for genetic and biological views of mental disorder because if a mental illness is regarded as an organic brain disorder, then it is presumably less likely that the individual will be blamed and stigmatized for the condition. It is no wonder that people often make prodigious efforts to show that their illnesses are really physical."[12]
—Allan Horwitz, PhD, sociologist

- "[Americans are] convinced that the origins of mental illnesses are to be found in biology, when, despite more than three decades of research, there is still no proof. . . . The absence of any well–defined physical causation is reflected in the absence of any laboratory tests for psychiatric diagnoses—much in contrast to diabetes and many other physical disorders."[13]
—Charles E. Dean, MD, psychiatrist

- "There are no external validation criteria for psychiatric diagnoses. There is neither a blood test nor specific anatomic lesions for any major psychiatric disorder . . . . Psychiatry has been almost completely bought out by the drug companies. The APA could not continue without the pharmaceutical company support of meetings, symposia, workshops, journal advertising, grand rounds luncheons, unrestricted grants, etc., etc. Psychiatrists have become the minions of drug company promotions."[14]
—Loren R. Mosher, MD, psychiatrist

- "Despite research that discredits genetic bases for human behavior, [the biological view] of mental illness has become solidly entrenched over the past several decades, not just within psychiatry and the medical profession, but within the general public as well."[15]
—Ellen M. Borges, PhD, sociologist

- "At the present time there is no proof that biology causes schizophrenia, bipolar mood disorder, or any other functional mental disorder."[16]
—Colin A. Ross, MD, psychiatrist

The Evidence

Though numerous researchers have rejected the theory that mental problems are caused by some disease or chemical imbalance, the American Psychiatric Association, most physicians and most of the American public continue to hold to this belief. The evidence for the theory is found in studies that are commonly discussed not just by the drug manufacturers' literature but by the textbooks used to educate psychologists, nurses and medical doctors.

So ideological is the position of the genetic/chemical imbalance advocates that they often talk in terms of the "proofs" rather than the evidences for their position. The "proofs" are found in four areas of research:

(1) studies linking prenatal exposure to influenza and schizophrenia, (2) studies which find depressed people have too little serotonin and schizophrenics have too much dopamine, (3) studies which find abnormal brain activity in those with mental problems as evidenced by brain imaging and (4) studies which show genetic links among those with mental problems. Each area of research can be very convincing and is presented in many different forums in hopes of winning the public and the profession to the biological/chemical imbalance view. This chapter will consider all four areas of research and, I believe, will provide many surprises for most of you.

"Proof" #1: Viral (Influenza) Exposure

The popular viral explanation for schizophrenia which suggests schizophrenia can arise from a brain damaged by a virus is supported by a number of correlational findings. The viral theory proposes that damage occurs before birth when the victim's mother catches the flu during the middle of her pregnancy. Consider the following facts taken from one of America's most widely used psychology textbooks:[17]

- During those years which have particularly bad flu epidemics, the number of new babies who will eventually develop schizophrenia increases.[18]

- Babies born during winter and spring (those exposed to influenza during the fall to winter flu season) are at greater risk of eventually developing schizophrenia.[19]

- Babies born in southern hemisphere locations where the flu season is opposite the flu season in the northern hemisphere also have increased risk patterns that are opposite those of the northern hemisphere.[20]

- Mothers who report having had influenza during their pregnancy are more likely to have children who will eventually develop schizophrenia.[21]

This area of research points to a biological explanation for one of the most serious of brain disorders. If the brain could be so damaged prior to birth that eventually the victim loses his or her mind, then surely anxiety, obsessive–compulsive disorders and depression could also result from viral damage and, if that is the case, the drug companies may be right: it is no one's fault.

The Obvious Overlooked

Clearly a baby's brain can be damaged prior to birth. Alcohol is such a common cause of prenatal brain damage that it has its own name—fetal alcohol syndrome. The baby is born mentally retarded with a small head, widely spaced eyes, and other facial abnormalities. But the condition is apparent the day the baby is born—not 20 years later. To assume that influenza damages the brain but that no brain damage (schizophrenia) can be measured for two decades would make this a unique disease among diseases. No, there is actually a much more rational explanation for the correlations. Here it is: Being exposed to the flu during pregnancy causes neurodevelopmental disorders,[22] thus increasing life stresses. Few realize that up to 71% of dyslexia cases are associated with flu exposure in utero.[23]

Consider the effects of dyslexia for a child attending public school— teasing, ridicule, poor academic performance, lowered career opportunities and financial status, lowered self–esteem and, for some children, increased social isolation. These do not necessarily occur, but they are more likely for those who cannot read as well or perform as well in school. In other words, some children who have dyslexia are likely experiencing extreme amounts of stress which may eventually lead to schizophrenia.

Babies who experience prenatal malnutrition are also eventually more likely to develop schizophrenia.[24] The same is true for babies who experience oxygen deprivation during birth.[25] Babies who are born prematurely are more likely to develop schizophrenia.[26] One research team calculated that a child who suffers brain damage prior to or just following birth is seven times more likely to develop schizophrenia.[27] Once again, a damaged brain means life will likely be more difficult and more stressful. Many other studies have also reported schizophrenia to be associated with trauma or disease during pregnancy.[28]

Though it has often been suggested that it is the flu virus that mysteriously damages the brain, it is not mysterious, and the damage can come from many different sources. In 1964 the U.S. experienced a German measles (rubella) epidemic. Thousands of mothers caught the disease and exposed their unborn babies to measles during pregnancy. Those who were thus exposed were more likely later to develop schizophrenia and other psychotic disorders than were those not exposed to the disease.[29]

Of course, many explanations could be suggested for the traditional viral theory. Perhaps because of the flu the mother is more likely to take medications that could harm the developing baby. Perhaps mothers who are more likely to catch the flu are more likely poor and in work environments where larger numbers of people congregate. All this is speculation, but to assume a simple, direct relationship between influenza and schizophrenia cannot be justified. Add to this the fact that 98% of women who get the flu during pregnancy give birth to children who never develop schizophrenia (as do 99% of those who do not get the flu), and the viral explanation loses all its force.

"Proof" #2: The Serotonin/Dopamine Imbalance

The standard line still voiced by countless physicians is that depression results from too little serotonin, schizophrenia from too much dopamine. That message is found in every psychology text I have ever adopted. Today they will sometimes mention other neurotransmitters as well (norepinephrine, especially in depression), but the role of neurotransmitters in causing depression, schizophrenia or other mental disorders is still taught throughout the nation. Here is a typical comment from an introductory text I used:

Drugs that relieve depression tend to increase norepinephrine or serotonin supplies by blocking either their reuptake
(as Prozac, Zoloft, and Paxil do with serotonin) or their
chemical breakdown.[30]

Or, concerning dopamine and schizophrenia, one popular textbook
author writes that a biochemical key is involved, and the "key to schizophrenia involves the neurotransmitter dopamine."[31] Another widely used textbook makes the following succinct statement concerning serotonin: "Too
little is linked to depression."[32]

If you took a psychology class while in college, you may be surprised
that I would suggest these "facts" are not considered true today and haven't
been for a long time. But you will likely be even more surprised to learn
that it was nearly four decades ago that the top researchers in the field,
including Dr. George Ashcroft, whose work led to the theory that depression
may result from low serotonin, had rejected the theory. Dr. David Healy, an
academic physician who has a doctor's degree in neuroscience and has written 13 books dealing with psychopharmaceuticals, discussed this fact in his
book *Let Them Eat Prozac*:

> By 1970 Ashcroft had concluded that, whatever was wrong
> in depression, it was not lowered serotonin. More sensitive
> studies had shown no lowering of serotonin. Indeed, *no
> abnormality of serotonin in depression has ever been
> demonstrated* (emphasis mine) . . . . A gap opened up
> between the science base and public understanding—a gap
> crucial to the later development of media talk about low-
> ered serotonin levels.[33]

Surprised? You should be. If you are an active reader, you have likely
read over and over and over that mental problems are tied to one or more
neurotransmitters. The idea is so widely perceived as established fact that

dictionary definitions sometimes mimic the standard line. Here is the *American Heritage*'s "politically correct" definition for schizophrenia:

> Any group of psychotic disorders usually characterized by withdrawal from reality, illogical patterns of thinking, delusions, and hallucinations and accompanied in varying degrees by other emotional, behavioral, or intellectual disturbances. Schizophrenia is associated with dopamine imbalances in the brain and defects in the frontal lobe and is caused by genetic, other biological, and psychosocial factors.[34]

You might also be surprised to learn that those first few neurotransmitters which we once thought controlled mental health and emotions are not the only neurotransmitters. Amazingly, new neurotransmitters are still being discovered. The first neurotransmitter to be identified, acetylcholine (ACh), was discovered in 1921. Norepinephrine was discovered in 1946, GABA in 1950 and serotonin in 1954. Dopamine followed a couple of years later (1957). Endorphin was not found until 1973.[35] These are the neurotransmitters most commonly mentioned in discussions of brain chemistry in psychology textbooks. What is not mentioned?

The answer is a host of facts that makes it clear that the complexity of the human mind is far greater than portrayed by textbooks. Neurotransmitters are far more numerous and how they operate is far more complex than ever imagined when the serotonin–depression or the dopamine–schizophrenia relationships were first suggested. By the beginning of our new millennium, approximately 75 neurotransmitters had been identified.[36] Today over 200 neurotransmitters have been found.[37]

Add to this the fact that there are many different types of receptors associated with these neurotransmitters. Serotonin alone has a minimum of 15 different receptor types.[38] How many receptor types are there for other neurotransmitters? To what degree do these almost innumerable combinations of neurotransmitters and receptors interact? Today the honest answer is still "No one knows."

In fact, whenever brain function and chemistry are considered, the principle that has emerged seems to be that the more we learn, the more we will realize how little we know. Neuropsychologist Elliot Valenstein understands this. In discussing neurotransmitters and their relationship to mental problems, he said, "Integrating all this new information and relating it to mental states grows more, rather than less, formidable."[39] However, we have learned enough to be very leery about taking drugs that change brain chemistry. Here are just a few facts worth pondering. (Study these fully referenced facts carefully. I have never seen a comparable listing. When added all together, they point to the absurdity of the chemical imbalance theory.)

- Even people with no history of any mental problems may have very high or very low levels of various neurotransmitters.[40]

- Supposedly low serotonin levels cause depression and high dopamine levels cause schizophrenia, yet some people with depression have high levels of serotonin and some people with schizophrenia have low levels of dopamine.[41]

- Drugs aimed at just one neurotransmitter (serotonin or dopamine generally) may affect numerous neurotransmitters.[42]

- Stress by itself can dramatically change brain chemistry—causing dopamine levels to rise[43] and causing serotonin levels to fall.[44]

- Stress in early life is correlated with high dopamine levels during the college years.[45]

- Massages raise dopamine and serotonin levels.[46]

- Eating can cause dopamine levels to rise.[47] Just seeing or smelling food we like causes dopamine levels to rise.[48]

- Exercise can keep dopamine levels from declining and keep serotonin levels high.[49]

- Serotonin levels vary between different sleep cycles.[50]

- Listening to music with a slow rhythm does not significantly increase epinephrine levels in the listener, but listening to fast rhythm music does.[51]

- Getting cold (a physical stressor) causes dopamine levels to rise, though staying cold for days reduces dopamine levels.[52]

Get the point? To assume, as most textbooks and advertisements still do, that unexplainable changes in a neurotransmitter level are what cause mental problems is absurd. It is a view that caught on and is still repeated daily, but it should have been buried many years ago. In fact, over two decades ago we learned that both serotonin and dopamine receptors diminish with age.[53] If the traditional (but wrong) explanation were correct, *all* old people should be depressed—and *none* should be crazy! If it were not for the millions of dollars spent each year by drug companies to keep this drug–promoting idea alive,[54] it would be an essentially unknown concept today.

Your logical objection to this set of documented facts should be "Hold on. You quoted numerous researchers earlier in this chapter who insist that we cannot measure neurotransmitter concentrations in living people. Now you have cited a number of studies that say neurotransmitter levels are changed instantly by being stressed or by eating or simply by smelling food we like. You are contradicting yourself." Good for you if you picked up on this "contradiction," but the fact is, there is no contradiction. The explanation is rather simple actually, though I eventually decided I could not discover the explanation on my own. I needed help. I describe that search for help and what I found in Box #2–1 (Is It Possible to Measure Serotonin and Dopamine Levels in the Brain or Not?). Related research follows in the section below as well.

"Proof" #3: PET Scans

PET (positron emission photography) scan photographs which show a difference in the brains of the depressed and the non–depressed or the schizophrenic and a healthy person are found in every psychology textbook, in nearly all the brochures on antidepressants or antipsychotics left by the drug reps in doctor's offices, in psychotropic drug ads in magazines, and in the literature of all the organizations that promote a drug approach to solving mental or behavioral problems. These colorful scans seem so scientific that they are convincing.

In truth, PET scans do not prove depression or schizophrenia or other mental disorders result from chemical imbalances or a defective brain. Thinking logically about the most basic pairs of questions should make this clear.

> **First question:** If a person gets depressed, is he/she apt to sleep better or not?
> **Second question:** What is the effect of sleep deprivation on PET scan results?

> **First question:** Are those taking illegal drugs more likely to get depressed?
> **Second question:** What is the effect of illegal drugs on brain function?

> **First question:** Could the lack of appetite associated with depression lead to reduced brain activity?
> **Second question:** Could the decrease in physical activity associated with depression have an impact on brain activity?

BOX #2-1

Is It Possible to Measure
Serotonin and Dopamine Levels or Not?

What you are about to learn is not understood by as many as 1 in 100 physicians in private practice or 1 in 100 practicing psychiatrists. (Evidence that the drug prescribing experts know very little about the mind drugs they prescribe is presented in the next chapter.)

For years I did not understand the measurement issue I am about to explain. I read the leading researchers declaring that serotonin or dopamine levels had never been measured in a living person's brain. (Both are easily measured following death by removing some brain tissue and doing chemical analysis of the tissue.) If that were true, then all the drug companies' literature and advertising claiming depression and other mental disorders were caused by too little serotonin (depression) or too much dopamine (schizophrenia) were false claims. Yet, I had read hundreds of articles which reported changes in neurotransmitter levels relative to various events (the many findings I report on pp. 55–56 being examples). These articles all seemed to say that those who claimed neurotransmitter levels could not be measured were simply ignorant. But these were research giants. How could they be ignorant of the hundreds of studies I was reading? You see the dilemma.

I tried to reconcile the two positions but could find nothing that did so, not even books and articles on neurotransmitters or PET, SPECT, MRI or fMRI imaging. The frustration was real when I finally decided there was only one option left. I had to prepare a letter which carefully described the apparent contradiction, quoting the authorities on both sides, and send the letter by email to about 30 of the world's leading authorities—those publishing research most closely related to my question. Approximately half the letters went out with the subject line being "Question from an Ignorant Psychology Professor." I was, but I was determined not to stay ignorant. Many of those publishing neurotransmitter research using positron emission tomography (PET) or other imaging technique research frankly admitted they did not know the answer (which was a surprise), but some were very gracious and referred me to others whom they believed might know. Others had no difficulty explaining. Here is what I learned.

(1) *Relative* levels of dopamine can be measured in the living brain. Thus, we can measure whether dopamine levels increase or decrease when a cigarette is smoked, a person is frightened, or a favorite food is smelled compared

to a baseline established for that person hours earlier. However, we cannot measure an *absolute* level of dopamine in the brain of any living person. Only brain tissue analysis following death can determine *absolute* levels of dopamine (and acetylcholine).

(2) Serotonin measurements in the brain are even more problematic than dopamine measurements. Whereas PET imaging and single–photon emission computed tomography (SPECT) imaging are used for relative dopamine measurement, cerebral spinal fluid taps are used to measure serotonin.

(3) Chemical analysis of brain tissue following death allows us to compare serotonin levels in depressed and non–depressed subjects and dopamine in schizophrenic and non–schizophrenic subjects. Those studies find that depressed individuals may have high or low serotonin levels, and schizophrenics may have high or low dopamine levels.

(4) Animal studies (where the animals can be put to death immediately before or after sleep or just before or after eating) find that eating, sleeping and other normal activities as well as stress–inducing events can raise or lower serotonin levels. It appears likely that anything we do—eat a large lunch, take a brisk walk, get upset, become bored, have an interesting conversation . . . anything we do—will affect our constantly changing brain chemistry.

(5) *Indirect* measurements of neurotransmitters are made in many ways (measuring synthetic enzymes, metabolic enzymes, and receptors), but even these indirect measurements have serious limitations. The most serious of these is that readings are susceptible to common drugs such as caffeine and nicotine and that the brain is regularly exposed to radioactivity (having dental xrays or taking an airline flight).

The bottom line is this: Despite the comments in psychology textbooks, explanations in the literature of non–profit mental health organizations (funded by drug companies), and what most doctors and the public have come to believe, the "chemical imbalance causes mental problems" philosophy is marketing, not science. Denmark's leading researcher in this field put it to me like this in 2005: "Today we cannot quantify the absolute amount of any neurotransmitter in the living brain, but research will probably eventually succeed in doing it if enough time and money is invested in the project." He then sarcastically added, "It would probably require that perhaps 5% of the United States military budget be put into brain scanning research."[1]

Questions like these could be asked all day long. Is it even possible that the very medications that many take for depression or schizophrenia influence PET scans? In fact, medications do affect the brain in dramatic ways.[55] Even smoking a single cigarette can greatly alter brain chemistry.[56] In other words, PET scans describe what is happening. They say nothing about the causes of depression or any mental disorder. Yet, the most extraordinary implications are sometimes suggested. The caption under one set of PET scan images in a psychology textbook from which I taught read, "PET scans illustrate reduced activation in a murderer's frontal cortex—a brain area that helps brake impulsive, aggressive behavior."[57]

This is inexcusable. When impressionable college freshmen and sophomores, all of whom lack the research background to properly critique these comments, are in effect told that even murder may be due to a brain disorder when no evidence exists for such claims, the textbook author or editor demonstrates either she has been badly fooled or she is not concerned about fooling others.

There is one other fact about brain imaging that demands that we discount the exaggerated stories we hear of brain image differences between schizophrenics or depressives compared with those with good mental health. It is the fact I shared with you in the last section—smiling, feeling pleasure or fear, and seeing someone who is angry, as well as smoking, drinking or using amphetamines, not only changes brain chemistry but changes it immediately.[58]

I was out walking before dawn recently when someone quietly came up from behind me and grabbed my leg. Actually, it wasn't a person; it was a large dog I didn't hear approaching, and she didn't really grab me. She was quite friendly and came so close that she bumped my leg. Of course, for that one second I thought it was a person who grabbed me, and I felt the result. All over my body I instantly felt a tingle. Goose bumps emerged. My heart immediately began racing. My muscles tensed. Chemical changes occurred suddenly. Why should we think it would be any different with the brain? The nine studies cited in the previous endnote make it clear

---

BOX #2-2

A Flaw in Chemistry?

John Hinckley shot President Reagan in 1981. His devastated parents began the American Mental Health Fund, his father becoming its chairman and president. One of their publications, "What You Don't Know About Mental Illness Could Fill a Booklet," begins with these words:

> Mental illness is a medical disease. You wouldn't blame someone for getting a physical illness, like cancer or heart disease. And it's just as illogical to blame someone with a mental illness. Because, like cancer or heart disease, mental illness is a medical illness. It is not a personal weakness.[1]

The booklet continues, "Don't blame the sick person for causing worry, embarrassment or family problems. It's no one's fault."[2]

The National Alliance for Research on Schizophrenia and Depression publishes a booklet which has the title "Depression: A Flaw in Chemistry, Not Character." It mimics the standard line:

> People with cancer aren't expected to heal themselves. People with diabetes can't will themselves out of needing insulin. And yet you probably think, like millions of people do, that you or someone you know should be able to overcome another debilitating disease, depression, through sheer will and fortitude. For untold decades, it has been thought that depression is the symptom of a weak character or underlying laziness. In reality, nothing could be farther from the truth. Recent medical research has taught us that depression is often biological, caused by a chemical imbalance in the brain. We've even found that depression has a genetic link.[3]

These publications, like most put out by the organizations that advocate prescribing drugs for mental problems, all receive large amounts of funding from the drug companies who manufacture antidepressants and antipsychotics. And these publications are full of photographs showing brain CAT scans or PET scans or have diagrams showing dendrites, axons or other brain parts. These publications look scientific, but they are not.

---

that the brain does respond instantly to all kinds of emotions, behaviors and drugs.

The point is this: There are literally thousands of studies today that prove brain chemistry can be changed instantly by what we experience and what we do. That means we can predict. We can predict that if we show a humorous film clip to subjects, frighten them or give them a drug, we will be able to measure a change in their brains. But I do not know of a single study that goes in the other direction. In other words, there are no studies which take frequent functional MRIs (fMRIs) or PET scans of healthy subjects and then, based on changes in brain chemistry, predict that person A will become depressed, person B will become schizophrenic and person C will begin stealing pencils.[59]

Why do advertisements ignore this most basic simple fact? Because those ads are paid for by drug companies that want you to believe that your brain chemistry may be messed up and that taking their $150 per month pills will fix your problem. I can understand why they promote that idea. However, I cannot understand why psychology textbooks continue to promote the unfounded assertion (what we can fairly call a myth) that because of genetic predispositions some individuals experience brain chemistry changes that then cause mental problems. In the face of so much contrary evidence, it is amazing that the myth endures.[60]

"Proof" #4: Genetic Studies

The research I will review in this section deals with schizophrenia because that research is old and abundant. Schizophrenia was considered a genetic disorder long before depression was said to be genetically influenced. Today, however, depression, schizophrenia and all other mental problems are seen as chemical imbalance problems that have a genetic link.

One of the world's largest drug manufacturers, Pfizer, publishes the *Pfizer Journal*. In an article entitled "Understanding the Family Connectedness in Mental Illness," what is commonly believed and what the industry continuously promotes is described:

> It was hard enough for Clea Simon to watch her two older siblings descend into schizophrenia in their adolescence and, as she says, "become wildly, uncontrollably ill." It

was harder still to later lose her brother to suicide. But it was even harder when she thought about having her own children: "I soon learned that any children of mine would indeed have an increased risk of developing the illness that destroyed my siblings' lives."

Clea Simon is just one of millions of people who have close relatives with a serious mental illness, and who are aware that this implies that the illness could be transmitted to subsequent generations. For now they can do little more than worry about this. But a hopeful development is on the way. The great advances in human genetics are now making it possible to actually identify the gene variants that are responsible for this hereditary susceptibility for some illnesses. It is even possible that scientists will one day use this knowledge for prevention and improved treatment.[61]

As evidence for a genetic link, the article notes that among identical twins the chance of both becoming schizophrenic is about 50%, not the 100% which would be expected if the condition were wholly a genetic disorder. This statement suggests both a genetic and an environmental influence, but a careful examination of the evidence reveals that this is another myth built on a foundation of distortion and dishonesty. Yet such thinking is in nearly all psychology and psychiatric nursing textbooks. Consider the two following comments from the last general psychology textbook I used.

Concerning depression: "We have long known that mood disorders run in families. . . . If one identical twin is diagnosed as suffering major depressive disorder, the chances are about 1 in 2 that at some time the other twin will be, too."[62]

Concerning schizophrenia: "Might people also inherit a predisposition to certain brain abnormalities? . . . The nearly 1 in 100 odds of any person's being diagnosed with schizophrenia become about 1 in 10 among those who have an afflicted sibling or parent and close to 1 in 2 among those who have an afflicted identical twin."[63]

The daily search for the "bad gene" continues. Though it is assumed that the gene causing or predisposing a person to depression is not the same gene causing or predisposing a person to schizophrenia, the mechanism is the same. This textbook also has a box which discusses the Genain quadruplets.

The Genain Quadruplets

The Genains constitute the single most famous case cited in support of a genetic basis for schizophrenia. Several of the psychology textbooks from which I have taught over the years show a photograph of the four sisters with a caption indicating the impossible odds of four quadruplets all developing schizophrenia if there were no genetic influence. The following caption accompanies the photograph in one of the textbooks.

> The odds of any four people picked at random all being diagnosed with schizophrenia are 1 in 100 million. But Nora, Iris, Myra and Hester Genain all have the disease. Two of the sisters have more severe forms of the disorder than the others, suggesting the influence of environmental as well as biological factors.[64]

An article in *Schizophrenia Bulletin,* a publication of the National Institute of Mental Health, suggested the odds were one in 1.5 billion.[65] But whether the odds are 1 in 100 million or 15 times greater than that, this virtually proves a genetic basis for schizophrenia. Or does it?

The Story Textbooks Will Not Tell

I allowed thousands of students to pass through my psychology courses without telling them facts about the Genains that are not mentioned by textbooks. For many years I did not know those facts myself. It was not until I began plowing through the "official" report that I learned the shocking truth. Many of these truths are not pleasant to consider, but since the

Genains have been a standard "proof" for the genetic basis for mental illness for decades and still are, you need to know the truths which are still hidden from college students.

Born in the 1930s to Henry and Mary Genain,[66] the Genain quads were identical quadruplets and were famous from birth. But the attention they received did not save them from lives of daily abuse. Both parents had extreme problems. Mr. Genain was an overweight, alcohol–abusing diabet-ic who treated both his wife and his daughters with incredible cruelty. Even when the girls were babies, Henry Genain showed he cared more about him-self than his family. Rather than protecting his daughters from an abnormal life resulting from the media's attention and the public's interest, Mr. Genain charged anyone who wanted a glimpse of the girls a 25–cent fee. This only came to an end when he began to become concerned about their possible kidnapping.[67]

Henry Genain often kept a gun in his pants pocket. That fact, combined with his acting "raving mad" when drunk and his direct threats of murder, caused his family to fear his drinking. Sometimes when drunk he would patrol their property with his loaded gun, arguing that he was sure someone might try to break into the house. He often abused his wife, behavior wit-nessed by the children. Behind closed doors he would sometimes bite her on the face during sex. Henry's mother lived with his family for six years. She was also cruel and unstable and would at times spit in the face of her daughter–in–law.

Mr. Genain allowed his wife almost no relationship outside the home. Her own mother came only twice—the second visit when the girls were seven—but was so unwelcomed that she never came again. Mrs. Genain would write to her mother, but never could a letter be sent until it had been read and approved by Mr. Genain. When Mrs. Genain's mother died, Henry would not allow his wife to attend the funeral.

At one point in their marriage Mrs. Genain became depressed and suici-dal, but in a surprising act of courage, she told Henry she was going to leave him. He told her that if she ever left, he would find her and kill her. Such a threat was not necessarily just talk. When a local man was murdered, the detectives immediately came to Henry and though he was never charged, even Mrs. Genain suspected her husband. (Immediately after the time of the murder he had run into their home, very upset and covered with bruises. And Mr. Genain had had an extramarital affair with the dead man's wife.) In light of the situation, Mrs. Genain's fear of her husband seems only reasonable.

Mr. Genain also sought to have complete control of his girls' lives. The girls attended public school, but they were not permitted to socialize with other children or participate in school activities. They always wore the same outfits and were literally forced to march to school. The girls' teachers reported that the girls not only were socially isolated but seemed fearful. One teacher related that the girls did not laugh like the other children and, though well behaved, seemed to have no curiosity. Two of the girls, Nora and Myra, were better students than Hester and Iris. The two girls who did the best were also the two that became Mrs. Genain's favorites. They received more attention and favorable treatment than the other two.

Hester and Iris were also the two girls who masturbated, a fact that greatly bothered both parents. The girls were taken to a physician who suggested clitoral circumcision. The girls pleaded not to be cut with the scalpel which infuriated the doctor. (The doctor was reported by another physician to be "a ruthless surgeon. He operated for a fee rather than for indications."[68] He eventually lost his rights to perform surgeries without obtaining the approval of another physician which forced him to quit his practice and leave town.) The official account is almost too startling to believe:

> Both girls resented the operation and broke their stitches in the hospital. Mrs. Genain reported that when Iris broke her stitches, Dr. Booth said that he would "fix her now" and would "cut all the flesh out." Dr. Booth ordered the girls' hands tied to the bed for thirty nights. When Mrs. Genain

realized the girls did not like this, "I did it just the same." During this month the girls were given sedatives to keep them from crying at night. They wet the bed two and three times a night and became so nervous they could not eat.[69]

Henry Genain's sexual abuse of his daughters was of the most extreme type. He demanded that they dress and undress in front of him. He is known to have had sex with at least two of the girls, a fact that Mrs. Genain was well aware of but chose to ignore. When the girls reached puberty, Mr. Genain insisted on watching them change their sanitary pads. He was obsessed with their sexuality and was convinced that they would try to have sex with someone against his wishes. In fact, it was Mr. Genain who was sexually promiscuous, having regular affairs and getting at least two other women pregnant. But for the quads, boys were off limits. No attention could be shown to any boy, and the girls knew it. They had often witnessed their father's fear–instilling behavior.

Throughout their high school years, various physical problems were manifested by each of the girls. All the girls had bed–wetting problems until adulthood. Hester developed gastrointestinal problems during her high school years and before her senior year became so mentally disturbed that her parents kept her at their home. The other three girls were told not to allow anyone to know what had occurred, but it was obviously most diffi-cult to keep the family secret when everyone knew that one of the quads was no longer attending school. The other three sisters all graduated and then took office jobs.

Their father continued to forbid any involvement with boys. Dating was not an option. And he continued to spy upon each of the girls and make false accusations about their sexual desires. Nora was the next to begin manifesting serious emotional problems. She quit her job and began spend-ing large amounts of time in her bed. She grew progressively worse until at 22 years of age she became fully schizophrenic and was hospitalized. Iris was the next to receive that diagnosis. She had developed a spastic colon, suffered from insomnia and vomited often. When a man showed some interest in her, she became greatly distressed. In fact, at the time, her father was likely sexually abusing her. Finally she very suddenly manifested severe symptoms of insanity. She began screaming at night, hearing voices and drooling. She began an entirely liquid diet, being unable to eat solids.

Myra was the last to lose her mind. She was 24 when she completely fell apart mentally. Her breakdown also followed an incident in which a man showed her some interest. Her symptoms were very similar to Nora's. She was not sleeping well, had panic attacks and would wake up at night screaming. When she was admitted to the hospital, she was unable to think clearly or even to distinguish reality from her distorted thoughts. She, like her three sisters before her, was diagnosed as having schizophrenia.

Many of you reading this book have taken psychology courses and learned about the Genain case there. You did not learn all I have shared with you here, however. Most of the story is either simply not told or the more sordid details are purposely overlooked. I find it most offensive that most of the psychology textbooks from which I have taught have cited this case as proof of a genetic basis for schizophrenia without sharing some of the abuse these girls suffered.

One abnormal psychology textbook that did include some of these details nevertheless concluded with these words:

> The fact is that we have four genetically identical individuals, all of whom became schizophrenic within a period of six years—three of them within a period of some two years. Is this not a compelling case for genetic determination? It is, and indeed there is ample evidence, in the family background of at least Mr. Genain, that he harbored some very pathogenic genes that were probably passed on to his daughters.[70]

Such a conclusion is infuriating. How could these girls not lose their minds even if they had perfect genes? How could these authors, all highly educated individuals, write such words? The answer is that they chose to follow the pattern set forth by nearly all textbooks. They simply accept the conclusions written by those who preceded them and, in the case of the Genains, the conclusion of the Genain investigators who carried considerable clout from working under the auspices of the National Institute of Mental Health.

David Rosenthal was the editor of the book *The Genain Quadruplets: A Study in Heredity and Environment in Schizophrenia.* Though Rosenthal was aware of the environment in which these quadruplets were raised, his extreme prejudice for genetic explanations led to inexcusable conclusions. Peter Breggin who is one of the real heroes in the fight to end the biological model of depression and mental disorders uses the strongest language in discussing Rosenthal and his work:

> The book presents one of the most tragic chronicles of child abuse recorded anywhere. Yet, at no time is the abuse discussed as such. In no place in the book is it summarized. The data is strewn throughout the six hundred pages in reports of the various professionals. Much of it is contained in footnotes . . . . To fail to underscore or to summarize the outrages perpetrated against the children constitutes intellectual complicity with the child abuser. To leave the reader to dig the abuse out of hundreds of pages is to invite the question, Why wouldn't this renowned NIMH geneticist face the facts directly? It's no surprise that Rosenthal's most famous and influential accomplishment—the Danish adoption study of schizophrenia—also was grossly oversold to the profession and to the public.[71]

Twin Studies

Twin studies are cited in every textbook I have ever used which addresses the issue of mental disorders. "The lifetime risk of developing schizophrenia varies with one's genetic relatedness to someone having this disorder.

Across countries, barely more than 1 in 10 fraternal twins, but some 5 in 10 identical twins, share a schizophrenic diagnosis."[72] Again, a genetic basis for schizophrenia may seem to be the only possible explanation. It is not.

Start with the basic fact that if twins are identical, they are both boys or both girls. Fraternal twins can be the same gender or different genders. But even when same–sex fraternal twins are born, they are less likely to be treated identically as identical twins would be. They are less likely to be clothed in identical outfits. They are less likely to participate in the same activities and pursue identical interests. And identical twins are more likely to be influenced by the experiences of each other since they have often been told they are identical. Identical twins are both more likely to have high or low IQs, poor eyesight or good eyesight, high physical attractiveness or low physical attractiveness (and so on) than are fraternal twins. (See Box #2–3, Comparing Apples and Apples?)

Those are just a few of the rather obvious critiques which must be made about textbooks' assumption that fraternal twins have environments which are just as similar as identical twins. That assumption (called the equal environment assumption) is essential to textbooks' common conclusion that genetics must be responsible for any greater incidence of schizophrenia in identical twins compared with fraternal twins. But when a more careful examination of the research is made, it becomes clear that this is another house of cards in the search for a genetic explanation for mental disorders.

The advocate of genetic causes would probably like to interrupt me here and object, "But with twin research we can isolate genetic versus environmental influences by examining those identical twins who have been raised apart." That would be a rather powerful research design if we actually had research studies involving identical twins that were truly raised apart. The most famous studies which claimed to have done so were those by British psychologist Sir Cyril Burt who died in 1971. Burt published studies in 1943, 1955 and 1966 which compared the IQs of identical twins raised apart

---

BOX #2–3

Comparing Apples and Apples?

Research which has examined the lives and characteristics of identical (monozygotic) twins has found that they differ from fraternal (dizygotic) twins in many ways. These facts can be found in many psychology textbooks from the 1950s and 1960s, but once biological psychiatry (chemical imbalances caused by genetic predispositions) took over, psychology textbooks removed discussions of monozygotic (MZ) and dizygotic (DZ) twin differences. (I suspect these discussions were removed because knowing these twins do not have equivalent environments invalidates the use of MZ–DZ studies as "proofs" for the biological view.) Here is just a sampling of how identical twins are more alike than fraternal twins:

(1) They are more similar in appearance.[1]
(2) They are more similar in height.[2]
(3) They are more similar in weight.[3]
(4) They are more similar in intelligence.[4]
(5) They are more likely to dress alike.[5]
(6) They spend more time together than fraternal twins.[6]
(7) Among identical twins, 47% are reported to have "very close attachment"—a level reported for only 15% of fraternal twins.[7]
(8) Identical twins are more likely to be "inseparable" during childhood (73%) than are fraternal twins (19%).[8]
(9) They are more likely to be raised as a unit.[9]
(10) They are more likely to experience "identity confusion" during childhood (91% vs. only 10% for fraternal twins.)[10]

---

with the IQs of identical twins raised together. That series of three studies provided strong evidence for the role of genes in determining intelligence.

I do not take issue with anyone who believes genes play an important role in transmitting height, skin color or intelligence. Even rat research has proved that "smarter rats" have smarter offspring—a fact we have known for many decades.[73] However, when Leon Kamin of Princeton University examined Burt's statistics, he concluded that Burt's statistics were not credible. When Burt added new twin sets to his sample, the correlations remained the same—an impossibility.[74] Two years later the *London Times* printed an article declaring "Crucial Data was Faked by Eminent

Psychologist." The *Times* reported that not only were the statistics made up, but Burt made up many of the twins and even the names of his collaborators.[75]

But even the very small number of studies that do examine identical twins reared apart are not convincing. As Harvard geneticist Richard Lewontin observed, most identical twins who are raised apart involve a mother who has died or a drug abuser who is too poor to raise both the children. Parents or a sibling have typically raised one of the twins. Thus, they are not really raised apart at all. They share birthdays, holidays, vacations and, most importantly, the same family. Many may not be raised in their mother's home but may nevertheless spend much time with her. Lewontin's conclusion? "As a consequence of such biases, there is at present no convincing measure of the role of genes in influencing human behavioral variation."[76]

No convincing measure? Then why does every psychology textbook continue to argue that twin and adoption studies have proven a genetic link? And this is sometimes done despite other facts being presented which make such claims seem illogical. Consider the following three statements which come out of but four brief, connected paragraphs in a single introductory psychology textbook.

- "The genetic contribution to schizophrenia is beyond question."

- "Adoption studies . . . confirm that the genetic link is real."

- "Although there are *barely more than a dozen such known cases* [emphasis mine], it appears that an identical twin of a person with schizophrenia retains that 1–in–2 chance [of developing schizophrenia] whether the twins are reared together or apart."[77]

Even a college freshman should know that "barely more than a dozen such known cases" is too small a sample size to be so bold as to declare a

"1–in–2 chance" of anything. One must wonder if any of these few cases are legitimate and worthy of analysis. Some studies have defined "identical twins reared apart" as meaning they did not live together for at least five years before schizophrenia developed.[78] But by this definition they may have lived together until they left home as young adults. No psychology text from which I have ever taught pointed out this incredibly flawed research design.

Jay Joseph, a professor at the California School of Professional Psychology, has become the authoritative voice on the validity of twin research studies. He has noted that following "the most important critique of twin research ever published"[79] (a study published in 1960 by Don Jackson), those studies fell into such disrepute that they came to be viewed as "virtual pseudoscience." Jackson's studies "wrote the obituary of the classical twin method, even if the world has been slow in realizing this fact."[80]

No group has been slower to abandon these very deceptive studies than writers of psychology textbooks, but until that changes, there is likely very little hope of overcoming the chemical imbalance view of mental problems.

Adoption Studies

> So many studies have demonstrated the heritability of schizophrenia that most investigators do not dispute the issue. In one of the best studies, Kety, Rosenthal, Wender and Schulsinger (1968) examined Denmark's *folkeregister* which contains a lifelong record of Danish citizens.[81]

These words begin the discussion of the heritability of schizophrenia in Neil Carlson's *Psychology: The Science of Behavior.* Carlson identified this Danish Adoption Study as one of the best, and it continues to be identified as one of the most cited.[82] Okay, the Danish Adoption Study is *the* study to turn to if we really need "proof" that schizophrenia is inheritable. That is

---

BOX #2–4

In Search of the Holy Grail

"There are several promising avenues . . ."
"We are closer now than ever."
"We have now learned so much that very, very soon . . ."
"We are on the verge of finally . . ."

For as long as I have been an avid reader of the research, I have read comments such as these concerning the genes that are supposed to be responsible for mental problems. The pot of gold at the end of the rainbow is always almost within reach and getting closer all the time. The search has involved X–rays, CAT scans, PET scans, single–photon emission computed tomography (SPECT) imaging, MRIs, functional MRIs (fMRI), MRI sequences (blood oxygen level–dependent signal–sensitive sequences) and magnetic resonance diffusion tensor imaging (MR–DTI). Research expenditures have involved hundreds of millions of dollars.

Drs. Nadine Norton and Michael Owen, two true believers in a genetic cause for schizophrenia, noted that "the search for genes for schizophrenia has often been described as a 'search for the Holy Grail.'"[1] The Holy Grail, of course, has never been found though many false claims of its discovery have surfaced over the last 20 centuries. About this search for genetic links, Norton and Owen have written, "The quest for these, while difficult, is not doomed to failure and at last seems to be showing clear signs of success."[2]

That's the line (or one similar to it) that I've been hearing for decades and, I suspect, will continue to hear for decades. To their credit, however, when Norton and Owen assess the current state of what we actually know, they write, "Although we can say that genes are important and that there are likely to be a number of them involved, we cannot say how many there are, how much risk each one confers or how much they interact."[3] Amen.

---

what the textbooks teach, and that is what is still suggested in recent journal articles. In other words, we are continuing to be fooled!

In reality the Danish Adoption Study is junk science and does not prove schizophrenia is inheritable at all. But the study has been cited as *the* study so many times by so many textbooks and articles that it is hard even to believe that it is a hugely flawed study. That helps explain the strong reaction of one psychiatrist who researched and wrote about the Danish study:

When I located the original 1975 summary report on the
Danish study by Kety and his colleagues in the book
Genetic Research in Psychiatry, I was shocked by what I
found.[83]

What he found was that the most famous and most cited study to supposedly show a clear genetic influence in the development of schizophrenia
revealed just the opposite. The study's statistics revealed that there was *no*
increase in schizophrenia among close biological relatives. (I would suggest if you have taught psychology courses as many years as I have that you
read that sentence again.) It is hard to believe in view of what our textbooks
still teach. But then, read on and you will learn more of what the textbooks
do not share.

The research team, to prove their unfounded conviction that schizophrenia is genetic, reached out to find other relatives with schizophrenia and
then implied what more honest researchers could not have implied.
Psychiatrist Peter Breggin declared,

> [T]he whole genetics of schizophrenia rests on this house
> of cards. What hocus–pocus! . . . It discredits psychiatry
> that these studies have been used to prove the opposite of
> what they really show and that the public has been con-
> sciously propagandized with misleading information.[84]

Many other researchers have now criticized this study,[85] yet its conclusions will continue to be taught in psychology textbooks for many years to
come despite its terribly flawed design. So, specifically, what is wrong with
this very famous study? There are many problems (see the previous endnote for several articles and books that discuss the study's flaws), but I will
limit my list to the big three. These are easy to understand, and any one of
the three should be considered sufficiently serious as to invalidate the study.

The Danish Adoption Study Flaws: The Big Three

(1) Because fewer adoptees born to schizophrenics had schizophrenia than would be found in a sample taken from the general population (evidence that schizophrenia is *not* genetic), the researchers decided to make up a new diagnosis, "schizophrenia spectrum disorder," and let raters make a determination as to who had this disorder and who did not based on "their own understanding"—and the diagnosis was often made in five minutes while on an adoptee's front porch[86] *after* the data was already gathered in order to demonstrate a link between genes and schizophrenia. (It is universally considered dishonest to adjust definitions after the data is already in; and if Kety's research team had not used this very broad and very questionable label, no significant relationships would have been found!)

(2) Danish adoption agencies tried to place newborns into families that would closely match the birth mother's environment—and mental health status of the birth mother and the adoptees *was* considered.[87] In fact, the "matching" policy ensured that "less desirable" children (those whose mothers abused alcohol and drugs, for example) were more likely to be placed with "less desirable" adoptive parents (again, for example, those more likely to abuse alcohol and drugs). Since alcohol and drug abuse are risk factors for the development of schizophrenia,[88] we should expect to see more schizophrenia (or "schizophrenia spectrum disorders") in both the homes of those birth mothers who abused alcohol and drugs and in the adoptees' homes.

(3) Those with a "schizophrenia spectrum disorder" mother had a mother who was more likely to abuse alcohol and drugs. Alcohol and drug abusing mothers are more likely to have offspring who have neurological problems and low birthweight. These are associated with emotional, behavioral, social and language difficulties, academic failure and poor occupational opportunity[89]—sources of great stress and, hence, more schizophrenia.[90]

A sister study to the Danish Adoption Study is the Finnish Adoptive Family Study of Schizophrenia which the authors admit was very similar in

---

BOX #2-5

Hyping Genetics

Examples of genetic promotion are found throughout the research literature. Hannes Petursson and his colleagues published a paper with the title, "Genes for Schizophrenia Can Be Detected—Data from Iceland Implicates *Neuregulin* 1."[1] I read the article with great interest, wondering if this would be the first study which might utilize a fair design to actually uncover significant evidence for genetic causation.

However, when I got to the conclusion I read, "If *neuregulin* 1 is a schizophrenia susceptibility gene, its impact is unlikely to be limited to Icelandic or Scottish populations."[2] If? That's right. The paper's title is really just hype. The search will continue.

---

design to the Danish study.[91] It is also frequently cited by psychology textbooks.[92] One report of their work begins with these words which are almost amusing: "Earlier adoption studies have confirmed convincingly the importance of a genetic contribution in schizophrenia. The designs, however, *had not incorporated observations of the rearing–family environment*" [emphasis mine].[93]

The problems of the Danish study plague the Finnish study as well. (See Jay Joseph's *The Gene Illusion* for a full discussion of the study.) Dr. Joseph's research and analysis are excellent. His conclusion?

> Leaving aside all other problems, the evidence suggesting that the selective placement of adoptees occurred in these studies is reason enough to reject any conclusions about genetic factors. . . . Investigators such as Kety, Rosenthal, Wender, and Schulsinger were intent on confirming their strong genetic views. *As seen clearly in their published works*, they changed definitions, comparisons, and ways of counting to ensure that they would find what they were looking for.[94]

77

A Rational Conclusion

Once all the "evidence" for biological psychiatry is honestly evaluated, it is rational to conclude that it is a house of cards. It is also rational to conclude that "I've been fooled." We may hate to admit that we have been fooled, but we should recognize that being fooled is to be expected when the myth is so often repeated as truth. It is not hard to imagine drug company literature being biased, but we expect college textbooks to be believable. Yet, virtually every psychology textbook tells these same false stories. No psychology textbook author is a neuroscientist. These are generalists who write the same "facts" that are recorded by other psychology textbooks.

I suspect some authors have read enough to know that the genetic explanation is not scientifically sound and that the chemical imbalance theory is false, but their copyright–holding publisher would never allow them to disparage the conventional wisdom as it could result in a loss of sales. (One textbook author readily admitted to me that he could not tell the truth on another issue as the publisher would not allow it.) I will do what I can to change psychology textbooks. What I ask you to do is to keep reading and then share what you learn with others. As I stated at the beginning of this chapter, truth wins in the end, but it can take many years to get there.

3

"This is a really interesting question. This company has this high flying stock price. It's a very expensive stock. And yet, nobody seems to know how exactly the company makes its money. How strange is that?"[1]
— *Financial reporter Bethany McLean on Enron*

"If you were brave and said you didn't get it, he would turn on you. 'Well it's so obvious,' he'd say. 'How can you not get it?' So the analysts and investors would pretend to get it even when they didn't."[2]
— *Major investor on Enron president, Jeff Skilling*

HOW PSYCHIATRISTS AND DOCTORS ARE FOOLED

Gary's entire career was with a company purchased by Enron and with Enron itself. As a personal friend I was aware back in 2000 that Gary would be taking an early retirement in the not too distant future but by the end of 2001, the plunging value of his retirement account meant early retirement was not possible, and he would have to start all over. His retirement still won't come for many years.

Enron was America's seventh largest corporation one year before it suddenly began to collapse and had to file Chapter 11 bankruptcy. The mammoth $77 billion company began 2001 with its stock price at over $80 a share. By October the price was under $40.[3] But even then, 16 out of 17 stock analysts covering Enron had "buy" or "strong buy" recommendations on the stock.[4] Four months later its stock was worth only pennies. So the question becomes, How could the rating agencies, stock analysts, investment bankers and fund managers have all failed to accurately perceive Enron as a house of cards with a business model and financial structure that would insure its eventual collapse?

Bethany McLean and Peter Elkins's book *The Smartest Guys in the Room*[5] makes it clear that there were at least four dynamics (aside from the greed and some carefully planned deceit by Enron insiders) which kept almost everyone fooled right up until the end.

(1) Assumption: "Surely the company must be sound since the government's Securities and Exchange Commission (SEC) inspects the company's financial statements and requires regular quarterly reports that are made public for inspection by any consumer as well as the experts. If there were something wrong, we would all know it."

(2) Assumption: "Enron is regularly audited by one of the nation's largest accounting firms (Arthur Anderson). They can't have their books audited every year and pass those reviews if there is something amiss."

(3) Assumption: "A big corporation like Enron must have a lot of smart guys who have it all figured out. They know what they are doing."

(4) Intimidation: "Who do you think you are? We have smart people here who have done their homework and know this business. You just don't understand."

Common reaction: "Who am I to question these experts?"

Biological psychiatry (the chemical imbalance theory) has parallels to each of these dynamics.

(1) Assumption: "The government's FDA approves drugs to fix the chemical imbalance. There must be a chemical imbalance or the government would never approve the various mind drugs people have to take to deal with their mental problems."

(2) Assumption: "The textbooks all say there is a chemical imbalance responsible for depression and schizophrenia. The textbooks must be right. Professors all across the country use them. They wouldn't use those books if they were filled with errors."

(3) Assumption: "Psychiatrists are very smart people. They are doctors who do nothing but study the brain. They would know it if the chemical imbalance theory wasn't right."

(4) Intimidation: "We have an abundance of research today that proves mental problems are largely the result of chemical imbalances in the brain. It is a highly technical field of study using positron emission tomography and other imaging techniques that the average person simply cannot understand."

Common reaction: "Who am I to question these experts?"

Perhaps the single most important lesson we can learn from the Enron story is one which we all should see very clearly: Just because lots of experts agree, does not make it true. That lesson has great application as we discuss mind drugs.

Drug Companies' First Priority: Fool the Psychiatrists

There is a pecking order in the mental health profession. Psychiatrists (medical doctors who have completed a psychiatric residency after earning their MD degree) are on top. Psychologists are generally viewed as being next in line. Then come the licensed marriage and family therapists and the psychiatric social workers. An assortment of other counseling specialists follow. The point is, if you want to impact the entire field, the profession which is the most important to influence is psychiatry. Academic psychiatrists are the opinion leaders. They are considered the most important conference speakers. Many are actively involved in drug research. Psychiatrists are, generally speaking, the only mental health professionals who can prescribe drugs. The drug companies of America are keenly aware of all this.

There is an education to be found in looking through old issues of the *Archives of General Psychiatry*, America's leading psychiatric journal. I have done so, and I am impressed by how hard it would be for a psychiatrist not to be fooled into believing that mental problems are caused by biochemical malfunctions in the brain. Drug advertisements fill the journal's pages with "the most advanced science" revealing the "truth" about depression, anxiety, schizophrenia and other mental problems.

A 1979 ad had a photograph of an obviously depressed woman sitting at a desk.[6] She is surrounded by neurons. The caption reads, "Unraveling the mystery of depression . . . (Electron micrograph of human synaptic cleft*)." The asterisk takes the reader to the bottom of the page where we read in fine print similar to that found on a drug insert sheet, "*Postulated site of tricyclic antidepressant activity." I have great reading vision. I could read the fine print, though I'll admit that I almost missed the word "postulated" as it was printed in white against a white background! Here was a full–page ad that tried to convince the reader that "science" now understands depression is due to a biochemical problem, and then they try to hide the fact that this is only a guess—a guess designed to make them billions of dollars if psychiatry can be convinced.

One of the messages that must be recognized in these ads is that, even before the first serotonin drugs became available (Prozac was first released in January 1988), the chemical imbalance (biological psychiatry) concept was being actively promoted by the pharmaceutical companies in a host of ways. Virtually all psychiatrists who have graduated from medical schools in recent decades have been indoctrinated in biological psychiatry. So successful has been this effort that even suggesting that it may be stress or family conflict or drug abuse that weakens the brain and helps bring about depression or schizophrenia rather than some unmeasurable chemical imbalance in the brain can bring a strong emotional response.

The Ideological War

Colin Ross, a psychiatrist and former professor of psychiatry who is one of a small but growing number of dissenting voices, calls this an "ideological war":

> Undermining the psychosocial would not be necessary if the biological actually had a solid scientific foundation. If there actually was a scientifically established genetic basis to schizophrenia, there would be nothing for biological psychiatrists to be defensive about, and therefore no need to belittle psychosocial variables. The ideological war within psychiatry about the dogma of biological psychiatry is itself evidence of the pseudoscientific nature of biological psychiatry.[7]

To call biological psychiatry a pseudoscience is as strong a verbal attack as could be voiced. Pseudoscience is generally the term applied to those who "document" alien abductions (Harvard professor and psychiatrist John Mack has, he claims, through hypnosis, recovered countless abduction memories that had been repressed in his patients' minds[8]) or those who advocate superstitious rituals to insure success in life (baseball great Wade Boggs's chicken dinners, 7:17 p.m. sprints and other rituals being the best known example[9]). Could it actually be that the whole "chemical imbalance" idea is not supported by scientific facts?

Dr. Susan Kemker, a New York psychiatrist, has provided a description of her own training that gives credence to the charge that biological psychiatry is pseudoscience. She describes an education in which she was taught the chemical imbalance view as though there was no question about its truth. And then she read Alvin Pam's critique of biological psychiatry.[10] Dr. Pam's book proved to be shocking and somewhat devastating. As she read, she began to see how badly she had been fooled. Her educational experience had led her to believe that what were actually unproven ideas were scientific facts. Her own life illustrates how the educational system can "brainwash" highly intelligent people. And once the professionals are all convinced, fooling the rest of America isn't too hard.

Dr. Kemker's description is so clear and so representative of what I believe occurs in psychology and psychiatry programs everywhere that, despite its length, it needs to be quoted in full.

> When I read his work [Dr. Pam's book on biological psychiatry], I felt that my entire education as a psychiatrist was subject to question. Some of the studies being scrutinized were known to me as major contributions to the field. I was shocked to find not a single "landmark" study emerging as methodologically sound. Definitions of terms alone rendered many of their conclusions invalid. The twin studies began with very questionable definitions of "reared apart," "same environments," and even "schizophrenia." There were biases in patient selection and interviews. Results were almost invariably overstated, with much confusion between correlation and cause.

> With virtually no regard for the flaws described, these studies were cited to my class of residents as "proof"of genetics of such disorders as schizophrenia and alcoholism, as well as for such theories as the dopamine hypothesis. They laid the foundation for a "medical model" of mental illness, which espoused the comforting faith that medical solutions would be found. These studies were regarded as part of an effort to develop psychiatry as a science. They were presented to me in textbooks and lectures with much authority, and I took them in—not the studies per se but their "bottom lines": that mental illness was determined by genes and neurotransmitters, to be eventually conquered by precise pharmacology.

> How could I have accepted so much pseudoscience uncritically? How could I have learned so much by rote, as if

what I was learning was the truth rather than assertions to be questioned?[11]

To understand how devastating it could be to any psychiatrist to realize that the chemical imbalance "fact" is not a fact, you must ask what is the alternative? What is a psychiatrist with many years of training to do with all the clients he or she is paid to help? If drugs aren't the answer, and if the psychiatrist is aware of the growing concern about the limited effectiveness of talk therapy,[12] what options are left?

Even for those who are great believers in talk therapy, it is a fact that psychiatry has been so won over by the biological view that some psychiatric programs provide essentially no psychotherapy training at all. That's not illogical if mental problems are all biologically caused (chemical imbalances in the brain). In fact, eliminating any kind of psychotherapy training began to be advocated as America became convinced that mental problems truly are just chemical imbalance problems.

Peter Breggin has noted that one of the profession's more influential psychiatrists gave a presentation at a 1987 conference, the year Prozac was approved, suggesting it was time for psychiatry to move away from a psychotherapy model entirely.[13] A little over a year later Samuel B. Guze, another very influential psychiatrist, wrote his much discussed paper, "Biological Psychiatry: Is There Any Other Kind?" In Guze's opinion, even to suggest that alcoholism, schizophrenia or depression are not genetically determined brain chemistry problems represents a prejudice against his view of psychiatry "stemming more from philosophical, ideological, and political concerns than from scientific ones."[14] For Guze, "there is no such thing as a psychiatry that is too biological."[15]

Want To Be A Psychiatrist? Then You'd Better Agree!

The very first faculty hiring committee on which I sat taught me that PhDs can be as guilty of failures in objectivity as anyone else. We had nearly

100 applications for a single position within our college's Division of Social and Behavioral Sciences. I placed into one stack the most outstanding candidates, but the one application that came to the very top was a university president who wanted to get back to full–time instruction. He was heavily published, came with outstanding recommendations (including an oral recommendation from our institution's president), and his research interests were directly in line with our specific interests.

However, to my astonishment, the chair of our committee (now deceased) did not even want to offer him an interview. "Why? He meets every criterion we have in spades." "Yes," he responded, "but he wouldn't really enjoy teaching after being a university president." I quickly realized that there was either an intimidation factor or an ideology concern (the applicant was the president of a conservative Baptist university). Arguing on the applicant's behalf would not have secured him an interview or been appreciated. I set his application into the "not under consideration" stack.

Dr. Guze, who served for many years as the head of the Department of Psychiatry at the Washington University School of Medicine, freely admitted that a physician's ideology determined whether he or she would be admitted to the medical school's residency training program. His admission is shocking but speaks to how strongly the biological view is seen as the only view a physician can properly hold:

> It has been my custom to interview as many as possible of the medical school students applying for positions . . . . There is one subject I have selected from these discussions to talk about on this occasion, because it is an issue that has come up often and touches on a very important subject for psychiatry . . . our department's "strong biological orientation." . . . A favorite response of mine is to raise the question about how can one think about psychiatry and psychiatric disorders except in terms and concepts strongly rooted in biology. Naturally, and unsurprisingly given the situation, nearly all students smile at this point and nod their heads

to signify that they agree with me or at least that they are sufficiently skilled in such encounters not to disagree directly.[16]

Dr. Guze had been an early proponent of genetics being destiny. His adoption studies served to confirm his theory. Guze reported that Danish adoptees who had an alcoholic parent were much more likely to become alcoholics than were adoptees without a known alcoholic parent.[17] Despite the study being hugely flawed (see pp. 73–77), his much–cited study helped change the textbooks as well as the nation's thinking about this issue. But what he really did was to fool himself and hundreds of psychiatrists whom he trained. Today the genetic influence on alcoholism is widely believed, and the "proof" which is most commonly cited involves not only Guze's Danish adoptees but also the many Native American reservations where alcoholism is so pervasive.

Are Your Genes Your Destiny?

Today I always have at least a few students in my classes who are aware of the terrible alcoholism problem that exists on many of America's Indian reservations. And generally those students believe that Native Americans are genetically predisposed to alcoholism. "One drink, and they become hooked." It's an idea taught by textbooks:

> The American Medical Association maintains that alcoholism is a disease and that it is incurable. According to this view, even a small amount of alcohol can cause an irresistible craving for more, leading alcoholics to lose control of their drinking. . . . Some studies suggest a genetic factor in alcoholism and lend support to the disease model.[18]

Another text states, "Men with a particular gene (for which they can be tested) are likely to become alcoholics if they drink at all."[19] Though referenced, that statement is simply false. A quick check of the reference reveals that the study upon which the statement is supposedly based makes no such claim. Yet, the fact that this statement is found in a college textbook gives it great credence.[20] (For a discussion of this problem see Box #3–1, Textbooks Have Errors?)

I have a large collection of psychology textbooks dating from the 1950s until today. All the newer books note that genetics are at least partially or even primarily responsible for alcoholism. That is not what was uniformly being said 40 or 50 years ago. It is not that the causes have changed. The ideology has changed. Here is an example from an older textbook whose comments would greatly upset those trained to believe in "biological psychiatry"—which is nearly everyone today. The comments concern the high alcoholism rates found among the Standing Rock Sioux Tribe:

> The most significant data . . . related to why the alcohol problem is so much greater among American Indians than among their white neighbors. In this regard the data suggested, first of all, that pressures to drink are greater . . . . The second factor that seemed to account for the higher incidence of alcoholism related to the absence of sanctions against drinking. If a man spent all his money on alcohol, his parents might feed him and his children, even though they disapproved of his behavior. Such disapproval, incidentally, was generally not overt. If a man were put in jail by the police for drunkenness, his relatives would even sell their own household goods, in many cases, to provide his bail. A wife could not leave her husband for any reason, including chronic drunkenness, but if she did, leaving the husband was more strongly disapproved than the husband's drunken behavior.[21]

You can find similar comments in other psychology textbooks, but only if searching through textbooks from many years ago. Today it is widely believed that Native Americans are simply predisposed to become alcoholics. It seems to me that such an idea should be far more offensive than

BOX #3–1

Textbooks Have Errors?

Students are often surprised when I explain that I choose the best books I can find but that they are full of errors. Once I select a text, I do a careful reading for factual errors which typically results in the discovery of some 25–30 mistakes. Sometimes I find even more. One psychology textbook I adopted had three absolute errors and a fourth fact that was not wholly true . . . all on a single page![1] (The endnote gives those "facts" and evidence as to why each was wrong.)

This problem is not limited to psychology textbooks. The leading college precalculus textbook has so many errors that one math professor decided to post them on the web for his students.[2] One might think that in 2nd edition textbooks such errors would be removed. This error–filled precalculus text is in its 4th edition.

Neither are textbook errors limited to college textbooks. Until the year 2010 in Texas (and likely an even longer time in some states), many U.S. high school students will be learning:

(1) Columbus first reached North America in 1492.
    Fact: Columbus never reached North America. He explored the Caribbean islands and the northern coast of South America.
(2) James Monroe was the last president to have fought in the Revolutionary War.
    Fact: Andrew Jackson was the last president of whom this was true.
(3) The Fourteenth Amendment extended the right to vote to all 21–year–old males, including former slaves.
    Fact: It was the Fifteenth Amendment that gave blacks the right to vote.
(4) Before the Civil War, greenbacks were redeemable for either gold or silver coins.
    Fact: There were no greenbacks before the Civil War. They originated *during* the War with the 1862 Legal Tender Act.
(5) The Statue of Liberty is made of bronze.
    Fact: The outer structure is made of copper (hence, the green color).
(6) The equator passes through Texas.
    Fact: The equator is approximately 2,300 miles south of Houston, Texas.[3]

the research which found that environmental factors and personal values are primary culprits. The genetic view admittedly lessens personal responsibility, but it also says that Native Americans are born with a genetic flaw which keeps them from having as much control over their own lives (at least when it comes to alcoholism) as do the rest of us.

Genetic Predestination's Logical Endpoint: Silliness

Once the genetic predestination belief is fully accepted, as it is by most mental health professionals today, why should other human behaviors and personality variables not also be seen as being in large measure genetically controlled? (See Box #3–2, Biological Thinking Can Get Really Silly.) As you see, this gets absolutely silly, but a large body of research is dedicated to tracking down these links. Thus, we are told that those with a certain genetic make up are not just more likely to be alcoholics but are three times as likely to divorce. (It was the study that did more to convince Americans one can be born with strong alcoholic tendencies that also found those same individuals are far more likely to divorce—a less reported finding.)[22] We are also told that how much TV a person watches is significantly influenced by their genes.[23] So is their vocational choice,[24] whether or not they choose to smoke[25] and whether or not they become a criminal.[26]

Why Psychiatrists Accept the Biological View

Once the chemical imbalance/genetic destiny ideas dominated psychiatry, it simply was not critically questioned by psychiatrists. Everyone knew it was true, so why question it? The experience of a psychiatrist trained in Canada indicates that biological psychiatry crossed America's borders and entered Canadian medical schools as well:

> When I entered my psychiatry residency, I believed that research had demonstrated the genetic foundation of schizophrenia and had shown that schizophrenia is primarily a

BOX #3-2

Biological Thinking Can Get Silly

I am often amazed at how much absolute silliness gets reported as legitimate views by psychology textbooks. Biological psychology with its focus on chemical or genetic destiny seems particularly prone to silliness. Consider the following comments coming from just one page of one textbook:

> The biological perspective helps explain why we learn some fears more readily and why some individuals are more vulnerable. Human behavior was road tested in the Stone Age. We humans, therefore, seem biologically prepared to fear threats faced by our ancestors, and most of our phobias focus on such objects: spiders, snakes, closed places, heights, storms. (Those fearless about these occasional threats were less likely to survive and leave descendants.)[1]

The author then explains that people who pull out their own hair do so because our monkey or monkey–like ancestors practiced grooming and "grooming gone wild becomes hair pulling."[2] And why do some people develop a compulsion for repeatedly checking to be sure the doors are locked? "Checking territorial boundaries becomes checking and rechecking an already locked door."[3]

One more? We are told that the British, Japanese and German populations did not panic during WWII bombing raids on their cities. Why? "Evolution has not prepared us to fear bombs dropping from the sky."[4] Such silliness can only be believed by those who are convinced genes control our behavior.

biomedical brain disease. This view was almost universally accepted at my medical school, and I had never heard serious criticism of it while in training.[27]

I fully understand being fooled. I was fooled by a number of studies reported in my graduate school textbooks (and still reported in textbooks). Yet those who are critical readers of journal research have long known about these poorly designed studies and their erroneous conclusions. Don't most medical doctors in training to become psychiatrists realize this also? The answer is that they do not. Dr. Colin Ross in writing about this problem stated,

It was not surprising that medical students accepted the dogma of [chemical imbalances and genetically caused mental problems] uncritically: they had no time to read and analyze the original literature. What took me a while to understand, as I moved through my residency, was that psychiatrists rarely do the critical reading either.[28]

The "Real Doctors Prescribe Drugs" Complex

Dr. Ross has suggested another reason why psychiatry embraced the chemical imbalance idea. Psychiatry may be the least respected medical specialty.[29] Fewer and fewer medical students are choosing it as a career. Consequently, the average age of psychiatrists is continuing to get older.[30] Income is extremely low for psychiatrists compared with other medical specialties.[31] Many Americans are rejecting Freudian talk therapy as quackery. The whole field is lacking the kind of quality research (randomized, placebo controlled experiments) that now guides the rest of medicine. How can psychiatry even be seen as a legitimate branch of medicine?

I also saw how badly biological psychiatrists want to be regarded as doctors, and accepted by the rest of the medical profession. In their desire to be accepted as real clinical scientists, these psychiatrists were building far too dogmatic an edifice . . . pushing their certainty far beyond what the data could support.[32]

Prescribing drugs is one answer to this dilemma. Prescribing makes one seem like "a real doctor." It adds credibility in the eyes of the patient. This explains why the American Psychological Association's official policy for many years has been to pursue prescribing privileges for psychologists.[33] It also explains why their main opponent year in and year out has been the American Psychiatric Association.[34] If psychologists gain the power to prescribe, it will rob some power from psychiatrists. Indeed, psychologists are claiming that they are increasingly being marginalized because they cannot prescribe drugs.[35]

The Intimidation Factor

Dr. Guze knew how to intimidate the student physicians seeking a residency at Washington University's School of Medicine, but his article "Biological Psychiatry: Is There Any Other Kind?" surely had an even greater impact. Those with a business degree in marketing know that the "everyone is doing it" bandwagon ad is difficult to ignore. However, an even more intimidating strategy has been used by other biological advocates.

The chart below (Box #3–3, Comparison of Old and New Approaches) was created by British psychiatrist Julian Leff. It uses the "Surely you don't believe *that*, do you?" approach. Appearing in *Psychiatric Annals* where it would be seen by a large number of psychiatrists, the chart dichotomizes psychiatry into the "Old Approach" and the "New Approach." The old–fashioned, behind–the–times approach looks at the environment. Was there

---

BOX #3–3

Comparison of Old and New Approaches to Families of Schizophrenic Patients[1]

	Old Approach	New Approach
Disease concept of schizophrenia	A psychological response to family dysfunction	A biological illness that can occur in psychologically healthy families
Role of family	Implicated in the etiology of the illness	Not a causal factor; can influence the course of illness for better or for worse
Aim of therapy	To correct family dysfunction; the family is the client	To help family cope better with the illness; the patient is the client

Used by permission of *Psychiatric Annals*

---

sexual abuse? A hostile father? An alcoholic mother? Those background factors (which we *used* to believe to be so important) do matter but are not considered the most important factors in mental health. The newer, educated understanding is that schizophrenia is a disease, just like diabetes. There aren't many who can stand up against that pressure and, if they tried, they would receive some of the same wrath this book will incur. (Julian Leff has himself modified his views since creating the "Old vs. New" chart in Box #3–3. Though still a biological psychiatrist, he now believes family, social and cultural factors do play a role as well.)

The Benefits Factor

There may be many reasons for psychiatrists to adopt the biological view, but it is hard to ignore the benefits that come with going along with the conventional wisdom. "Going along" can result in free trips to Hawaiian or Caribbean conferences where other psychiatrists declare "chemical imbalances are behind all mental problems." It means free dinners, free symphony tickets and more from drug representatives who also provide free charts and literature that parrot the standard genetic/chemical imbalance arguments. It means consultancy fees and honoraria from the drug companies (see Box #3–4, The Benefits of Playing the Game). And it means a much larger, growing private practice as the hundreds of millions spent by drug companies on advertising bring patients to the office. There aren't many who can resist all the benefits.

How Other Doctors Become Promoters of Mind Drugs

If psychiatrists were all convinced of the effectiveness of mind drugs but general practice physicians, ob–gyns, internists and other doctors were not convinced, there would not be nearly as many people on these medications. Thus, drug manufacturers use every imaginable tactic to convince physicians that depression and other mental problems are primarily brain chemistry problems. In addition to massive amounts of advertising (discussed in the next chapter), the drug companies use company representatives who are regularly trained in how best to promote their employer's drugs.

⚹ "Drug reps" are so numerous that many physicians limit the number with whom they are willing to visit each day. These drug reps bring free food for office staff, free samples for distribution to patients (an important reason to see these drug reps),[36] free pens, free textbooks and other free gifts. The reps are sometimes authorized to provide free vacations for physicians who would enjoy spending a weekend with other physicians and hearing the latest "research" on the effectiveness of a given drug or class of drugs.[37]

⚹ Do these "marketing" efforts work? They work so well that there are now over 90,000 of these "drug pushers" walking the streets of America.[38] Since there are less than 600,000 office–based physicians in the U.S. today,[39] there is approximately one full–time drug rep for every six office–based physicians (which explains why the medical literature sometimes has articles on how to cope with their constant attention).[40] Of course, drug reps do not see themselves as "drug pushers." They believe their job is in large measure to educate doctors—98% saying so in one survey.[41] Most of this same sample did not believe that their main job was marketing, and 96% of them believed the information they provided the physicians was accurate.[42]

As you learn how drug studies are designed (mind drug studies being the most problematic of all), you will learn that these drug reps are wrong. The information they provide is often inaccurate. Furthermore, they are primarily marketers. This is not just a matter of being self–deceived. Drug companies know their armies of drug reps will have better morale and will be more convincing if they truly believe their role is to educate doctors.

Jerry Avorn, a Harvard Medical School professor and drug researcher who may be the leading authority on how physicians are educated about new drugs, states that drug reps may be close to the mark as regards their educational role. It is not something Dr. Avorn approves, but he acknowledges that most physicians have only minimal knowledge about drug studies. Few gather information through a careful examination of the medical

---

BOX #3–4

The Benefits of Playing the Game

Until recent years few journals asked authors to disclose financial conflicts of interest. A study out of Tufts University found only 16% of 1,396 scientific journals even had a policy related to the issue.[1] Because of this failure, the tobacco industry has been able to publish many scientific papers on smoking which found it relatively safe using company employees or university professors whom they paid as authors.[2] Findings such as that prompted more and more scientific journals to adopt conflicts of interest policies.

Nowhere is this more needed than in psychiatry since no profession of its size has so much money seeking to influence it. Now that some of the psychiatric journals have adopted conflict of interest policies, we can get some idea about whether or not there are drug industry ties to the drug research. Are there? "Wow!" is the best answer. Here is the brief "declaration of interest" for one *Psychiatric Bulletin* article:

> D. T. has received research funding from various manufacturers of atypical antipsychotics and the Department of Health, and consultancy fees and honoraria for presentations received from AstraZeneca, Janssen–Cilag, Novartis, Pfizer and Eli Lilly. S. M. has received consultancy fees and honoraria for presentations from Eli Lilly and Novartis; S. M. has received research funding from Pfizer; and E. W. has received honoraria for presentations from Eli Lilly.[3]

---

literature. So where do they get their knowledge about new drugs? Listen closely to Dr. Avorn's amazing conclusion:

> Pharmaceutical marketing is about the most important source of knowledge about new drugs for most physicians, and a major form of continuing conditioning as well.[43]

That is an absolutely startling admission, but perhaps we should not be surprised since the physician–industry relationship is established so early. During medical school students are showered with free gifts from the drug industry.[44] They attend presentations by pharmaceutical representatives

How profitable are some of these honoraria received for simply attending a medical conference and stating publicly (it may be a brief pronouncement or a full presentation) that a particular antidepressant or antipsychotic really works well? As an academic psychiatrist, E. Fuller Torrey has had many opportunities to "make pronouncements" and thereby profit handsomely. He has chosen to take the narrow road instead but is keenly aware of how common "kickbacks" are within his profession:

> There are colleagues of mine who have not only accepted tickets to football games, but been paid to go to football games, and then turn around and say this has not influenced them. . . . Ten thousand dollars is not an unusual amount of money to be paid to stand up and make pronouncements [at conferences]. . . . They are given future speaking engagements depending on how well they do.[4]

The Center for Science in the Public Interest (CSPI) is a non–profit organization whose purpose includes ensuring that the research found in medical journals is objective and honest. In an investigation into whether or not the journals with the best "conflicts of interest" policies were adequately monitoring the admissions of private industry ties, the CSPI researchers found they were not. Even at *JAMA* the CSPI researchers discovered that 11% of the articles were written by authors who failed to disclose their financial conflicts of interest.[5]

regularly (44% attend two or more each month).[45] This same study noted, "Students regard the pharmaceutical industry as one of their most important sources of pharmaceutical information."[46]

More and more medical schools are not even teaching pharmacology[47] and are allowing the drug companies to educate our future doctors through industry–sponsored lectures, meetings and lunches.[48] Indoctrinate them early, and most of them will be compliant for life. One critic of this system has declared, "Replacing medical education with industry promotion in the guise of scholarship causes demonstrable harm to trainees, the public, and the profession."[49] I agree, but the system is now in place and will likely continue well into the future.

The Medical Journals

The "mere–exposure effect" is a fascinating psychological principle. By repetitious exposure to anything new we will find our liking for it steadily increasing. That is why most of us prefer our own mother's cooking to someone else's cooking and why those who grew up in homes where classical music was appreciated nearly always like classical music. Experimental research has found that "mere exposure" increases our liking for various types of music, faces, geometric shapes—even nonsense syllables.[50] We even prefer the image we see in the mirror each day rather than its reverse as seen in a photograph, though our friends prefer the photo.[51]

Surprisingly, seeing without conscious awareness has a more powerful effect on us than does a more conscious recognition of what we actually see.[52] This has implications for anyone who reads printed medical journals. I just picked up a copy of the *New England Journal of Medicine* that was sitting on my desk and began counting how many pages of ads I had to pass over to get to the first article—31 pages. Pick up a copy of *JAMA* and you will have the same experience. Why do even the leading medical journals accept these drug ads (nearly all the ads are for drugs)? An editorial in the *British Medical Journal* gave a blunt but honest answer to that question: "The stark reality is that without pharmaceutical sponsorship many journals would not survive."[53]

Put the experimental research on mere–exposure effect with the reality that research and non–research medical journals are filled with drug company ads,[54] and we are forced to conclude that there is a daily, unconscious growth in appreciation for drugs among physicians. Many drugs save lives, fight infection or encourage healing, but there should always be a critical skepticism toward drugs. There is a multi–billion dollar interest by pharmaceutical companies to sell their drugs whether they work or not. And antidepressants are unique in both the boldness of their claims and their failure to pass honest efficacy tests. I'll ask you, the reader, to judge whether I am right or not in my judgment that there is a bias among physicians on behalf of antidepressants.

Here is an example of where I see bias. St. John's wort (hypericum perforatum) is taken by large numbers of Americans for depression. (A full discussion of the St. John's wort research is found in Chapter 8.) It makes sense to compare its effectiveness to the leading antidepressant pill (Zoloft) and to a placebo. A "Hypericum Depression Trial Study Group" was formed, research was conducted, and the results were published by the *Journal of the American Medical Association.*[55]

The experiment found that Zoloft, St. John's wort and the placebo all produced equivalent effects. However, the conclusion states, "This study fails to support the efficacy of *H perforatum* in moderately severe major depression." What did they not state? They neglected to state, "This study fails to support the efficacy of *Zoloft* in moderately severe major depression." Why did they choose to point out that St. John's wort only worked as well as a placebo but not point this out for the antidepressant? That may be the subtle, perhaps unconscious preference for advertised drugs which results from the mere–exposure effect. Of course I should point out that Dr. Davidson, the lead author, also

holds stock in Pfizer, American Home Products, GlaxoSmithKline, Procter and Gamble, and Triangle Pharmaceuticals; has received speaker fees from Solvay, Pfizer, GlaxoSmithKline, Wyeth–Ayerst, Lichtwer, and the American Psychiatric Association; has been a scientific advisor to Allergan, Solvay, Pfizer, GlaxoSmithKline, Forest Pharmaceuticals, Inc., Eli Lilly, Ancile, Roche, Novartis, and Organon; has received research support from the National Institute of Mental Health, Pfizer, Solvay, Eli Lilly, GlaxoSmithKline, Wyeth–Ayerst, Organon, Forest Pharmaceuticals, Inc., PureWorld, Allergan, and Nutrition 2 . . . and has received royalties from MultiHealth Systems, Inc., Guilford Publications and the American Psychiatric Association.[56]

The Specialty Which Refuses to Disclose Financial Conflicts of Interest

I hope you were startled by the research I shared a few pages back (p. 97) which found that medical school students (our future doctors) "regard the pharmaceutical industry as one of their most important sources of pharmaceutical information." I hope you were also stunned by the fact that Dr. Davidson has received money from nearly every major antidepressant drug manufacturer in America and Europe. We should expect objective research from an academic psychiatrist. Do you really trust Dr. Davidson to provide such?

Are physicians not aware of the influence drug manufacturers have on what is found in medical journals? Are physicians not aware of how biased the research is which is done on mind drugs? They are not. *JAMA* now demands financial disclosure (which allows readers to see how tied an academic psychiatrist is to the manufacturers of mind drugs). The psychiatric journals which publish a disproportionate number of articles on antidepressants and antipsychotics have many more pages of drug advertisements than the general medical journals. The *American Journal of Psychiatry*, the official journal of the American Psychiatric Association, will typically have over 50 pages(!) of drug ads before the articles begin. As you might suspect, they refuse to require authors who own stock in the drug companies whose drugs they research and write about to disclose these or any other financial ties.

No specialty has more financial conflicts of interest than does psychiatry. Allowing this system to continue as is is unconscionable. Yet, instead of being skeptical of any research appearing in the *American Journal of Psychiatry* or the *Archives of General Psychiatry* (as I am), I suspect many physicians assume that since these are the leading psychiatric journals, their articles should be seen as especially credible. Clearly, it would be easy for the average physician to be fooled.

How Much Do the "Experts" Really Know?

Psychiatrists should discount drug company information in favor of medical journal research and should even be cautious and critical readers of the medical research. Yet, something very strange is occurring in psychiatry today. Not only are many psychiatrists not very skeptical of the mind drug research; some apparently view reading journal research as optional. I suspect this is because a majority are now almost fully convinced that they cannot really help their clients other than by prescribing pills. Here is how one psychiatrist put it:

> Reading our current psychiatric journals is probably character–building and interesting for the sake of knowl-edge, but optional. I say this from feeling that the journals will not contain evidence to change expected clinical prac-tice and that most psychiatrists feel similarly.[57]

This absence of scientific skepticism is most apparent when we examine the health consequences of taking these drugs. I have long known that very few individuals taking mind drugs have any awareness of the brain damage and other side effects of taking antipsychotics or antidepressants. I learn that truth again every semester when lecturing to students on this subject. However, I was amazed to discover that psychiatrists, the medical specialty which should have the most intimate knowledge of this subject, are, as a group, just not aware of the research.

For example, two side effects of antipsychotics which have received much attention include significant weight gain[58] and the hugely increased risk (4 to 6 times) for developing diabetes.[59] Yet, a nationwide survey of 300 psychiatrists chosen at random found only half (51%) had any knowl-edge that taking antipsychotics can cause their patients to develop diabetes. Only a little over half (59%) were aware that these drugs cause weight gain.[60] Even more disturbing, only 2% knew that diabetic ketoacidosis, a condition that can cause a patient to enter into a coma or even cause death, can result from taking antipsychotic drugs.[61] All of these findings have been widely reported in the research literature.

I can understand how some general practice physicians may not know about these side effects, but I cannot excuse psychiatrists. This is basic to what most psychiatrists do most of the time. These findings tell me that psychiatrists, as a group, may be reading the literature the drug reps bring to their offices, but they are not reading the journal research.

Physicians Are Given "False and Misleading" Information

Of course, the health consequences of taking a mind drug are not facts about which the drug companies actually want to make psychiatrists keenly aware. That is apparent from examining some of the correspondence between the FDA and the drug companies (much of which is a matter of public record and available on the internet[62]). For example, when the FDA reviewed what is known as a "Dear Healthcare Provider" (DHCP) letter for Janssen Pharmaceutical's antipsychotic drug Risperdal (risperidone), they found Janssen's letter was clearly meant to deceive. (The FDA described it, in their usual language for such a deception, as "false or misleading."[63])

The FDA–approved package insert that comes with a prescription for Janssen's Risperdal reads,

> Hyperglycemia, in some cases extreme and associated with ketoacidosis or hyperosmolar coma or death, has been reported in patients treated with atypical antipsychotics including Risperdal. . . . Epidemiologic studies suggest an increased risk of treatment emergent hyperglycemia–related adverse events in patients treated with atypical antipsychotics.[64]

Translated, the FDA–approved warning states that if patients take Risperdal, they are more likely to develop diabetes, diabetic ketoacidosis and other high blood sugar problems such as eye, heart and kidney damage. But what did Janssen's letter to physicians (their DHCP letter) state?

> Hyperglycemia–related adverse events have infrequently been reported in patients receiving Risperdal. Although confirmatory research is still needed, a body of evidence from published peer–reviewed epidemiology research (1, 2, 3, 4, 5, 6, 7, 8) suggests that Risperdal is not associated with an increased risk of diabetes when compared to untreated patients or patients treated with conventional antipsychotics. Evidence also suggests that Risperdal is associated with a lower risk of diabetes than some other studied atypical antipsychotics.[65]

In other words, the DHCP letter sent to physicians and the package inserts that come with their drug have very contradictory statements. Only one can be true. The one that is true is the one with the very small print. This brought the warning letter from the FDA. That letter is most revealing. It indicates that Janssen purposely tried to deceive physicians into believing their drug was safe—in fact, particularly safe. Here is the FDA's response to Janssen's DHCP letter:

> The references cited in the letter do not represent the weight of the pertinent scientific evidence. That evidence, as explained above, indicates an increased risk of hyperglycemia–related adverse events and diabetes with Risperdal. In addition, this statement does not accurately describe the results of the cited studies. Two of the studies (1, 8) actually show an *increased* risk of diabetes and hyperglycemia with Risperdal.[66]

The FDA then criticizes Janssen for failing "to recommend regular glucose control monitoring to identify diabetes mellitus as soon as possible."[67]

It is inexcusable that drug companies are routinely guilty of downplaying, denying and hiding the adverse health effects of their drugs. Millions of people are putting their health at risk—and many are dying[68]—because their psychiatrist or physician is not aware of the dangerous health risks mind drugs pose.

One More Reason Physicians Prescribe Antidepressants

There is at least one more reason most physicians freely prescribe antidepressants—most sincerely believe they can work wonders. It is not just that the drug reps say these drugs can cure all kinds of mental problems. Most physicians have seen it with their own eyes. And so today these drugs are prescribed for depression, anxiety, stress related to marital problems, compulsive behaviors, eating problems, anger and sometimes even immorality. (See Box #3–5, Can Immorality Be Fixed With a Pill?)

I regularly hear stories indicating that antidepressants are prescribed even when they are not sought. Over and over friends or clients share comments, such as

- "I had not been sleeping as well as I used to. I had hoped he might give me something that would help. I was surprised that he gave me an antidepressant. I told him I wasn't depressed, but he said to give it a try."

- "When I went in for my annual check–up, my ob/gyn asked me if I ever feel tension before or after my menstrual periods. I said, 'Yes, but it has never been anything major.' Then she almost insisted that I try an antidepressant and just see how it worked for me."

- "My husband and I have some conflict occasionally. It isn't anything major, really, but when my doctor asked about my marriage and I told him it wasn't perfect, he felt certain that an antidepressant could help."

- "Recently our only child began college 500 miles away and about the same time I realized I was dissatisfied with my job.

BOX #3–5

Can Immorality Be Fixed With a Pill?

I had a couple come see me about their relationship. She had recently given birth to their baby but, though engaged, she wasn't sure she should marry her fiance. He was all for getting married, and he was the one to contact me when it looked like she was losing interest.

When it was time to find out why they were engaged but she was thinking about ending the relationship, I turned to her. "Tell me what your concerns are about marriage." This is what I learned. In addition to the sexual relationship he was having with her, he was in sexual relationships with a few additional women. He jumped in. "I don't want to keep having these other relationships. That's why I am here really. I just want to get some insight into why I keep doing this. I don't know if there are unconscious, unmet needs that I'm trying to meet or if this is due to an unconscious depression that is masking itself through sexual acting out. Maybe I need to take an antidepressant."

Could his problem have been caused by an unconscious depression? I did not offer him that out, but his very language indicated how successful marketing efforts have been. He was not the first person I have heard blame an immorality problem on the acting out of an unconscious depression. Others have confessed to angry outbursts and hitting or an unwillingness to help with family chores and then blamed it on an "unconscious depression." Far more have told me they began taking antidepressants for the first time after sharing a behavioral problem with their physician, and the physician suggested an antidepressant. Is a pill the answer to anger, abuse or immorality? That anyone can be convinced a pill has such power may be a testimony both to human gullibility and to the power of marketing. Or it may represent the human tendency to grasp for any excuse we can find to reduce responsibility for bad behavior.

I was really feeling blue when I went to the doctor, and he prescribed an antidepressant."

How is it that physicians see with their own eyes the powerful effects of taking an antidepressant when these drugs actually lack that power? To explain this mystery I will need to share an imaginary study comparing antidepressants, psychotherapy and exercise.

We will assume that for this study we randomly assigned 40 depressed subjects to each of our three experimental groups. After six weeks, we measured depression levels in each subject. Here are the results. Consider them carefully, and then I'll share how this relates to physicians seeing the benefits of antidepressants with their own eyes.

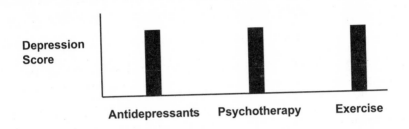

Now, if you were the physician and you knew the results of such a study, would you prescribe antidepressants, psychotherapy or exercise? You would likely suggest exercise because it relieves depression just as well as drugs or therapy yet, unlike these other options, it does not cost any money. Add to that the fact that exercise has physical (not just mental) benefits, and exercise wins hands down.

But, now, let's do that imaginary study again, except this time we are going to add a fourth group. The fourth group will be what is known as a control group. They will be measured for depression at the same time the other groups are measured for such, but they will be told that we will need to put them on a waiting list and we will get to them as soon as possible. Again, remember this is an imaginary study. But with that in mind, let's look at the results of our second study.

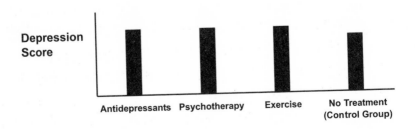

What happened? The "no treatment" group did not do as well as our other groups, but they did almost as well. How could that be possible? The answer could be related to the old saying, "Time heals all wounds." If people are most apt to visit their doctor when they are in a physical and an emotional crisis (and they are) and the doctor, believing that antidepressants really work well (whether they do or not) prescribes an antidepressant and then hears from the patient at the next appointment "I'm doing great now," they tend to assume the healing is due to the drugs (not that the trauma has simply passed). We call this confirmation bias. (See Box #3–6, Confirmation Bias.) Once we believe something to be true, we see and remember examples of its truth whether it is true or not.

If you are like my students and my clients, you will not be satisfied with an imaginary study. You want to know if there really has been research comparing exercise and antidepressants. There have been many studies. I will provide a full discussion of that research in Chapter 8 (Do Antidepressants Work?), but I won't leave you hanging. I will share with you the conclusion of those studies right now. Here it is: Exercise is not just as good as taking antidepressants. It is better! Were those studies designed and paid for by the drug companies? Of course not. No pharmaceutical company would allow its scientists to conduct such a study any more than they are apt to pay for advertising that tells the world that exercise is better than their drugs. No, these studies are independent of the drug companies and, thus, far more credible.

If you are a medical doctor and are feeling put down by the suggestion that you have been fooled by the drug companies, I have two comments to make to you. First, you have been fooled. I make no apology for saying so. But, as I noted in my "Personal Note to Physicians" (p. 19), I am also very sympathetic. Dr. Jerry Avorn, the Harvard Medical School physician and academic scientist mentioned earlier, would be as well. "Studying drugs is what I do for a living, and I still have trouble finding a reliable way to compare a given medicine with its alternative in terms of effectiveness, safety,

---

BOX #3–6

Confirmation Bias—Why Doctors Increase Dosages and Try Other Antidepressants

The psychological principle known as confirmation bias states that once we become convinced something is true, we don't just see examples of it—we look for and remember supporting "proofs" and reject and forget evidence which does not support our belief. That is one of the reasons it is hard to change someone's opinion once they have an opinion (a psychological principle known as the belief perseverance phenomenon).[1]

For a physician who has become a believer in the effectiveness of antidepressants, which of the following examples will most likely be remembered?

Positive Report: Doctor, I do appreciate your encouraging me to take this antidepressant. I really didn't want to get on antidepressants. I had always doubted they even worked, but I was feeling pretty desperate. And now I'm doing better than I ever dreamed I could be doing. I'll surely never again suggest you can't fix depression with a pill. They gave me back my life.

Negative Report: Doctor, I think I need to get off these drugs. I've been miserable since starting them. I'm not sleeping any better and I'm having some sexual problems. I don't think I am any better than I was before. In fact, now I've got some new problems.

Once a physician is a true believer, he or she will assume that the patient with a negative report needs a larger dose (though larger doses have been shown not to help[2]) or needs to try a different antidepressant (though pharmacological differences are reported to be irrelevant[3]). That is the real world. I hear it on a regular basis. "They are trying to get my medication adjusted." In other words, the person still has problems, so perhaps another drug will work better. Often more than one medication will be prescribed.

Again, I will emphasize that there is no blood or urine analysis performed to determine if the drug or the dosage is actually raising or lowering a neurotransmitter level or anything else in the brain. No, this is a hit and miss proposition that will continue until the patient has a good report. That is the real world, but it should not be.

---

and price."[69]   He also confessed, "We know much less than our patients think we do about the drugs we use."[70] That from a researcher who has published over 200 papers on drugs and drug effects. Today finding the truth about a drug can be time–consuming and difficult. Most of you in private practice just do not have the time or the research design backgrounds needed to dig through and analyze design weaknesses in drug studies.

Second, I want to say, "Thank you." I can promise you that reading this book will educate you to some facts that will cause you to be more skeptical. That's not bad. That skepticism added to the information you will gain from reading the chapters which follow will help you do a better job of protecting and helping your patients.

4

"Human beings are absurdly easy to indoctrinate."[1]
— Edward O. Wilson
Harvard biologist

ADVERTISING WORKS

A question for married women: How would you have felt if your husband had presented you an engagement ring that had no diamond?

A question for married men: Did you even consider not purchasing a diamond ring for your fiancee?

We all know how most Americans would answer those questions, yet prior to 1939 diamonds almost never adorned engagement rings. Most people could not afford gems and, if they could, they typically wore rubies, sapphires or emeralds. But beginning in 1939 shortly after an executive with DeBeers, the diamond–mining syndicate, met with the N. W. Ayer and Son advertising firm in New York City, diamonds took on a new meaning. DeBeers provided diamond rings which were given to the early Hollywood movie stars. The stars were simply asked to wear them in their movies—especially in engagement scenes. Magazine ads showed a young man pulling out a diamond as he proposed to his future wife. And then, starting in 1948, the "A Diamond Is Forever" campaign was launched. After twenty years of promotion, the New York advertising agency contracted by DeBeers was able to report, "To this new generation a diamond ring is considered a necessity to engagements by virtually everyone."[2] (Isn't it amazing how a little advertising can dramatically influence our values and beliefs and behaviors? Advertising clearly works.)

In 1954 Marlboro cigarettes were a "mild as May" cigarette smoked by less than 1% of the nation's smokers when Philip Morris turned to a New York advertising agency in hopes of increasing sales. The cigarette never changed, but when the Leo Burnett Company came up with the "Marlboro Man," the brand went from a cigarette smoked by a small number of ladies to the best–selling tobacco product in the world.[3] Sales in 1955 rose 3,241% over 1954's pre–Marlboro Man levels.[4] The point? Advertising works.

Without advertising, Wham–O may never have left the garage where two friends started making 75–cent slingshots in 1948. Instead, they went from an almost unknown name to the makers of hula hoops, an old toy which needed the benefits of mass advertising. Within two months of entering the market, 25 million hula hoops had been sold, and before the year was over the number was approaching 100 million. First year profits exceeded $45 million—a fantastic sum in 1958.[5] The point? Advertising works.

In the South American country of Chile a marketing campaign was aimed at new and expectant mothers in hopes of getting them to use formula for their newborns. Breastfeeding rates plummeted from 90% in 1960 to less than 10% by 1968.[6] In 1960 it was known that the inferior "formulas" of that era were associated with higher infant mortality rates and more diseases and infections. Those medical facts did not matter, but advertising did. It works.

Advertising Directly to the Consumer

There are thousands of additional examples, each of which points to one simple fact: advertising works. It works for drugs as well. Yet, there was a time when "direct–to–consumer" (DTC) advertising was not legal in America and so promoting Robert Wilson's *Feminine Forever*, establishing non–profit foundations to send out free literature, distributing free samples to encourage drug use by physicians, and advertising to physicians were the methods employed by pharmaceutical companies, as well as dozens of other back–door strategies. That all changed in 1997. That was the year that drug

---

BOX #4–1

Don't Be Fooled— Don't Buy the Purple Pill Nexium

Drug patents are good for 20 years in the United States and elsewhere.[1] If a company's profits are strongly tied to one or two blockbuster drugs, they can lose billions when a drug's patent expires. The Swedish–British drug company AstraZeneca faced that situation when the $6 billion Prilosec was going off patent in 2001. So what did it do?

It made an equivalent drug (using the "left hand" version rather than a left and right hand combination), added three yellow stripes on one end of the pill, got a new patent, and began what was one of the largest drug advertising campaigns America had ever seen—a campaign that would not be legal in Sweden or in Great Britain. There is no more benefit from the new Nexium than the much cheaper generic forms of Prilosec, but unless AstraZeneca could get physicians to prescribe and patients to request the new Nexium, profits would plummet.

An astonishing $219 million was allocated just for direct–to–consumer advertisements; advertisements which claimed Nexium was even better than Prilosec.[2] Yet Nexium is the same drug, so how can it be better? It's not, but in order to prove that it is, the company set up clinical trials where patients were given small doses (20mg) of Prilosec and full doses (up to 40mg) of Nexium.[3] An unfair comparison? People ought to go to prison for this kind of dishonesty. (Remember, this isn't like a minor $10 million bank robbery; this involves taking billions from mostly older people when it is completely unnecessary.)

The rest of the story? Too many citizens were catching on, so in 2005 AstraZeneca reported it could not keep up with Prilosec sales (though sales were falling), and suddenly "shortages" of the then less expensive Prilosec emerged.[4] No such shortage for the more expensive (the patented Nexium) occurred!

companies were allowed to advertise directly to the consumer without having to list all the side effects of their drugs. (It actually became legal to do DTC advertising beginning in 1981, but the rules required full disclosure of all side effects. Drug companies knew that might hurt sales rather than help them, and listing all the harm that might befall users could consume most of a one–minute commercial.)

Drug companies from France, Great Britain, Germany, Canada and other nations joined with the U.S. pharmaceutical firms and pushed for changes in the FDA requirements, finally winning the battle. As long as they mentioned a few side effects and then said "For more information, see your doctor" or mentioned where the consumer could find additional information ("See this month's *Healthy Living* magazine for more information"), the pharmaceutical companies from France, Great Britain, Germany, Canada and other nations could do in America what they could not do in their own countries. In fact, America and New Zealand are the only developed nations in the world that allow direct–to–consumer advertisements[7] (and New Zealand is seeking to ban them altogether in 2006 despite a well–financed battle with the drug manufacturers[8]).

Once the FDA's policy changed, the money that went into DTC advertising was staggering, rising from $791 million in 1996 to $2.46 billion in 2000.[9] And it continues to rise.[10] Immediately requests from patients for drugs they felt they needed began to rise, with one out of four patients making such requests. A survey conducted by the FDA found that 85% of physicians reported that their patients asked either "often" or "all the time" for advertised drugs.[11] Yes, advertising clearly works.

The most requested drugs were those for treating impotence.[12] But antianxiety and antidepressant drugs were requested almost as often as those for impotence, and the mind drugs together were requested even more often. And mind drugs were sought more than twice as much as any other drug type including drugs for arthritis, allergies, high blood pressure and high cholesterol.[13] Yet the DTC ads, now a regular part of television viewing, account for only 15% of total drug promotion spending. Total promotional spending in 2001 amounted to over $19 billion,[14] an amount greater than the total gross domestic product of all but approximately 69 of the world's nations. Over 100 of the world's nations including Costa Rica, Panama, Uraguay, Bolivia, Honduras and most of the other Latin American countries have GDPs far below this amount.[15]

And where did the drug companies spend most of that vast sum? By a wide margin the largest amount was spent on antidepressant promotion.[16] Run the numbers, and you will find the pharmaceutical companies are spending $367 million dollars per week promoting their drugs.[17] That figure is correct, but I am just amazed when I consider it.

The next question needs to be "But is it working?" The answer is "Isn't it obvious?" Would drug companies spend $367 million per week if they were not certain that drug promotion increased drug usage? A government report found that in just one year the most heavily advertised drugs had prescription increases of 25%.[18] There is even a formula that generally applies to drug advertising: Each dollar spent on advertising increases drug sales by $4. So when AstraZeneca spent $108 million in one year advertising its purple heartburn pill Prilosec, it increased profits by about $432 million.[19] (As Prilosec was going off patent, promotional spending for its substitute "little purple pill" skyrocketed from these already lofty levels—which is another story. See Box #4–2, Would Your Physician Prescribe Nexium?)

Why It Matters

What does it matter if drug companies actively promote their drugs? Won't this inform the public about drugs which could benefit their health which they might never even know about otherwise? That is the standard view voiced by the drug companies. But there is another view. A study published in the *Journal of the American Board of Family Practitioners* reported that 49% of patient requests for drugs or other requests prompted by

BOX #4–2

Would Your Physician Prescribe Nexium?

As discussed in Box #4–1, Nexium is simply a much more expensive version of the now off–patent Prilosec. The two are equivalent drugs. So why would a physician write a prescription that costs $131.87 per month rather than $21.34 per month?[1] The *New York Times* reported a federal Medicaid–Medicare administrator told physicians at an American Medical Association conference, "You should be embarrassed if you prescribe Nexium."[2] Why? Because, as he noted, it costs far more but does not work any better than Prilosec. Yet physicians are prescribing Nexium more than ever.[3] Why would they do this to their patients? Consider Prilosec's formula, and then I will answer that question.

The Formula: 5–methoxy–2–[[(4–methoxy–3, 5–dimethyl–2–pyridinyl)–methyl]sulfinyl]–1H–benzimidazole inhibition of the H^+/K^{+4}

The Point: The formula is the International Union of Pure and Applied Chemistry's official name for Prilosec. The point is that it takes PhD chemists with specialized training to understand what is in a drug. In other words, most physicians do not have the background to understand the chemical composition and action of drugs or the time to investigate. Thus, they often rely on the information provided by drug reps and on what they see and hear in advertisements—little of which is balanced. They don't prescribe Nexium to get kickbacks from its manufacturer. But neither are they the only group in America that cannot be fooled!

P.S. The same basic story could be told about Claritin (off patent) vs. Clarinex, Prozac (off patent) vs. Serafen, and many other drugs.

DTC advertising were not clinically appropriate.[20] In other words, physicians did not believe the patient needed an antidepressant or a test or some other requested intervention.

What would you do if you had a patient who asked for a drug that you felt they didn't need and you knew had risks (as all drugs do)? Would you comply with their requests? I would have thought that most physicians would take the time to explain that the drug option is not the best choice and, even if the patient insisted, say "I'm sorry." Yet 7 out of 10 times, physicians gave in to the requests.[21] And that is by their own admission. If there is a small percentage of physicians not willing to admit that they write prescriptions or order tests which are unneeded, then the true number is even higher.

Other research also points to the power of direct–to–consumer advertising finding it is more effective than providing the physician free samples or even doing "detailing" (drug company representatives meeting and teaching physicians about the latest "research" on an antidepressant or whatever drug he or she is promoting on that visit).[22] In fact, it appears that DTC advertising may be the single most effective way a drug company can increase the number of people who are diagnosed with depression and will then begin taking antidepressants.[23]

But what if the patient's physician will not give in to a patient's request? Real life can be tough—a fact doctors have to face regularly also. It is not easy to be firm when the patient's initial reaction is to become upset if denied the desired drug. Research on the issue has found that some (about 15 out of every 100 patients) will, in fact, decide to start using a different physician.[24]

False Claims

The FDA's Division of Drug Marketing, Advertising, and Communications (DDMAC) is responsible for keeping drug ads from making false claims. Now that the ads go out to anyone who watches television, it is more important than ever to monitor advertisements. But it is hard to regulate an industry that knows it can increase revenues by tens or even hundreds of millions with one dishonest but effective ad.

The Government Accounting Office (GAO) which sometimes investigates other government agencies looked at how well the FDA was doing at keeping false and misleading ads from being disseminated and concluded that the "FDA's oversight has not prevented some pharmaceutical companies from repeatedly disseminating new misleading advertisements for the same drug, and some pharmaceutical companies have failed to submit in a timely manner all newly disseminated advertisements to FDA for review."[25]

And why should they? (They should for moral reasons, of course, but I'm being pragmatic in asking the question.) One large law firm which advises pharmaceutical companies has very publicly noted, "The agency–imposed consequences for most promotional labeling problems are usually relatively mild, in the form of a Warning Letter or an untitled letter."[26]

Who Files Complaints

There are a lot of consumer protection groups in America, but most of the complaints made to the FDA's DDMAC do not come from these groups. In fact, most complaints come from the very group one might expect to be the last group to file a complaint—drug manufacturers.[27] Writing to the industry which pays its fees, the same law firm that admitted penalties are "relatively mild" when given noted, "Frequently, your competitor will send FDA copies of your promotional materials, advertising and labeling to provoke FDA into taking action against you for an alleged violation of the advertising and promotion rules, e.g., false or misleading claims or comparisons."[28]

Drug manufacturers must pay attention to their competitors' ads since an ad which states, "Five clinical trials have found our drug works better and has fewer side effects than does their drug," regardless of whether or not it is true, could absolutely decimate sales. Companies know they will get stopped if they go down that road, but they might not get stopped until great harm has been inflicted on the competitor.

BOX #4–3

A *British Medical Journal* Editorial:
Direct–to–Consumer Advertising

"No country has been successful at regulating any type of direct to consumer advertising to ensure the public obtains reliable balanced information on drug benefits and risks. Repeated breaches by companies speak for themselves."[1]

The FDA issued four letters to Pfizer for violations related to unfounded Lipitor claims including the assertion that Lipitor could reduce heart disease and was safer than competitors' rival drugs. But, as a GAO investigation reported, "Many television DTC advertisements are on the air for only a short time—about one–fifth of them for one month, about one–third for two months or less."[29] Yet, the FDA's warnings would take up to 78 days to issue—long after the ads may have stopped being shown anyway.[30]

It was not the fact that Pfizer claimed Lipitor could reduce heart disease that bothered Pfizer's competitors. It was that Pfizer claimed their product was safer than their competition's product. An inspection of FDA Warning Letters makes it clear that more warnings are related to "comparison issues" than to false statements. Zoloft continues to claim the following:

> Although the way Zoloft works for depression, panic dis-order, OCD and PTSD is not completely understood, what is understood is that Zoloft is a medicine that helps correct the chemical imbalance of serotonin in the brain.[31]

As I explain in detail in Chapter 2, there is no scientific basis for claim-ing that any antidepressant "helps correct the chemical imbalance of sero-tonin in the brain," though it has now been said so often that most Americans assume it is true. Advertising works! Yet the FDA still allows these claims to be made. If they decided to tell drug manufacturers to stop making this and related claims, it would make it to the evening news, and suddenly millions of Americans would believe they had not been told the truth. Sales of antidepressants would likely begin to slide. Pharmaceutical companies would lay off employees. It sounds dramatic because it would likely have a dramatic effect.

No one should be surprised that drug makers sometimes make false claims or even promote drugs known to be harmful. In the 1800s heroin was advertised by Bayer as a nonaddictive cough suppressant,[32] and there have been numerous examples during each succeeding decade of drugs being actively promoted that later proved to be unsafe. But drug stories and even their once–famous names are quickly forgotten as they go off patent protection. (There is no point in promoting a drug which won't make a lot of money—unless the public's benefit was truly the purpose of advertising.)

In 1988 the top–selling arthritis drug in the world was Voltaren (diclofenac), a name most of you probably don't remember any more. It became the top–selling arthritis drug in the U.S. as well, thanks in part to the drug's promotion by the famous but retired baseball star, Mickey Mantle. Mantle made numerous television appearances during the year and casually mentioned that growing older brought some additional aches and pains, but, fortunately, Voltaren was available. No one knew at the time that these appearances were bringing Mickey Mantle a substantial amount of money from CIBA–Geigy, the drug's manufacturer. What was known (by the manufacturer, not the public generally) was that Voltaren posed greater liver damage risk than did Voltaren's competitors. It was promoted anyway.[33] We now have enough history to know that this is the pattern.

Why Antidepressants Are So Heavily Advertised

Most Americans do not think of themselves as a little crazy, mentally unstable or completely insane. Neither do most of those who are a little crazy, mentally unstable or completely insane. So don't look for an abundance of direct–to–consumer television ads directed at this group. There is a lot of money spent in marketing antipsychotics, but that money goes towards physician "education." Conferences are sponsored where well–paid, drug–promoting psychiatrists and professors speak. Millions of dollars go to medical journal advertising. More millions go for the distribution of drug samples. Marketing dollars also fund research studies which, due to the study design, are very likely to yield positive results. Another effective marketing strategy is to ask a very large number of practicing physicians to participate in "research studies" which are never really designed to be published but tie the physicians personally to a drug.

Marketing departments also fund patient advocacy groups which use leading academic psychiatrists as consultants and board members. These groups support the use of mind drugs.[34] Private practice physicians and psychiatrists know they are not experts in neurotransmitters and neurochemistry, so they must listen to these expert consultants. In other words, antipsychotics are marketed primarily to physicians, not to the public.

When it comes to mind drugs, direct–to–consumer television ads are antidepressant ads. Unlike schizophrenia, there are great numbers of Americans who will freely admit they have had periods of serious depression, and nearly everyone will admit to having had at least some emotionally difficult time in their lives. If drug companies could convince a substantial number of us that these difficult times are due to a chemical imbalance in the brain, they would have a huge market. That's exactly what they have accomplished.

The next step was to convince lots of us that if we had depression or another mental disorder, a pill could fix the problem. Zoloft has been not just the nation's best–selling antidepressant in recent years; as its sales soared, it was also the most advertised antidepressant. To reach that top spot, Zoloft decided to expand its potential market by claiming Zoloft could fix more and more mental problems. So now, if you go to Zoloft's official website (www2.Zoloft.com), you will find Pfizer claims Zoloft can not only help overcome depression but can help with Social Anxiety Disorder, Posttraumatic Stress Disorder, Panic Disorder and Obsessive–Compulsive Disorder. (Another success which the drug companies have helped foster is that what used to be viewed as the normal emotional ups and downs of life is now viewed as one of many new disorders or diseases. For more on this, see Box #4–4, Isolated Explosive Disorder.)

Click on Social Anxiety Disorder, and Pfizer will inform you that "Social Anxiety Disorder is a real medical condition."[35] And how do you identify it? To help you determine if you have this disorder, a description is provided. It does not focus on blood cell counts or even serotonin, norepinephrine or

BOX #4-4

Isolated Explosive Disorder

For many years I have introduced students to the American Psychiatric Association's *Diagnostic and Statistical Manual* and its mental disorders by presenting case studies and asking them to find the diagnosis. (Each student is given a short list of mental disorders with brief criteria for determining a correct diagnosis.)

Case One goes like this: Before class begins a student is sitting at his desk, playfully twirling a pencil while quietly waiting for class to start. As the student continues playing with the pencil, another student initiates a conversation and says with a smile, "That's an awfully small baton," at which the first student stands up, shouts, "Shut up," pushes the other student, and then walks angrily out of the classroom. What is the diagnosis?

In the past we might say, "That guy has problems" or "Wow, he has a temper" or "He must have something bad going on in his life." No more. Today bad behavior has been "psychologicalized." The correct diagnosis in this case is "Isolated Explosive Disorder" if this is the first time, and "Intermittent Explosive Disorder" if he has had other angry outbursts.[1] New diagnoses come and others go on a regular basis (whenever the American Psychiatric Association meets to vote on diagnostic labels).[2]

Kids who are disruptive, who refuse to obey and who like to argue (kids who used to be called brats) are likely to be diagnosed with Oppositional Defiant Disorder.[3] Those who are lazy and refuse to do their schoolwork may have Academic Underachievement Disorder.[4] Those who steal things probably have Undersocialized Conduct Disorder.[5] Those who are clumsy have Developmental Coordination Disorder (Clumsy Child Syndrome).[6] Adults who foolishly gamble away their earnings will likely be diagnosed with a Pathological Gambling Disorder.[7] Those who smoke may have Nicotine Use Disorder.[8] Men and women who are very insecure and fear being rejected by others, consequently staying away from people and social events, may have Avoidant Personality Disorder.[9]

Giving medical labels to problems makes it possible for these people to receive insurance coverage when treated by psychiatrists, medical doctors and psychologists. Many of these diagnoses also commonly lead to an antidepressant prescription. That is, of course, why the drug companies spend untold millions to promote these "mental disorders." The fact that so many have so readily accepted these labels as legitimate is just one more evidence that America has indeed been fooled.

GABA concentrations. No, to determine if you have this "medical condition" you must simply ask yourself whether or not "you are afraid of making a mistake or looking like a fool." Do you know anyone who does not mind looking like a fool? They continue, "It feels like everyone is watching you and judging you." Do you know any junior high girls or boys who do not feel self–conscious? Do they all really have Social Anxiety Disorder and need Zoloft?

This is crazy, but some doctors have been so fooled that they freely write prescriptions. To continue—we are told, "You may even avoid certain people, places or social events." I have taught classes full of college students since 1982 and frequently speak to large audiences, but *I* am uncomfortable at some social events. But how many Americans reading such a prescription are fooled into thinking they may have a medical condition? The Zoloft ad then declares, "Social anxiety disorder is a serious illness. It can cause real problems in your life. Like any health condition, it needs to be treated." Next follows a list to help further clarify if you have this disorder and need Zoloft.

Social anxiety disorder can make you fear or avoid:
- Meeting new people
- Talking to your boss—or anyone in charge
- Speaking in front of groups
- Drawing any attention to yourself[36]

Based on my experience working with college students I would guess that, using Pfizer's criteria, Social Anxiety Disorder affects not just 5% of the population,[37] but something more like 90% of the population. Is it surprising that drug manufacturers now spend more dollars each year promoting their drugs than U.S. medical schools do educating their students?[38] (Yes, the total combined cost for all U.S. medical schools.) No dollars are more effectively spent than the direct–to–consumer advertising dollars. Advertising works!

5

ANALYZING AN ANTIDEPRESSANT AD — Effexor® XR

I recently made a visit to my physician's office. For want of anything else to read while waiting, I picked up a medical journal. As I flipped through the journal, I came across a four–page ad for Effexor, a drug aimed at overcoming not just one, but three common mental problems: Major Depressive Disorder, Generalized Anxiety Disorder and Social Anxiety Disorder. It caught my attention because the focus of the ad was on the data that supports Effexor's usage. Knowing what I know about the ineffectiveness of antidepressants and other mind drugs, I decided to read carefully what the advertisement had to say.

Page 1 was a photograph of a woman without a smile. The boldly printed words at the top of the page read, "See depression." The large words at the top of Page 2 read, "See the data." Page 3's headline declared, "See a

See the data.

Proven to achieve remission
of symptoms in 32 double–blind
comparative trials
with over 7,000 patients[2,3]

Proven to resolve emotional and
physical symptoms[4,5]

Proven tolerability with
once–daily dosing[2,3,6]

References: **1.** *Diagnostic and Statistical Manual of Mental Disorders.* 4th ed. Text rev. Washington, DC: American Psychiatric Association; 2000:349–356. **2.** Nemstein GE, Entsuah R, Willard LB, et al. Comprehensive pooled analysis of remission (COMPARE) data: venlafaxine vs SSRIs. Presented at the European College of Neuropsychopharmacology; September 20–24, 2003; Prague, Czech Republic. **3.** EX110. Data on file, Wyeth Pharmaceuticals Inc., Philadelphia, Pa. **4.** Entsuah R, Zhang J. Remission of depressive symptoms in patients treated with venlafaxine or SSRIs. Presented at the World Congress of Women's Mental Health; March 17–20, 2004; Washington, DC. **5.** EX114. Data on file, Wyeth Pharmaceuticals Inc., Philadelphia, Pa. **6.** Effexor® XR (venlafaxine HCl) Extended–Release and Effexor Immediate–Release Prescribing Information, Wyeth Pharmaceuticals Inc., Philadelphia, Pa.

difference," and yes, there was the woman again, this time surrounded by friends and laughing as she and an attractive male arm wrestled.

But back to Page 2 and "See the data." I contacted Wyeth Pharmaceuticals, maker of Effexor, to seek permission to reproduce the ad. Wyeth's Deputy Chief Counsel for North America notified me that Wyeth would not allow me to do so. However, they cannot legally keep me from providing an exact quote of a portion of the ad. The exact words as well as the ad's general appearance are reproduced on the previous page. Read it carefully. Note that "proven" appears in bold type three times. **Proven** by "32 double–blind comparative trials" is most impressive and, of course, that is the key point of the ad——to convince medical doctors that there can be no doubt that this drug really works. The ad really only proves that, though Wyeth's marketing department may know that most physicians are very intelligent, they also know that most physicians either lack the research background needed to critique the research or are unaware of how misleading and dishonest research associated with mind drugs tends to be.

The First "Proof"

Two references are associated with the first "proof." Looking at the bottom of the ad's second page, we find the studies which support the claim that "32 double–blind comparative trials with over 7,000 patients" have proven Effexor eliminates symptoms of depression, Generalized Anxiety Disorder and Social Anxiety Disorder. How many of these 32 studies were published in peer–review journals? Not one. In fact, the first reference is to a psychiatrist (whom I promised not to name, the name "Nemstein GE" in the ad being a substitute) who received data from Wyeth and then presented it at a conference in the Czech Republic—a conference Wyeth helped sponsor; i.e., Wyeth money helped pay for the conference. Wyeth also assisted this psychiatrist with travel expenses. And, yes, this man has served as a paid consultant to the company.

I did not ask him how much Wyeth might pay him for various services. I didn't have to. It is now a matter of public record that professors of medicine with significant influence can be paid as much as $9,000 "for an hour's talk about a drug they have no experience using." This incredible fact was revealed in testimony before a health committee investigating drug company influence.[2] Many receive stock options, company stock, research funding and sponsorship of prestigious studies.

You also need to know the following fact. The study's second author, Richard Entsuah, is a Wyeth employee who is the "second" author for other published studies on Effexor as well. The lead author of other studies may be from Canada's University of Alberta, Department of Psychiatry, from England's Imperial College School of Medicine, London, or from the United States Neuroscience Education Institute in California. It does not really matter where they are from as long as it sounds prestigious and each study has a different lead author so that the impression can be made that Effexor is being researched all over the world by psychiatrists with no ties to the drug's manufacturer. That impression is false and misleading.

Examining the second fine print reference for these "32 double–blind studies" we find the following information: "EX110. Data on file, Wyeth Pharmaceuticals Inc., Philadelphia, Pa." In other words, not a single one of these "32 double–blind studies" is found in a published medical journal which could be inspected. This is almost criminal. People's lives and well–being are at stake and, yet, the "32 double–blind studies" turn out not to involve even one independent study.

I again contacted Wyeth. This time I asked to be able to examine this "data on file." Again their attorney notified me that I could not have access to the studies mentioned in their ad.[3] Without the studies being available for inspection, it is not possible to determine if they were fairly conducted or even if they actually found what they report they found. Since Wyeth owns and controls the data, we cannot prove and we cannot disprove that the studies or the data have been manipulated. We need independent studies.

Do independent studies exist? They do. And what do they find? They find these drugs do not work! But more on that in Chapter 8. First, let's look a little more closely at the one study they cite which is not just "data on file at Wyeth." Again, it was not a peer–reviewed, published study but a presentation at a conference. The conference was the 16th Congress of the European College of Neuropsychopharmacology (ECNP). To the average private practice physician, this sounds both legitimate and impressive. They would be less impressed if they knew this was not a college but an organization whose funding comes primarily from the pharmaceutical firms and whose purpose is "the promotion of psychopharmacological thinking, research and information exchange."[4]

In fact, the funding is so generous that the ECNP provides free or subsidized accommodations and travel expenses to a huge number of participants by way of "Fellowship Awards," "Travel Awards" and "Exchange Awards," among others. To qualify for a Fellowship Award, one must have an MD or PhD, be under 50 and "be engaged full–time in clinical or basic research, training or teaching activities in neuropsychopharmacology or closely related disciplines." A Travel Award simply requires that the applicant (1) submit a paper for a poster presentation and be a student in a related degree field or (2) have a PhD and be within the first four years of employment with that degree or (3) have an MD and be in a residency.

When all this is boiled down, we find that almost all future decision makers in areas of teaching or practice who are concerned with mental problems are eligible for awards. (Yes, I will admit that if I were offered a free or subsidized trip every year or two to Paris, Vienna, Hawaii or Rio, I would not be inclined to turn it down.) This is one of the reasons the conviction that drugs are the best hope for overcoming mental disorders is so widespread. Thousands of young college professors and psychiatrists attend these conferences (thanks to drug company money) and then are further propagandized. The drug manufacturers host symposia where their drugs are praised by psychiatrists and others who have been associated with the drug companies for years.

Because any "neuropsychopharmacology" organization which is established will be generously funded by the pharmaceutical firms, these groups are now located all over the world. On our part of the globe we find the American College of Neuropsychopharmacology, the Canadian College of Neuropsychopharmacology and the Mexican College of Neuropsychopharmacology. Over in Europe there is the Austrian Society of Neuropsychopharmacology and Biological Psychiatry, the Belgian College of Neuropsychopharmacology and Biological Psychiatry, the British Association for Psychopharmacology, the Czech Neuropsychopharmacological Society and on and on it goes. The Estonians, the Finns, the French, the Germans, the Hungarians and an alphabet of other countries now have organizations whose purpose is to promote "psychopharmacological thinking" (i.e., to promote mind drugs). And why not, when there is so much money to be made?

This would be denied by all of these groups. Most have policies which state they will not be unduly influenced by drug manufacturers. I have read a number of these policy statements. But I also contacted many of these organizations to inquire concerning how much of their funding came from drug companies.[5] Not one of the "independent" bodies was willing to share that information.

The Second "Proof"

The Effexor advertisement's "See the data" page then makes the following claim: "Proven to resolve emotional and physical symptoms." Once again there are two references to the fine print at the bottom of the page. The first of those two references is to another presentation at another conference. The two presenters whose names appear in the reference are Richard Ensuah (yep, the #2 author for the reference discussed above) and J. Zhang, another Wyeth employee, though there is no mention of their relationship with Wyeth in the advertisement. The conference at which they made their presentations also received funding from Wyeth, and of course, Wyeth paid for them to attend. The second reference for "Proof" #2 is once again to data in Wyeth files, "EX114. Data on file, Wyeth Pharmaceuticals Inc., Philadelphia, Pa."

The Third "Proof"

The third proof, "Proven tolerability with once–daily dosing," has three references. The first two are to the same "32 double–blind comparative trials" we have already discussed. The third reference is not to a study at all. It simply states, "Effexor® XR (venlafaxine HCl) Extended–Release and Effexor Immediate–Release Prescribing Information, Wyeth Pharmaceuticals, Inc. Philadelphia, Pa."

Bottom line: This ad does not reference even one published article indicating that their drug works. And yet this is one of, if not the single most seen drug ad in the world's top medical journals in the last two years.[6]

Not Unique

Unfortunately, the Effexor ad is by no means unique. I have investigated a number of these ads recently and found that the research behind most of the mind drug ads I checked was just as phony. Even when studies are conducted by non–employees and published in the best medical journals, the financial ties between the authors of studies and the drug companies are so great that the studies consistently fail to use research designs that would be utilized by those who were unbiased and objective.

One example of the ties that commonly exist brought a much discussed editorial from Dr. Marcia Angell, who was at the time the editor of the *New England Journal of Medicine*. The *New England Journal of Medicine* adopted a policy demanding that authors fully disclose any financial ties that existed between themselves and any drugs for which they submitted articles for publication. It seemed like a good idea, and it was. But when

Martin Keller, a psychiatrist at Brown University, and his colleagues published a study of an antidepressant manufactured by Bristol–Myers Squibb,
the conflict–of–interest disclosures were so extensive that Dr. Angell concluded she could not print the entire list in the paper version of the journal.
Instead she put the information on the *New England Journal of Medicine*'s
website and then wrote an editorial with the stinging title "Is Academic
Medicine for Sale?"[7] Eleven of the 12 principal authors had financial ties
with Bristol–Myers Squibb as did most of the study's 17 secondary authors.
Two were employees of the company. Nearly all the authors received
income from the drug manufacturer in one or more ways—as consultants,
advisory board members, or as honorarium or grant recipients. The study
itself was paid for by Bristol–Myers Squibb.

That is not the end of the story. By 2002 the *New England Journal of
Medicine* found that obtaining reviewers without financial ties to drug companies was so difficult they felt it necessary to change their conflict–of–
interest policy. Today it no longer states that there cannot be any financial
interest in the drugs being evaluated. Today the policy states that there cannot be any "significant" interest, meaning amounts exceeding $10,000 per
year. Former editor Angell, in discussing the problem, noted that financial
ties with makers of antidepressants are especially significant.[8]

If the existence of such extensive financial ties between drug manufacturers and those who are conducting and publishing the research in independent journals causes you to react with some degree of indignation, then
I can virtually guarantee you will be amazed and angered at some of the
other facts associated with mind drugs today. This is a scandal, and the
financial ties are only the tip of the iceberg. In the next two chapters I will
discuss "ghostwriting" and explain how drug studies are conducted.
Unfortunately, you are going to learn that the Effexor ad has not been the
only effort to deceive. You will shortly become aware of how much of the
antidepressant drug research is truly fraudulent.

6

"Most studies are now sponsored, designed and analyzed, in addition to being efficiently written, by pharmaceutical companies."[1]
— **British Journal of Psychiatry**

GHOSTWRITING

My students have often been surprised and impressed that most of the published drug studies have not one or two authors but ten or twenty or even several hundred.[2] (See Box #6–1, Guess How Many Authors Wrote This Article.) If the authors' affiliations are noted, it can be found that they typically come from many different parts of the country and sometimes from all over the world.

The *New England Journal of Medicine* article mentioned at the end of the last chapter with its 29 authors is not unusual. The first 12 authors came from ten different states and even those in the same states came from different cities. It is hard to imagine how a group of psychiatrists (nearly all of them are psychiatrists) from all over the nation can write a single article. And, of course, they don't. What commonly occurs is that a single individual writes an article (not necessarily the lead author), and then everyone who participated in the research in even minor ways will be given a chance to have their names attached. Having numerous academic MDs gives the research a very impressive appearance, and it is a benefit for all the academic researchers who must publish to receive tenure and promotions. Unfortunately, many published studies concerned with mind drugs are actually written by an author employed directly or indirectly by the drug company which makes the drug being studied. This is a fact that few private practice physicians are apt to realize. But those on the highest levels of academic mind–drug research are keenly aware of this fact and are keenly aware of what is meant by the term "ghostwriter."

BOX #6–1

Guess How Many Authors Wrote This Article

I have always sought to provide my psychology students with various "experiences" rather than just prepare a course of facts. You can learn by hearing or reading facts, but if you want to remember something for the rest of your life, you need to "experience" the facts. I want to provide you with an experience that will make an impression you won't forget. The requirements are quite simple.

(1) Go to the National Institutes of Health medical literature search engine on the internet. (The easiest way to do so is to Google "PubMed Medline"; i.e., go to http://www.google.com, put "Entrez Medline" in the search box and press your keyboard's "enter" key.)

(2) Enter three last names—"Aubert Barate Boutigny"—into the search box and press "enter."

(3) Guess at the number of authors which are listed for the first ten articles. (See Chapter 6, endnote 2 on p. 447 for the answer.)

Ghostwriting is the practice of having articles composed by professional medical writers who are employees of a pharmaceutical firm or by medical writing agencies hired by a drug company which are passed on to medical journals as research supposedly produced by independent academic psychiatrists and researchers. One might think that academic psychiatrists would be unwilling to allow their names to be used despite the benefits arising from being much published. And likely they would be unwilling to do so if they were not paid so handsomely for this service.

How Much Is Your Signature Worth?

A study conducted by the Stanley Medical Research Institute of Bethesda, Maryland, found that psychiatrists in America typically receive between $3,000 and $10,000 per signature. Executive Director Fuller Torrey declared, "Some of us believe that the present system is approaching a high–class form of professional prostitution."[3] The acting editor of the *British Medical Journal* declared that the amount of money sometimes made for allowing one's name to be used is even greater. "We know that gift authorship happens, and the nature of the gift may vary from a pat on the back and anonymity to a *six figure sum* [emphasis mine]."[4]

A Man of Honor Tests the System

Guess which articles have the greatest impact on physicians in private practice, ghostwritten or non–ghostwritten. It appears ghostwritten articles win in a big way. An analysis of 96 Zoloft articles published between 1998 and 2000 found 55 had medical writing agency involvement, and 41 did not. But the study also found that agency–written articles had more listed authors, were longer, were cited by other papers more often and were more likely to be found in the most prestigious journals.[5]

Dr. David Healy is a psychiatrist and researcher and is recognized as one of the world's foremost authorities on mind drugs, having authored over 100 peer–reviewed articles on psychopharmaceuticals. Having his name attached to a published study could clearly increase drug sales. He discussed one of the ghostwriting experiences he had in his book *Let Them Eat Prozac:*

> Usually, ghostwritten articles arrive with a covering letter authorizing me to alter the piece in whatever way I see fit. One such letter arrived linked to a meeting aimed at promoting Wyeth's SSRI Effexor. This Laguna Beach meeting came complete with honoraria, expensive travel and accommodation provision, and the opportunity to have

one's article ghosted, in this case by CMED, a medical writing agency based in Toronto.[6]

Healy decided he could not simply attach his name to the glowing report for Effexor. He was aware of the research indicating an increase in suicide risk for those on SSRI antidepressants. He was also aware that Effexor's claim to be superior to other antidepressants was false. But instead of notifying the writing agency that he did not want his name on ghosted articles, he decided to test the system. He accepted the article, inserted what he termed "two viruses," and then returned the article without making any other changes.

The first "virus" was a statement that Effexor was not superior to another drug, Remeron. The second "virus" simply reported the increase in suicide risk for some individuals on SSRIs. The medical writing agency asked Healy to remove the Remeron statement. He wouldn't. So did the agency decide not to publish the article? No. They simply reworked it and published it—with the Remeron and the suicide risk comments removed—under the names of some new "authors."[7]

This is not a rare event. There are numerous ghostwriting agencies composing and publishing articles in medical journals. As a result of a lawsuit against Pfizer, documents were made public which revealed they had used a New York ghostwriting agency to produce nearly 90 articles for their antidepressant Zoloft. By 2001, 55 of the articles had been published, many in well–respected journals such as *JAMA*, the *New England Journal of Medicine*, and the *Archives of General Psychiatry*.[8]

Determining Which Articles Are Ghostwritten

It is impossible to know how many articles in medical journals have been ghostwritten. However, in testimony before a British Parliament health committee, David Healy testified that he believes that "at least half of articles on *drug efficacy* that appear in the *British Medical Journal,* the *Lancet* and the *New England Journal of Medicine* are ghost–written by pharmaceutical companies and that 'the most distinguished authors from the most prestigious universities' put their names to them *without ever seeing the raw data* [emphasis mine]."[9]

I sought to interview individuals at some ghostwriting agencies, but, as you might expect, they did not want to discuss their businesses. However, following the publication of a *British Medical Journal* issue whose theme was "Time to Untangle Doctors from Drug Companies,"[10] Susanna Rees, a former editorial assistant at a medical writing agency, sent a letter to the *British Medical Journal* editor in which she revealed some of the secrets of the trade, including how her agency disguised "the true authorship from the editorial boards of journals." What she termed "standard operating procedure" included removing "names of the medical writing agency or agency ghost–writer or pharmaceutical drug company." Those names were then replaced with "the name *and institution* of the person who has been invited by the pharmaceutical drug company (or by the agency acting on its behalf) to be *named as lead author*, but who may have had *no actual input* into the paper [emphasis mine]."[11]

Even the *New England Journal of Medicine* cannot identify which articles are truly independent and which are not. Despite having policies aimed at insuring the integrity of the articles it publishes as well as an editorial board that is more concerned about drug company influence than many other medical journals, not long ago it had to retract an article that was authored by eight respected researchers. It was only when one of the researchers, a cardiologist who supposedly helped write the article, contacted the journal and informed them that he had never even seen the article before it was published that they realized it was a ghosted article.[12]

The retraction noted that a majority of the authors did not get to see the article before publication (meaning that at least 5 of the 8 authors did not know what the article said until after it was published). The *New England Journal of Medicine* now requires authors to certify that they "have seen and approved the final manuscript."[13] The *New England Journal of Medicine* has been a leader in promoting a higher degree of accountability than required by any journal associated with psychiatry. Yet this is, nevertheless, a corrupt system. Simply certifying that one has "seen and approved" is not the same as being involved in the actual research. We need a system in which we can feel confident that an article's listed authors were actually involved in the research and are not listed just to give credibility where credibility is not justified. And we need to know if the authors are employees or beneficiaries of the drug companies. Research should ideally be published by those who are fully objective. But when research is published by ghostwriters or ghostwriting companies working for and receiving huge fees from drug companies, the end result is not objective science.

What Gets Published

Nor do we get objective science if those studies which find data that would be harmful to a drug's sales do not get published. Dr. Peter Wilmshurst, a cardiologist and researcher, testified he has been offered large financial bribes not to publish results that were unfavorable to the drug under investigation. He also testified before the government committee that he was familiar with a case in which three other professors of cardiology did not publish their findings after the sponsoring drug manufacturer saw the unfavorable results.[14]

I would suggest that you read that last paragraph again. It contains startling facts. They call out for intervention. As you will learn in the chapters dealing with the adverse health effects of antidepressants and antipsychotics, these drugs cause permanent brain damage, serious health effects and shorten lives. Drug studies should not be allowed to be buried just because the results show a drug has no benefit or causes harm—a problem that is more acute now than it was in the past. (The government funds fewer trials today, so drug companies now have greater control over drug trial data.)

I believe it is fair to say that most areas of medical research and publication are not so plagued with problems as is research and publication associated with mind drugs. An insulin shot lowers my wife's blood sugar level. There is no debate about it. We can measure the change. Antibiotics do indeed kill bacteria. A blood test can confirm that as well. But what is your serotonin or dopamine level right now? No one knows, but as long as conjecture, theory and myth reign over psychiatry, marketing in its many forms will be effective.

7

*"Folks everywhere—the shrewd, the simple, the powerful
and the weak—have been taken in by hoaxes and scams
since the beginning of recorded time."* [1]
— *Carl Sifakis*
Author, **Hoaxes and Scams**

TRICKS OF THE TRADE

In 2004 New York's activist attorney general, Eliot Spitzer, brought suit against the British pharmaceutical giant GlaxoSmithKline. The suit centered around five clinical trials of the company's antidepressant Paxil. Seeking to expand sales, the company conducted a series of clinical trials using children who seemed anxious. The attorney general charged the drug maker with fraud for releasing only one of the five trial results—the one showing mixed results—which was then spun to indicate Paxil was the drug of choice for treating nervous children. The unreleased studies found not only was there no mental health benefit, but each of the four studies found suicide related events rose for children on Paxil compared with a placebo.

Many Americans heard media stories concerning suicide risk for children on antidepressants. But behind the main story there are often many other "sub–stories," some of which make for some interesting reading and some which make one want to exclaim, "Well, that's strange!" The Paxil–suicide risk data had been in the hands of several British regulatory agencies long before the story entered the newspapers. However, the suicide risk found in these studies had been hidden by Glaxo. It was not hard to do. They simply called suicidal thoughts and behaviors "emotional lability," a term which few people actually understood. (Well, that's strange. Why would they use a term that almost no one knew?)

When American journalists later saw the term and made inquiries, it caused the British authorities to reexamine the data in their files. That is when they discovered the suicide risk and proceeded to issue a warning against use by children.[2] That action prompted further response in America by journalists, lawyers and regulators. This is where the story really took on some drama.

The American College of Neuropsychopharmacology Contradicts the British Authorities

In January 2004 the American College of Neuropsychopharmacology (ACNP) decided they had better issue a report in support of antidepressant use by children. (No group is more tied to the drug companies than the ACNP. Their annual meetings, by invitation only, are hugely subsidized pleasure trips to Puerto Rico [2004], Hawaii [2005], Florida [2006] and other locations where guests hear presentations by psychiatrists given large fees by "big pharma.") The FDA had called a hearing on antidepressant use in children for February, and if the agency said children should not be on antidepressants, it would be a black eye on the members of all the neuropsychopharmacology organizations and could greatly harm sales. The ACNP task force's report went to the major media outlets and was heard across the nation.

Time magazine noted that the ACNP, "having reviewed the data, says the link to suicide is weak and that the drugs' benefits outweigh the risks."[3] The published report[4] did not mention that (1) all but one of the report's authors received income from the makers of antidepressants; (2) three of the report's authors had actually been the researchers who worked on the Paxil study which was released (the only one that did not report an increase in suicide); (3) those three authors had published much of the total body of research on antidepressant use by children and had never issued any warnings about suicide and (4) (perhaps the strangest fact of all) the report included this sentence: "The ACNP Task Force emphasizes that its findings and recommendations are preliminary because it did not have access to all the data held by regulatory agencies and pharmaceutical companies."[5] How strange is that? Here are the leading proponents and researchers for antidepressant use in children, but they have not been allowed access to the data coming out of their own research?

My questions are: Why are you issuing a report that you have portrayed to every media outlet as saying, "Antidepressant use by children is safe"? Why would you try to usurp the effect of the British warning when they did have the data (and they did)? Why would you make a preemptive strike just days before the FDA panel examines the issue? And why did you use a term like "emotional lability" (instead of "suicide ideation," "suicide behaviors" and "suicide," the standard terms) in your Paxil study? Why use a term which means nothing to most of us?

All of these questions are troubling, but it gets worse. It was later reported that the ACNP Task Force was not the author of their own report. It was actually done by GYMR, a ghostwriting agency out of Washington, D.C.[6] The listed authors were not the authors at all. Think about this: Here we have a report about a life and death issue which made the news all over the world saying that highly trained British medical authorities had it wrong. That pronouncement was not coming from actual drug researchers, but from people who may not have had more than a bachelor's degree in English who happened to work for a Washington, D.C., public relations firm.[7] It just couldn't get much stranger! Well, I take that back. I guess it could.

Dr. Andrew Mosholder Gets Gagged

Dr. Andrew Mosholder, an FDA drug safety officer, was aware of various studies which indicated that antidepressants could increase suicide and aggressive behavior. In view of the growing number of users, Mosholder contacted drug manufacturers and requested that they provide additional data from their drug trials. When he completed his study, he was convinced that the British had it right. The drug companies' own data revealed the dangers which most physicians simply did not know existed. He was to present his findings at an FDA advisory committee meeting scheduled for February 2004. However, when his superiors learned of the conclusions he was going to share, they would not allow him to make his presentation.[8]

That decision angered someone at the FDA although no one knows who contacted the *San Francisco Chronicle* which reported on these events the day before the advisory committee was to meet. (Dr. Mosholder later signed a statement indicating he was not the one who contacted the newspaper.)

The data used in Dr. Mosholder's study was then given to another FDA scientist for reevaluation. Seven months later that scientist confirmed Mosholder's original conclusion. FDA officials may have hoped this reevaluation of Dr. Mosholder's analysis would stay out of the media. It did not. The *Washington Post* was more than willing to tell the story.

Congress Calls for Hearings

When Congress learned of these events, they called the FDA to the hill. The congressional committee's ranking member declared, "The FDA has handled the decisions involving questions of both the safety and efficacy of these drugs in adolescents in such an unscrupulous manner that it is very hard for anyone to accept that objective science is the basis of the agency's conclusions."[9] Another congressman wondered aloud if the FDA was guilty of "sheer ineptitude or something far worse."[10] He pointed out that the FDA

144

had failed the public since they had known of the suicide risk for many years.

I have entitled this chapter "Tricks of the Trade." I believe you understand why. Within this short story we see two tricks. Relabeling can hide facts that would be quickly seen otherwise. Calling suicidal thoughts and behaviors "emotional lability" allowed the trials to be filed with the British authorities without anyone noticing a problem. The even more common trick is to "count successes only" which will be the first of the tricks of the trade I want you to know about. But first, let's consider the proper way to design a study.

Doing It Right

Drug trials randomly assign study participants to research groups and utilize a double–blind design. A double–blind design requires that one group of subjects be given the actual drug being studied and the other group be given a different drug or a placebo. However, if members of either group know whether they are getting a real drug or just a "sugar pill," the responses subjects give could be dramatically affected. Therefore, the subjects are not told what they are receiving. They are "blind" to what the pill they swallow actually contains.

But even researchers may have a bias which can impact what they perceive. If a researcher "knows" vitamin C cures colds, he might see improvement in those taking vitamin C but not in those taking a sugar pill—even if there is no change in anyone. Thus, it is best not to allow even the researcher to know who is getting the vitamin C and who is getting the placebo; i.e., the researcher should also be kept "blind" to that information until all the data is collected. Then the envelope which reveals who got what (kept by an independent assistant) can be opened, and the results can be analyzed.

That is a double–blind design, and it is the gold standard for doing drug research. Such a design is required for the approval of any new drug, including all antidepressants and antipsychotics. In fact, it is more needed when doing research with mind drugs than for other types of drugs since improvement using mind drugs is measured so subjectively. The ten "tricks of the trade" included here are not all that could be mentioned, but these ten should increase your skepticism and make it plain that if a drug company was not simply interested in truth, they could distort it or keep it from being discovered. It is my opinion that since the knowledge learned in pursuing academic degrees is based on research studies, no skill is more important to college graduates than an ability to critique research studies. I think you will understand why I feel so strongly about this before you finish all ten tricks of the trade.

Trick One: Count Only Successes

It would seem blatantly dishonest to count only the studies which yielded favorable results and to exclude all those which did not. It is clearly dishonest, but this is the standard procedure used by mind drug manufacturers. If "32 double–blind studies" found Effexor worked well, it is likely that approximately 38 double–blind studies found Effexor did not work better than a placebo or found that the placebo was more effective than the antidepressant. I base that estimate on information gained from an analysis of all drug studies submitted to the FDA which were responsible for the approval of various SSRI drugs.

The Freedom of Information Act became law in 1966. That law forces government agencies to release information which the drug companies do not want the public to know about. In 2002 a Freedom of Information Act request led to the discovery that the drug companies (who must submit all their drug studies to the FDA) had been sharing only their "successes" with the public in their antidepressant advertising.[11] That is no more fair than a major league baseball player not having to count strikeouts in calculating his batting average.

Trick Two: Alter the Dose

If a drug is being compared with the competition, simply increasing the competitor's dose to a level that is higher than what would be optimal will insure that the competitor's drug will have an increase in adverse side effects. Most of the antidepressants and anti–anxiety drugs prescribed today are SSRIs. They are very similar chemically and all act in essentially the same way. The best selling point for many of these drugs is that they have a "safer profile." Of course, this works in reverse as well. If you want to demonstrate that your drug is safe, you can cut the dosage which will reduce the number of adverse side effects. In Chapter 9, The FDA Drug Approval Process, I will note that when Merck was ready to do a large trial with Vioxx, they gave patients only half the dosage used in an earlier trial—a trial which had resulted in a large number of heart attacks and strokes.[12]

Trick Three: Use a "Placebo Washout"

When comparing a new drug to a placebo, researchers face a dilemma. A large number of those given a sugar pill respond very favorably to the pill. A sugar pill won't destroy a cancerous tumor or the bacteria causing a sore throat, but it has been found to do wonders for problems that are subjectively evaluated. Many on placebos will report great improvement in their depression after taking the sugar pill for only a week or two. In fact, some on a placebo will respond even better than those on an antidepressant.

All the large drug manufacturers are not only aware of this but they also use a research design that takes advantage of this fact, something that is not done in oncology (cancer), cardiology (heart), dermatology (skin) or any other area of medical research where the disease can actually be objectively measured. The technique is known as a placebo washout. When the study begins, every participant is given a placebo. Those who have the best response are then removed from the study. This is not a needed trick in oncology, cardiology or dermatology because the drugs in those areas of research are either genuinely effective or they are not. But without this trick, antidepressants and, to a lesser degree, antipsychotics, do not compare well with placebos. Psychiatrist and drug research authority Peter Breggin shared that "this is done in every study I have ever seen used for FDA approval of antidepressants."[13]

Trick Four: Break the Blind

Another trick is almost the opposite of the placebo washout. Once those who respond very favorably to a sugar pill are removed from the study, subjects will be divided into a group getting the real drug and a group getting a placebo. One might think that once those who responded very favorably to a placebo are eliminated, any positive response must be due to the drug. That would be an erroneous assumption.

The reality is that drugs have side effects. Antidepressant drugs have lots of side effects. Thus, after a few weeks, some of those on antidepressants will have experienced or will still be experiencing insomnia, nervousness, tremors, nausea, weakness, dry mouth or other common symptoms.[14] Those who respond positively just because they took a pill are gone, but having symptoms indicates one is taking the "real medicine," and knowing that fact will lead to placebo effects even in those who are less easily influenced. Knowing one is on a real drug means the blind has been broken, even if the study's administrators never reveal to the subjects which pill they are getting until that part of the study is concluded. A more fair comparison would put the mind drugs up against placebos that are neutral except that they produce some of the same adverse symptoms——insomnia, nervousness, tremors, nausea, weakness and dry mouth.

Trick Five: Add a Sedative to the Drug Trial

I find it incredible that *over half* of all drug trials submitted to the FDA in seeking approval for the leading SSRI antidepressants allowed a sedative to be given to study subjects. Kirsch and colleagues reported, "In most trials, a chloral hydrate sedative was permitted in doses ranging from 500mg to 2000mg per day. Other psychoactive medication was usually prohibited but still was reported as having been taken in several trials."[15] This may increase the likelihood of the blind being broken, but even more disturbing, it assures that we cannot know exactly how the antidepressant may impact study participants. The motivation for giving a sedative stems from the concerns over side effects common to antidepressant drugs. But if a drug causes nervousness or insomnia or agitation, we need to know it.

Giving a tranquilizer is unfair for another reason. If participants report feeling more relaxed and less depressed, we need to know what drug, if any, is responsible. If both an antidepressant and a tranquilizer are given to study subjects, we cannot know.

BOX #7–1

What is a Tranquilizer?

Most of the drugs we sometimes call tranquilizers are more precisely known as benzodiazepines. Prior to the development of benzodiazepines in the 1950s the drugs most commonly used to aid sleep and sedate were the barbiturates. Barbiturates were first created in 1903. They very quickly became popular as a sleeping aid, a relaxant and an anesthesia for surgery. They worked by depressing the central nervous system, but they were inherently dangerous—if too much were taken, coma and death could result. Furthermore, many patients loved the relaxed feelings the drugs provided and quickly became addicted. Consequently, drug companies sought to develop a new drug that could depress (dull) the mind without depressing the entire body.

Thorazine was the first drug to do this effectively. However, its effects were too dramatic. Thus, an effort to develop a drug that was less effective than the "major tranquilizer" Thorazine was pursued. This resulted in the "minor tranquilizers"; for example, the benzodiazepines which are often called anti–anxiety drugs today. The best known of the benzodiazepine drugs are Valium, Xanax, Halcion, BuSpar, Serax, Librium and Tranxene.

Trick Six: Be Unfair in Choosing Study Participants

Ideally, whenever a study is set up, a sample of people similar to those who will be using the drug once it is approved should be selected. If an antidepressant is eventually going to be given to those who are at high risk for suicide, have bipolar disorder, have an eating disorder, are obsessive–compulsive, are antisocial or experience general anxiety, then those people should not be purposely excluded from an antidepressant drug trial. But they are.[16] Those designing these trials are not looking for subjects who are the most like those who will be prescribed their drug. They are not looking for participants who have a problem that has gone on for years and are less likely to respond. They want people who just recently indicated they are depressed and are the most likely to be over the depression soon whether they take an antidepressant or not. If those in charge of a study find out that a person did not respond favorably to the antidepressant in a previous study, that person will be excluded from the new study. If he has been to a therapist and reported that it did not help, he will be excluded.[17]

None of this is fair, but that is not as offensive as what I consider the most offensive trick of all—eliminating those study participants who are not responding to the new drug and replacing them with new participants. In other words, researchers will give their new antidepressant to 100 depressed people. After two weeks, those who do not indicate they are now less depressed will simply be eliminated from the study and replaced with other depressed individuals. They will not report in their drug packaging insert that "20 of 100 participants were replaced with new study subjects." They will pretend that the additions had been a part of the study from day one and then report the percentage of the 100 participants who were helped as though no substitutions had ever occurred. It doesn't seem that such a trick would ever be allowed by the FDA, but substitutions after two weeks are very common.[18] It is an obviously unfair tactic, but it does increase the percentage of those who are responders to the drugs under investigation. That meets the needs of those who want to increase drug sales, but it deceives more than it reveals truth.

Trick Seven: Hire a For–Profit Company to Conduct Research

Historically, much of the medical research was conducted and paid for by the federal government or by universities. Eventually drug companies began funding research at federal facilities and university laboratories. This made sense. The drug companies could, in effect, hire the nation's top scientists without having to fund some of the graduate students, libraries, research equipment or many other expenses associated with drug research. This saved the drug companies huge sums and resulted in better funding for bioscience in universities all over the nation.

I am not arguing that this was a good development. The evidence indicates that this system did, in fact, compromise objective science. However, today drug company research dollars go more frequently to an even less objective source—private, for–profit research companies.[19] Studies of "for hire research" have found it consistently to result in unobjective, pro–industry results.[20]

Trick Eight: Use Invalid Measures of Success

A study of the antidepressant Serzone (nefazodone) which appeared in the *New England Journal of Medicine* used as poor a research design as I have ever seen.[21] Yet appearing in the *New England Journal of Medicine* silently implies the research must be of high quality. Perhaps that is why it has been termed a "landmark study"[22] and has been often cited.[23] The study began with 681 patients who had a history of depression. The patients were randomly assigned to an antidepressant group, a psychotherapy group or to a group which received both antidepressants and psychotherapy. No placebo only group and no placebo with psychotherapy group were included in the study. This alone means whatever results would be found would be meaningless.

But then the study's authors made a shocking admission. "Of the 681 patients, 662 attended at least one treatment session and were included in the analysis of response."[24] Did you catch that? Those who attended only one therapy session were still included in the analysis though all participants were expected to attend psychotherapy for 12 weeks. Why would anyone go only once or stop before all scheduled sessions were completed? (We don't know how many dropped out after two sessions or three sessions, etc.) Likely the most common answer would be that they did not feel the therapy was helping and was wasting their time. Others may not have cared for their therapist. Now, how will these "drop–outs" rate the effectiveness of their psychotherapy experience? If only those who *completed* psychotherapy had been compared with antidepressant users, the antidepressants would not have fared nearly as well. More to the point, just because the drug–only users and the psychotherapy–only users had comparable outcomes does not indicate the antidepressant drugs worked.[25] To imply the drug worked since it was as effective as the psychotherapy is using an invalid measure of success.

Trick Nine: Count (and Market) Studies With Completion Rates Below 70%

Year in and year out I have emphasized to my students that if a study has a low response rate, the results are likely meaningless. Some famous sex surveys have had response rates of only 7%,[26] 4.5%,[27] and 3%.[28] When such a small percentage of people respond, it makes one wonder if those who responded are very different than most of the people in our society. For example, perhaps these responders (1) are *not* offended by weird sex questions, (2) have a preoccupation with sexual issues or (3) have fewer inhibitions sharing about sexual topics than most people. Whatever the reason, the results cannot be applied to the entire population.

BOX #7–2

Investigation: How Much Research Is Published By the Drug Companies?

If you would like to increase your awareness of how much research is published by the drug companies, it will take you just a couple of minutes. Here are the instructions:

1. Go to http://www.Google.com or any other search engine.
2. Enter PubMed or Medline. The first choice will likely be "Entrez PubMed." Click on it.
3. Enter the names for each of the following drug companies and note how many articles (items) are found for each. (I have done the first one, AstraZeneca, for you.)

- AstraZeneca – 1,495
- Aventis
- Ayerst
- Bayer
- Bristol
- Ciba
- Glaxo
- Hoffman–LaRoche
- Johnson & Johnson

- Lilly
- Novartis
- Parke–Davis
- Pfizer
- Pharmacia
- Roche
- Schering–Plough
- Warner–Lambert
- Wyeth

As you just learned, all the major pharmaceuticals have teams of scientists who regularly publish articles in the scientific journals. Do you believe the drug research coming out of these companies is apt to be disinterested, unbiased and objective? Common sense demands that we ask questions such as the following:

Question 1: If a scientist suspects a drug his company makes may cause cancer, is he apt even to research the issue?

Question 2: If a scientist does research a drug's effects and discovers the drug has unexpected adverse effects, will he consider not publishing the finding?

Question 3: Are university drug researchers commonly supported by grants from the drug companies? Do they frequently serve as consultants to these drug manufacturers? Could this influence their objectivity?

Survey results vary with the nature of the subject and the population being studied. However, if the researcher is willing to make sufficient effort and has enough money for the investigation, I believe response rates in excess of 80% are very achievable for most studies.

Completion rates involve a similar principle to response rates. If a large percentage of subjects drops out of the study, the data will ultimately become meaningless. Drug studies should have completion rates of 80% or better in my judgment. The FDA lowers the bar somewhat and seeks a 70% completion rate. Amazingly, few of the SSRI drug studies submitted to the FDA to get the leading antidepressants approved met the 70% standard.[29] When less valid studies are accepted and treated as if fully valid then when advertising for the drug begins, the pharmaceutical companies can seriously distort the truth about a drug.

Trick Ten: Be Dishonest With the Research

There are many other ways to manipulate study outcomes. This last one does not require any manipulation of the study itself. Instead, when the study is completed, the public and physicians are simply told that the study found certain facts—even though it is not true. One easy way to do this is to cite trial data located in company files and then not let anyone ever see the data. (The Effexor ad discussed in Chapter 5 likely used this trick.) It is a common practice. In fact, drug advertisements found in medical journals cite their own research 58% of the time.[30]

The other way to deceive is to cite the research found in published articles which does not actually support the advertised drug. One leading medical journal, the *Lancet*, published a study examining advertisements which cited medical research supporting the advertised claims.[31] They found 44.1% of claims were not supported by the cited reference. The number would have been much worse except the researchers counted any study, no matter how poor the design, which supported the advertised claim. They concluded, "Doctors should be cautious in assessment of advertisements that claim a drug has greater efficacy, safety or convenience, even though these claims are accompanied by bibliographical references to randomised clinical trials published in reputable medical journals and seem to be evidence–based."[32]

Is Change Coming?

Is change coming? There is a movement in all of medicine to require that studies use superior designs. Randomized, clinical trials that are placebo controlled and double blind will eventually become the enforced standard. So, yes, change is coming. However, this change will likely have an ironic effect. It will result in drug advertising that will get progressively worse. When the tricks of the trade are no longer used for advantage, the advantage will be sought in even more false advertising claims.

Television networks could use a committee of medical advisors to review all ads for truthfulness. That will not happen. I say so knowing that medical journals are run by physicians who are far more aware of these problems than are television executives, and they will not even monitor advertising claims. The *British Medical Journal*'s official policy on advertisements is an embarrassment (see Box #7–3, *British Medical Journal* Policy on Advertisements). The editor of the *British Medical Journal* defended the journal's policy by noting the benefits for his journal as well as for other leading journals:

> Doctors in Britain receive the *BMJ* free in part because of the support the journal receives from pharmaceutical advertising. . . . Because of advertising the *New England Journal of Medicine* is sent free to many hospital doctors in Britain and *JAMA* to many doctors in the United States.[33]

He also noted that the American edition of the *BMJ* was being sent to 90,000 U.S. physicians "paid for entirely by advertising."[34] The American Medical Association's advertising policy is not any better, though it is less blunt than the *BMJ* policy[35] (see endnote 35). Change is coming, but it will not all be change for the better. The ability to read and critique research studies will continue to be important, and an even greater skepticism of advertised claims must be adopted. The desire for money, whether it be by the drug companies or by those willing to accept their often misleading advertisements,[36] is still the root of all kinds of evil.

BOX #7–3

British Medical Journal
Policy on Advertisements

"At the *BMJ* we don't attempt to review the claims made by advertisements. We do review advertisements for taste but rarely turn any down. . . . This policy is against the backcloth that we want the income from advertising. Like many editors, we believe that, paradoxically perhaps, such income buys us independence. Advertisers have little power to influence what is published—partly because there are many of them. But if owners have to support a journal financially they will want the journal to promote their view of the world. We also know that if readers are given a choice of paying for a journal without advertising or receiving free a journal with advertising, nearly all opt for the free journal."[1]

8

"The results of that analysis surprised us."[1]
— *Irving Kirsch, PhD*
Professor Emeritus
University of Connecticut

DO ANTIDEPRESSANTS WORK?

"Warnings About a Miracle Drug: Reports of Suicide Attempts in Prozac Users Raise Doubts About the Popular Antidepressant"

That was the title of a *Time* magazine article 14 years before the antidepressant–suicide link again became a hot media topic. Most of the stories in 1990 were focused on suicide among adult users of antidepressants. Children were rarely prescribed these drugs in those days. However, in 2004 it was the antidepressant–suicide link among children that became the center of attention, and that led to congressional hearings on that issue. The congressional hearings were originally scheduled by Congressman James Greenwood, chairman of the House Energy and Commerce Subcommittee on Oversight and Investigations, to begin Tuesday, July 20, 2004. The hearings were a clear danger to the pharmaceutical industry. If the drug trials had generally found antidepressants to be of no value or even harmful and the drug manufacturers knew those results but (as reported) had buried each of the studies that came to these conclusions, the publicity could damage sales and bring lawsuits.

On Monday, July 19, the day before hearings were to begin, they were abruptly cancelled by Congressman Greenwood. Then on Tuesday, the very day hearings were originally scheduled, the congressman announced that he would be resigning from Congress in order to become president of an industry group called BIO (Biotechnology Industry Organization), the industry group to which drug manufacturers belong.[2]

After the controversial cancellation of the July 20th hearing, it was rescheduled for September 9, 2004. The purpose was stated most succinctly by Vice–Chairman Greg Walden when he declared, "It's time to ask the tough questions. Are America's kids being prescribed drugs for depression that are no better than sugar pills yet may nearly double their risk of suicidal behavior and thought? Are the companies selling these drugs adequately disclosing the results of their trials in ways that allow parents and physicians to get all of the facts?"[3]

Between 1999 and 2001 Pfizer had conducted two studies to determine the effectiveness of the antidepressant Zoloft in treating depression in children. Neither study found that the drug worked any better than a placebo. Nevertheless, in 2002 the drug company petitioned the FDA to grant approval for the use of Zoloft by children. The FDA refused to do so. Meanwhile, as a result of its various marketing efforts, physicians all over America began prescribing Zoloft and other unapproved antidepressants for children anyway. (It's foolish, but not illegal.) Over 10 million of these "off–label" antidepressant prescriptions were written for children in 2002 alone.[4] Pfizer knew their drug Zoloft was not shown to help but was found to harm children. The FDA also knew these facts, but neither Pfizer nor the FDA ever revealed to the public the results of the research[5] (except for data released by the FDA under Freedom of Information Act requests).

Then something truly mysterious occurred. Pfizer combined the results of the two studies, juggled the statistics and published an article which found Zoloft *was* effective in treating depression in children. This article appeared in one of the world's most prestigious journals, the *Journal of the American Medical Association).*[6] Greg Walden, the congressman from Oregon, was clearly skeptical. He asked the Pfizer representative to explain how two individual studies which found that the drug did not work could suddenly, when combined, find that the drug worked very well.

> **Walden:** And is it correct that neither study showed efficacy?
>
> **Pfizer:** It is correct that neither study showed a statistically significant difference between Zoloft and placebo.[7]

Walden then read from the *JAMA* article that announced Zoloft "was found to be more effective than placebo."[8] "How do you arrive at this conclusion?" Walden asked. The Pfizer representative tried to explain why this was not illogical, but Walden didn't buy it. Neither did Henry Waxman, the congressman from California.

> **Waxman:** So it is not true that you pooled two negative studies and published them as positive.
>
> **Pfizer:** That is true, but that was a scientific decision that was made before we knew what the outcome would be.[9]

The tension was building when Waxman asked the FDA's representative at the hearings the following pointed question: "When manufacturers choose to publish only the positive studies and to withhold the negative studies, or worse, to portray negative studies as if they were positive and FDA knows about missing or distorted data, does FDA have any responsibility to the medical community?"[10] The FDA spokeswoman's response was, "We have long tried to deal with this issue . . . this is a conundrum for the agency. It is often difficult for us to explain our actions to the public when we are constrained from revealing the data upon which our opinion is based."[11]

Joe Barton, chairman of the subcommittee, was angry. "The conduct by the FDA has only reinforced my past sentiments that the Food and Drug Administration stands for 'Foot Dragging and Alibis.'"[12] Barton's words were uttered as he held in his hand a memo sent out of the FDA's Office of Legislation which instructed employees not to provide the congressional investigation some of the documents they desired. "If we have to, we will send our staff people, if necessary, with the Capitol Police to the FDA . . . and we will go through the files ourselves."[13]

BOX #8–1

More on the *JAMA* Article—Mystery Solved

The study in *JAMA* which reported Zoloft (sertraline) "is an effective and well–tolerated short–term treatment for children and adolescents with major depressive disorder"[1] posed a mystery. How could the *JAMA* article come to such a conclusion when it was based on two studies which found Zoloft was not superior to placebos? This could hardly be explained in the past.

Fortunately, *JAMA* now requires that authors reveal financial ties and associations with the drug manufacturers they serve. Consider the ties that were revealed about that study's principal author, Dr. Karen Dineen Wagner:

Dr. Wagner has received research support from Abbott, Bristol–Myers Squibb, Eli Lilly, Forest Laboratories, GlaxoSmithKline, Organon, Pfizer, and Wyeth–Ayerst; has served as a National Institute of Mental Health consultant to Abbott, Bristol–Myers Squibb, Cyberonics, Eli Lilly, Forest Laboratories, GlaxoSmithKline, Novartis, Otsuka, Janssen, Pfizer, and UCB Pharma; and has participated in speaker's bureaus for Abbott, Eli Lilly, GlaxoSmithKline, Forest Laboratories, Pfizer, and Novartis.[2]

The study's principal statistician was Dr. Ruoyong Yang. Both he and another of the study's authors, Dr. Christopher Wohlberg, are employees of Pfizer, the company who makes Zoloft. And both have stock options for Pfizer stock. Such ties do not guarantee a lack of honest analysis, but . . .

The Emperor's New Drugs

In 2002 a team of researchers published the results of their investigation of antidepressants compared with placebos. Their article carried the provocative title, "The Emperor's New Drugs: An Analysis of Antidepressant Medication Data Submitted to the U.S. Food and Drug Administration." The lead author, Dr. Irving Kirsch of the University of Connecticut had begun his study of antidepressants as a part of his ongoing research into placebo effects. He later reported that when he and his co–author began their study, "We did not doubt that antidepressants are pharmacologically effective. Our intent was to evaluate the placebo effect. The results of that analysis surprised us."[14]

They were not surprised by the powerful placebo effect. An abundance of research over a period of many decades has demonstrated that the placebo effect can be dramatic. What surprised these researchers was the very small effect of the actual drugs. They expected the drugs to have a very real impact. In fact, they found that most of the effects produced by the medications included in their study were actually placebo effects. This discovery led to the title of a subsequent article, "Yes, There *Is* a Placebo Effect, but Is There a Powerful Antidepressant Drug Effect?"[15]

To answer that question Dr. Kirsch and his colleagues submitted a Freedom of Information Act request. They wanted to see the data the drug companies submitted for gaining FDA approval for the six antidepressants which were most widely prescribed between 1987 and 1999—Prozac, Paxil, Zoloft, Effexor, Serzone, and Celexa. The FDA released to the researchers the data for the 47 clinical trials used for gaining approval for the six antidepressants. From this information at least five facts were learned that I believe would greatly surprise most Americans and most physicians.

> **The following "surprises" may sound familiar as they involve some of the standard "tricks of the trade" which were discussed in the previous chapter. How many can you find?**

The First Surprise

First, these were not studies that lasted many years. Though millions of Americans take these drugs year in and year out, the clinical trials lasted only weeks. The very longest studies lasted 8 weeks, most lasted 6 weeks, and some ended after only 4 weeks. This is a shocking fact when we recognize that repeatedly over the last several decades it has been conclusively demonstrated that many drugs appear to be safe for months and sometimes years but then are found to cause great harm and even death further down the road. (See Box #8–2, How Safe Are New Drugs? It Takes Years To Know.) Consider the following three examples:

BOX #8–2

How Safe Are New Drugs?
It Takes Years to Know

After a new drug goes through three phases of testing it is released to the public. However the number of human subjects who have taken the drug during clinical trials is always a tiny fraction of future users. That smaller number of human guinea pigs must be healthy. They are excluded if they have medical problems which might be complicated by the new drug. In the real world, once a drug is released, it is taken by many people with various health problems, typically taken at higher doses, and often taken for years or even for life, not the 6 to 8 weeks common to initial drug trials. Put it all together, and it becomes apparent why new drugs should always be considered riskier than drugs that have been on the market for many years.

The research on how long it takes for new drugs to begin causing serious health problems is another reason to view drugs with great caution. Over 10% of drugs approved between 1975 and 1999 were eventually withdrawn or given a "black box" (a box warning that serious dangers are associated with the drug's use).[1] But realizing the drug's dangers generally takes years. "Only half of serious ADRs [adverse drug reactions] are detected and documented in the *Physicians' Desk Reference* within 7 years after drug approval."[2] To assume, as many do, that once a drug has received FDA approval it can be considered safe reveals a fundamental ignorance of the drug approval process and the dangers of drugs. It can take years before a "safe" drug is found to damage the heart, kidneys or liver or cause other unanticipated harm.

---

(1)   A ten–year study of men with high blood pressure who were all 68 years old when the study began found that 35% of those on medications (mostly diuretics or beta–blockers) experienced cardiac–related deaths, but only about half as many (18%) of those not taking any medications had died from cardiac–related events. The cardiac–related death rates were especially high among those on medication with diastolic blood pressure less than or equal to 90mmHg when the study began compared with the equivalent group not taking medication.[16] Sometimes such a startling finding will only emerge after many years, and yet few studies last as long as ten years. FDA approval is based on studies lasting weeks, not years, and "post–marketing surveillance" which will hopefully improve in the future has been very inadequate in the past. This fact should be seen as a warning not to take any newer drug for which an older equivalent is available.

(2)   The Bristol–Myers Squibb antidepressant Serzone (nefazodone) was first made available to both U.S. and Canadian citizens in 1994. Numerous drugs that have been approved for use by the FDA were later found to cause liver damage. (All drugs are, in one sense, poisons. It is the liver's job to filter out and break down any "poison" such as alcohol and illegal or legal drugs. Hence, regular intake of any of these has the potential to harm the liver and to a lesser extent, the kidneys, the body's other filter.) But the warnings about Serzone were particularly clear. The same year Serzone was approved the first of several studies appeared in the medical literature which would voice concern about Serzone's effect on the liver.[17]

By 2000 half a dozen articles had appeared whose titles were blunt and pointed such as "Nefazodone–induced acute liver failure"[18] and "Acute liver failure ascribed to nefazodone."[19] Health Canada warned its nation's physicians that Serzone could cause liver failure in 2001. They removed the drug from the Canadian market in 2003. The Dutch Medicines Evaluation Board (CBG) announced in 2002 that because of the danger of liver failure Serzone was going to be removed from the Dutch market.[20] Other European countries followed suit, but the FDA never removed Serzone from the U.S. market. However, the antidepressant could not withstand the media reports which decimated sales and increased lawsuits. The company claimed their decision to remove their drug was due to declining sales, not safety concerns.[21] However the drug went off patent in 2003, and the steep price drop which that event always triggers combined with headlines such as "Teen death stirs fresh debate about depression medication; Bristol–Myer's Serzone, despite removal elsewhere, is still available in the U.S." made the profit–lawsuit risk equation very unattractive.[22]

(3) The Redux debacle is perhaps our nation's best known example of a drug being approved by the FDA and then later having to be recalled. Redux was the first half of the famous combination of two diet pills, Redux (dex**fen**fluramine) and **Phen**termine—hence, fen–phen.[23] Most Americans have heard of the heart–valve damage and primary pulmonary hypertension which occurred in thousands of fen–phen users.[24] The resultant lawsuits will cost Wyeth, the manufacturer of Redux, an estimated $21.1 billion.[25] Few realize that Redux almost never made it to market. An FDA advisory committee voted 5 to 3 in September of 1995 to keep the drug off the market because animal studies found it could cause brain damage in animals. But because every drug which is approved is approved based on a risk–benefit analysis, the advisory committee reversed itself later in 1995 by a 6 to 5 vote.[26] The vote, like many advisory committee votes, reflects the fact that drug approval is often not a black or white issue but is dependent on each member's opinion.[27]

Only the smallest fraction of Americans would have put their health at such risk if the public and physicians had not been fooled by the media stories and advertising hype which proclaimed these drugs silver bullets against obesity. No study had ever been published on the potential health dangers of combining the two drugs when the fen–phen craze began.[28] The FDA approved Redux in 1995. It was on the market by April 1996. Wyeth agreed to withdraw Redux in 1997 after a *New England Journal of Medicine* article reporting the link with heart valve damage made national news.[29]

The FDA does a tremendous job on many levels, but Baycol, Rezulin, Ephedra, Lotronex, Propulsid and a host of other approved but later recalled drugs make it clear that adverse events may not show up for months or even many years after FDA approval is received. In view of such experiences, it is hard to believe that the FDA approved all the SSRI antidepressants with no more than 8 weeks of clinical trial data.

The Second Surprise

A second surprising fact: not only are the clinical trials far too brief, but the studies had such high drop–out rates that they became essentially worthless for demonstrating the effectiveness of the drugs. Imagine that you wanted to find out whether or not your class of college students had been completing their reading assignments. You ask your assistant to go to your class and announce, "We are going to take the first 15 minutes of class today to take a quiz over your reading assignment." As soon as the announcement is made a student says, "I think I'll wait outside until this is over. I think I would rather Dr. Scott not know whether or not I read the assignment." Out he goes, and then 29 more students also walk out. Would the 70 who are left give you a valid statistic concerning how many of your 100 students did the reading?

You will see the point of the illustration. Out of the 47 studies which were submitted to the FDA and used by the FDA to give approval to the nation's six leading antidepressants, only 4 had as many as 70% of the study participants stay in the studies until the end.[30] How did those who stayed in differ from those who dropped out? Were they the kind of people who are more eager to please? Were they less depressed than those who dropped out? We do not know the answers, but for research that will lead to billions of dollars in sales as well as harmful side effects for users, we should expect studies with far more quality than that.

The Third Surprise

The third surprise, even if you have never taken a research–design course, should hit you as a gross violation of what should be objective science. For a number of studies the researchers removed those patients who were not improving after two weeks. These individuals were replaced by other depressed patients whom the researchers obviously hoped would do a better job of improving.[31] Were those who were removed counted as study drop outs? No, they were replaced, and everyone pretended that the substitute had been in the study from the very beginning! If you have ever taken Prozac or Zoloft, I think you should know the kind of science that is behind your antidepressant.

The Fourth Surprise

The fourth surprise was so egregious you may find it difficult to believe what I am going to share here is even true. (Fortunately "The Emperor's New Drugs" was e–printed in an American Psychological Association online e–journal and will likely be available online for many years. In the endnote referenced at the end of this sentence I share how you can easily find and read the original article for yourself.[32])

Here is the fourth surprise: in most of the studies (25 of the 47 clinical trials), the subjects were not just given a placebo or an antidepressant—they were also given sedatives! Rather than simply provide an antidepressant, the researchers, who did not want to take any chances that no measurable change might result from taking their yet–to–be approved antidepressants, rigged the studies. The researchers for the various drug companies who make America's leading antidepressants usually used the same sedative (a chloral hydrate) which makes it rather apparent that they are keenly aware of one another's research designs and what tricks have to be played to make a drug look effective.

If you do not find that dishonest, then I would wonder about your sense of morality. If you want to ask, "Why would they do that?" I have an easy answer. The end result is the potential to make millions of dollars each day. If you ask, "Why would the FDA allow the drug companies to design their own drug studies and then accept these studies?" I have no easy answer. But I think you are getting a clearer understanding of why I felt compelled to write this book.

The Fifth Surprise

The last surprise I will mention is that despite all the drug companies' manipulation of their own clinical trials, they still could not prove antidepressants are effective. In fact, in 4 of the 47 studies the placebos helped those with depression as much or more than did the antidepressants to which they were being compared.[33] For another 9 of the 47 trials the drug companies submitted the studies without reporting mean improvement scores. Why would they not report how much the drugs worked? The answer is that "no drug effect was found."[34]

So for four studies, the placebo is the better pill to take. For nine studies, no mean was reported because no change occurred. That leaves 34 studies in which the antidepressant edged out the placebo. But that should not impress you. Real drugs nearly always have a slightly greater effect even if they are ineffective for treating the problem at which they are aimed. This is because real drugs often cause drug side effects which convince the user the drug is powerful—dry mouth, dizziness, sleepiness, and so forth—and thus trial participants tend to report greater change.

In these FDA submitted studies which are responsible for the antidepressant industry in America and the rest of the world, the antidepressants came out exactly as would be expected if they had no real benefit for overcoming depression. Specifically, for the 34 remaining studies the antidepressants

BOX #8–3

The Emperor's New Drugs: A Biological Psychiatrist Objects

One of the commentaries that accompanied Dr. Kirsch's article, "The Emperor's New Drugs," was by Dr. Michael Thase, an academic psychiatrist who has published extensively on antidepressants. I believe he provides an example of how we can be blinded by long–held beliefs (the belief perseverance phenomenon). His article states he "does not dispute" the basic findings of Kirsch and his colleagues.

However, "The Emperor's New Drugs" points out that not only are antidepressant effects modest, but those only modest effects emerged from studies that generally lasted only six weeks, often allowed subjects to be on a sedative during the trials, used a placebo washout procedure, sometimes removed subjects not responding to antidepressants, may have frequently broken the blind and were all paid for and designed by the drug manufacturers. An objective conclusion would be that these studies cannot possibly be seen as proof that antidepressants work—even if only modestly.

Yet Thase does not arrive at the objective and, I would add, obvious conclusion. I won't question Thase's motives. I have visited with too many physicians who genuinely believe in the chemical imbalance/drug rebalancing theory. But I will note that I am also aware that Dr. Thase has had close financial ties to Wyeth and likely numerous other drug companies for many years.[1]

Thase writes concerning "The Emperor's New Drugs," "The authors appear not to appreciate the public health impact of relatively small therapeutic effects on conditions that afflict millions of people."[2] Thase believes that even if "for every 10 patients treated with an active SSRI (instead of a placebo), one more

did only slightly better than the placebos—the placebos accounting for over 80% of the antidepressant drug effect.[35] Yet, if it were not for the Freedom of Information Act, no one would imagine that even the drug studies responsible for Prozac, Zoloft, Paxil, Effexor, Serzone and Celexa receiving FDA approval found these drugs work only slightly better than a placebo. It is clear why this research team from the University of Connecticut and the George Washington University School of Public Health and Health Services chose to entitle their study, "The Emperor's New Drugs."

patient would remit," the drugs should be prescribed. Of course, Thase here assumes again that the question of whether or not these drugs have any real ability to overcome depression has already been settled. But let's grant him, for the sake of further discussion, that his "1 in 10 patients" is helped. The following questions must then be asked:

(1) Can we justify giving millions of Americans SSRIs when 9 out of 10 users are not helped?

(2) Can we justify giving millions of Americans SSRIs when 9 out of 10 users are not helped and yet are put at risk for the many harmful side effects of SSRIs including permanent brain damage, tardive dyskinesia, upper GI bleeding, sleep disturbance and suicide risk?

(3) Can we justify giving millions of Americans SSRIs when we still do not know all the health consequences of being on these drugs for many years—consequences which may some day cause these drugs to be removed from the market?

Dr. Thase answers these questions in the affirmative. I find this amazing and, frankly, do not find it to be a rational position. Again, his criticism of the article by Dr. Kirsch and colleagues states, "The authors appear not to appreciate the public health impact of relatively small therapeutic effects on conditions that afflict millions of people." I would turn it around and state, "Dr. Thase appears not to appreciate the public health impact on the 9 out of 10 Americans on SSRIs who will receive no benefit but face many known and, perhaps, many unknown health consequences." The Hippocratic Oath still declares, "First, do no harm." I doubt if Hippocrates would have allowed an exception for mind drugs.

To return to the question about why the FDA approved these drugs based on studies that lacked scientific merit or honesty, answers are difficult to provide. However, once the first drug was approved, the precedent was set. Listen to what one FDA scientist wrote (another Freedom of Information Act discovery). After acknowledging that the evidence as to whether or not the antidepressant had any true effect on depression, he wrote, "It is difficult to judge," but then made a terrible admission. "Similar findings for other SSRIs and other recently approved antidepressants have been considered sufficient to support the approvals of those other products."[36] (My interpretation: "We helped out Pfizer, Merck and Wyeth. We can't say no to Forest Labs just because their research is garbage also.")

Not a New Finding

"The Emperor's New Drugs" was not the first study to report that antidepressants appeared to have little real value. Nearly a decade earlier another study sought to determine how effective Prozac was compared to a placebo. Roger Greenberg, a professor in the Department of Psychiatry and Behavioral Science at the State University of New York, led that investigation. Greenberg and his colleagues were aware that some studies which claimed to have double–blind designs (neither patients nor researchers know who is getting an antidepressant and who is getting a placebo) were sometimes not fully "blind." They allowed the researchers or the patients to know (or accurately guess) who was getting what. By simply controlling for the "degree of blindness" (analyzing the results of studies in which neither the depressed participants or those rating the participants' level of depression knew who was getting Prozac and who was getting a placebo), the power of what the media reports were daily heralding as a magic pill suddenly disappeared. In fact, "the average person treated with placebo did better than roughly one–third of the patients taking [Prozac]."[37]

Previous research had already found that the "degree of blindness" is a major determinant of study results.[38] Even previous studies of antidepressants had found that "the degree of blindness is crucial . . . the blinder the study participants are to who is getting the active drug and who is getting the placebo, *the more modest the advantage for antidepressants becomes* [emphasis mine]."[39] That was the conclusion of an analysis of 22 antidepressant studies which controlled for degree of blindness. In fact, when just patients' own ratings of their depression were considered, the placebos did just as well as did the antidepressants.[40] This absence of effect (beyond the placebo effect) was consistent regardless of age, gender, dosage levels and treatment duration.

Objective, Honest Reporting Failures

The point is: if you take out the placebo effect, antidepressants just don't work. But as the medical literature is read, it is clear that this fact often pains the researchers, and they commonly seek to explain away their own findings. For example, a study published by the *American Journal of Psychiatry* examined the effectiveness of antidepressant use by the elderly by comparing an antidepressant and a placebo. Their results forced them to admit "medication was not more effective than placebo for the treatment of depression."[41] (Medication response rates ranged from 18% to 82%. Response to placebo ranged from 16% to 80%.) However, immediately after sharing the no–difference finding, they suggested that "given the considerable psychosocial support received by all patients, the placebo condition represents more than the ingestion of an inactive pill."[42] In other words, the placebo worked as well as the antidepressant, but please don't believe the placebo actually did any good. After all, the patients received a lot of support and attention during the 8 weeks the study lasted, and that probably explains the improvement. (Of course, the researchers explaining away the placebo's benefit does not explain why the antidepressant did not yield a better outcome, a fact completely ignored by their article.)

The researchers then stressed that the antidepressant did work better than the placebo for those who were the most depressed. However, they are again unfair to the placebo. They did not point out that, if the most depressed respond better to an antidepressant, it also means that those who are not as severely depressed respond better to a placebo. Also they fail to note other studies finding active drugs bring the best response during the first several weeks, but that placebos tend to *catch up and even surpass* active drugs in longer trials.[43] They also should have emphasized that adverse events were so much more common in the antidepressant group that they were ten times more likely to drop out of the study (10.7% vs. 1.1%). This fact alone could explain any difference seen in those who were more seriously depressed.[44]

In recent years many others have also found antidepressants have little advantage compared with a placebo in overcoming depression.[45] The *Archives of General Psychiatry* published a study in April of 2000 with many similarities to the Kirsch study. Using a Freedom of Information Act request, the authors of the study obtained information from the FDA on clinical trials submitted to that agency by the drug manufacturers for seven leading antidepressants. Though there was a specific interest in suicide and suicide attempts among those on antidepressants compared with those on placebos, their study also looked at the ability of the active drugs to provide "symptom reduction." When the data was analyzed, the symptom reduction was only slightly better for those using the active drug than for the placebo and like the Kirsch team, they found that placebos sometimes actually outperform antidepressants.[46] They also made another discovery—a slightly lower incidence of suicide for those on a placebo compared with those on antidepressants.[47] I can guarantee that few physicians writing antidepressant prescriptions daily are aware of this research. Let's look at some other lines of investigation, and you will find the pattern continues.

Depression and Exercise

If you haven't skipped any chapters, you know I already let the cat out of the bag back in Chapter 3 (How Psychiatrists and Doctors Are Fooled) concerning what the exercise vs. antidepressants research discovered. Nevertheless, it is important to look at this research. If you can avoid the expense and the potential health consequences of being on antidepressants, you have made a smart choice.

One such study was done by the Department of Psychiatry and Behavioral Sciences at Duke University. The researchers used 156 men and women age 50 or older who had been diagnosed with major depression and then randomly assigned them to an exercise only group, an antidepressant only group (they received the antidepressant Zoloft, the most prescribed antidepressant in the U.S.) or an exercise plus antidepressant group. Those in the exercise only group were to get 30 minutes of exercise three times each week.[48] After 16 weeks when depression levels were again assessed, it was found that the exercisers had improved as much as the other two groups.[49]

But this is not the end of the story. At ten months (six months after the first study was concluded), depression was assessed once again. The researchers were surprised to find that the group who was asked to exercise had made more improvement than either of the other groups.[50] And not only were the patients who engaged in exercise alone far better off emotionally at 10 months, they were far less likely to have had a relapse back into serious depression. The high relapse rates associated with antidepressants are not advertised, so you may not even be aware that it is not at all uncommon.

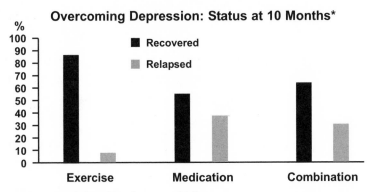

*Used by permission of *Psychosomatic Medicine*

Why would exercise alone prove to be even better than exercise and Zoloft? The researchers admitted that they were very surprised by this unexpected finding. "It was assumed that combining exercise with medication would have, if anything an additive effect."[51] It didn't. Exercise by itself proved to be the best cure. But why? The researchers speculated that taking antidepressants might actually have undermined an important aspect of overcoming depression. As they put it, instead of patients thinking, "I was dedicated and worked hard with the exercise program; it wasn't easy, but I beat this depression," they lost the benefit of feeling they made an important accomplishment without drugs and thought instead, "I took an antidepressant and got better."[52]

Turn on the Lights (or Ions)

People throughout the world are using "light exposure therapy" to overcome depression. Researchers at the National Institute of Mental Health are sometimes credited for the idea that perhaps more people are apt to become depressed during dark, dreary winter days than on bright, crisp spring days because they are not getting enough light.[53] Today we even have a name for these wintertime blues—Seasonal Affective Disorder (SAD).[54] However, light therapy is also used for major depression at any time of the year.

Beginning the day sitting in front of a fluorescent light box that typically emits about 10,000 lux units of light has helped many people who might otherwise struggle with depression throughout the day begin and end it with a smile. Does it actually work for major depression? It does, according to numerous research investigations.[55] But there is a problem with these research studies. It is not possible to keep someone from knowing whether they are being exposed to very bright light or the placebo (dim light). Could those getting bright light simply assume that the bright light should make them feel good? To put that possibility to the test Columbia University researchers decided to compare the light condition to a non–light condition in which patients would be exposed to negative air ionization. The results were very exciting because, as they reported in the *Archives of General Psychiatry*, "bright lights and high–density negative air ionization both appear to act as specific antidepressants in patients."[56] Antidepressants had long been options, but here were two non–drug options that worked. You can see why there was much excitement over this research.

Other studies were being conducted at the same time in other laboratories. One of those studies also assigned depressed patients to morning light, evening light or a negative ion generator.[57] After four weeks of exposure, morning light proved to be the most effective means of relieving depression, though the negative air ionization also helped the patients. That was a very interesting finding since, for this study, the researchers never even plugged in their black and shiny negative ionization generator!

The significance of these studies for us is that they indicate that bright lights (and sometimes negative ionization generators) help people overcome depression—just like antidepressant drugs. The biological psychiatrists (again, the true believers in depression being a pill–fixable, chemical imbalance) would object, "It may be there are many ways to reduce depression, but those should be used *in addition* to antidepressant drugs." But any biological psychiatrist who would make such a comment would be wrong. Let me quote from another study published in psychiatry's *American Journal of Psychiatry*: "Bright light as an adjunct to antidepressant pharmacotherapy for nonseasonal depression was not effective." It doesn't help to add antidepressants to the daily routine of bright light exposure. But then the authors added, "Bright light for nonseasonal depression [was effective] with effect sizes equivalent to those in most antidepressant pharmacotherapy trials.[58]

Don't miss this point. The conclusion was that bright lights work as well as standard antidepressants. Or, maybe I should say antidepressants only work about as well as bright lights. Should you go purchase a bright light box? It would be cheaper than buying antidepressant drugs, and it would undoubtedly have fewer side effects and less long–term health risks.

What is your judgment now that you know the results of the research? I will give you my opinion. I believe bright lights work for many people, but I also believe it is still impossible to determine how much of their beneficial effect is because the depressed person sitting in front of the light expects it to do some good. (It will never be possible to keep the person exposed to the light "in the dark" as to what treatment he or she is receiving. Thus, measuring the non–placebo–effect portion of bright light's benefits, if any, is impossible.)

Acupuncture

Acupuncture involves inserting thin needles at strategic points (acu-points) in a patient's body to stimulate nerves in the skin and in muscle tissue. The practice originated in China over 2,500 years ago but was almost unknown in America until 1972. That was the year President Nixon made his historic trip to China. With him was a *New York Times* reporter who developed appendicitis. Following an emergency appendectomy he wrote an article describing the almost miraculous relief from pain he experienced as a result of acupuncture.[59] As the popularity of acupuncture has grown in America and the West, so has the body of research examining its effectiveness. Today many double–blind, placebo–controlled clinical trials have reported acupuncture can be effectively used to treat several common medical problems including lower back pain,[60] post–operative pain,[61] post–operative nausea,[62] and chemotherapy–related nausea.[63]

Can it help with depression? It can. In fact, studies sometimes find acupuncture works better than antidepressants. One study reported 70% of patients treated with electro–acupuncture were either cured or markedly improved compared with 65% of those on amitriptyline, still a favorite tricyclic antidepressant for some physicians.[64] That is not the norm, however. The norm is for acupuncture to perform just as well as antidepressants. The *Cochrane Database Systematic Review* (the gold standard for medical research reviews today) came to just such a conclusion. "There is no evidence that medication was better than acupuncture in reducing the severity of depression," they announced.[65]

Of course, we always have that problem of the placebo effect. Like bright lights, acupuncture is difficult to accurately assess since it is impossible to provide a truly equivalent placebo. (Either you are stuck with needles or you aren't.) Several sham studies have stuck needles in non–acupuncture points assuming this is an adequate placebo, but those patients were still being stuck. The best placebo control studies use a fake needle which feels like it penetrates the skin but never does. It does appear to enter the skin, though, as it can be made "shorter" as the fake penetration occurs. (That's pretty close to an equivalent placebo.) Comparing the real with the fake, researchers found acupuncture worked, but so did the fake placebo needles.[66]

St. John's Wort (Hypericum)

St. John's wort is an herb that can be used to make tea, or the "active ingredients" within the herb can be extracted and put in capsules. In Europe St. John's wort is widely prescribed as an antidepressant. No prescription is required in the United States, and many Americans use St. John's wort instead of antidepressant drugs. Pharmacies all over America—CVS, Osco, Rite Aid, Save–on, Walgreens—all stock various strengths and bottle sizes.

Those who choose St. John's wort over antidepressants save lots of money, but the question should always be, "Does it work?" Many studies have reported that St. John's wort does work, including many double–blind, placebo–controlled studies.[67] Yes, it works, but then we should ask, "How does it compare to Celexa, Lexapro, Zoloft, and all the other antidepressants?" There are numerous studies that have examined that question, and what they find is that St. John's wort works as well or better than standard (synthetic) antidepressants. For example, compared to Paxil, depression scores fell more (56.6% vs. 44.8%) and side effects were less.[68] Similar results were found for Prozac.[69] A comparison with Zoloft found St. John's wort again performed as well as the antidepressant drug without as many side effects.[70] Other studies with other antidepressants find this same pattern.[71] Should you consider using St. John's wort if you are depressed? The number of adverse effects is minimal, being essentially equivalent to taking a placebo.[72] So, here is an herb that can be purchased in any city in America, is much cheaper than antidepressant drugs and has fewer side effects than standard antidepressants. You can see why it has so many fans.

The medical establishment is confused today about what its position should be. The *Cochrane Database of Systematic Reviews* posted its most recent review of the research during July 2005. Their conclusion is now seen as the most authoritative statement in the medical world, and it will not likely be revised again until 2010. Their conclusion needs comment:

> Current evidence regarding Hypericum extracts is inconsistent and confusing. In patients who meet criteria for major depression, several recent placebo–controlled trials suggest that Hypericum has minimal beneficial effects while other trials suggest that Hypericum and standard antidepressants have similar beneficial effects.[73]

The research, however, should not be called confusing or inconsistent. St. John's wort works. It works only a little better than a placebo, but it works. It works as well (or better) than standard antidepressants. All of this is what we should expect if standard antidepressants work only because they are expected to work. Antidepressant drugs also enjoy the benefit of a placebo effect. But physicians and psychiatrists are so convinced that antidepressants do work that a survey of all the research seems inconsistent and confusing.

Any pill which can cause some physical symptoms (a caffeine pill would be great) would be convincing and would do slightly better than a sugar pill placebo. Any pill that causes physical symptoms breaks the "blind" somewhat ("I have a dry mouth. I must be taking the real drug.") Some researchers correctly argue that placebos should not be sugar pills but should be "symptom–matching pills."

Personal Testimonials

On a very regular basis I find myself in a conversation with someone who says, "Believe me, I wish I could get off my antidepressant, but I just can't. They help me get through the day. On the days I get away from home without taking my pill I start feeling sad or angry within hours." Another common testimonial goes something like this. "I never had depression in my life until about a year ago. When it hit me I could hardly function. So I went to my doctor and he prescribed Cymbalta, and I started feeling better within days."

Testimonials such as these reveal why some people get angry when someone suggests antidepressants work but do not work much, if any, better than a placebo. They believe those antidepressants gave them back their lives, and in some cases, even saved their lives. But the same loyalty can be found for bright lights, St. John's wort, acupuncture and negative ion generators. In just minutes on the internet I found several examples. (See Box #8–4, Antidepressant Testimonials.)

Many of you will find it offensive if I suggest your overcoming depression was because the antidepressant worked as a placebo. You shouldn't. The placebo effect is powerful. It can even bring about physiological changes. I will share that research shortly. But let me also suggest that your getting over depression might not be related to the placebo effect at all but to something equally as powerful—time.

Regression Toward the Mean

Even in an introductory psychology course I give some attention to some important statistical concepts which must be understood if we do not want to be easily fooled. One of the most important of these concepts is called "regression toward the mean." "Regression toward the mean" applied to real life says that if we are angry today, we are less likely to be angry tomorrow. With time on our side we are apt to move toward the norm (mean)

BOX #8–4

Antidepressant Testimonials

Do antidepressants work? Personal testimonials from users are hard to refute. And there are literally millions of Americans who will testify to their power to heal. How can any of us refute their personal experiences? Even if antidepressants don't work for every person who has ever tried them, they clearly can and do work for many. Here is proof.[1] (In each case a different antidepressant was used. The antidepressant to which each refers in the testimonials is printed upside down at the bottom of the box on the opposite page.)

1. "Starting the 3rd week of October, I was already starting to feel lethargic, sad, hopeless and overwhelmed. On Oct. 23 I used _____ and felt immediately better. Today is the 3rd day and I feel strong, energetic, capable, and happy. . . . I'm beginning to have pleasant dreams where I wake up feeling a sense of happiness. I sleep more deeply. My immune system seems to be improving . . . . Most importantly, I have more energy during the day. . . . I did not think it possible to experience this much improvement in my mood within such a brief period of time."

2. "I began to take _____ and I could tell the effects immediately! Well actually it took about 2 days. It gave me energy, a new outlook on life and a goofy happiness. I guess that is just the way I am when I feel good. I could not believe this happened

---

which, hopefully, is not anger. The same is true for depression. If we are the most depressed we have ever been today, we should anticipate moving away from depression (moving closer to the mean) in the days and weeks ahead.

I have counseled countless men and women who were in the process of divorcing or had recently divorced who felt as if they could hardly go on. And yet they did. Crises involving marriages, children or other close relationships can be emotionally draining. That's not hard to see. But what about depression that seems inexplicable? I will discuss that phenomenon in Chapter 16 on avoiding and overcoming depression. For now, let me simply state that even the inexplicable type of depression can come and go.

so rapidly so I decided (after about 2 months) to stop using it for about a month. Slowly the depression came back and I decided that I would continue to take _____. Why not? A few days after I began to take it again, the great outlook I had came back, and that is why I am here."

3. "I was always upset, angry, crying, couldn't sleep well and tired . . . . Now I can work 60–plus hours a week, I am always full of energy, I sleep a lot better, and I don't cry any more. I've never felt better."

4. "I've suffered from SAD for 14 years and winters have been very tough for me. This one was worse than most . . . . After doing a lot of research at the National Library of Medicine and asking quite a few questions, I decided to [use] _____. The result for me was almost immediate. I began feeling better within the first day and was back to my normal self within three."

Once you hear even a few of these personal testimonials concerning the life–changing power of antidepressants, it is easy to become a believer. You are most likely to hear from those taking synthetic drugs because the huge sales force, the massive advertising budgets and the government stamp of approval all encourage widespread use. But drugs are not the only antidepressants.

1. light therapy 2. St. John's wort 3. acupuncture 4. a negative ion generator

If you can accept that as true, then you can see why so many attribute their healing to a drug. When are they most likely to go to their physician? When they feel fine or when they feel depressed? So at the bottom of a depression low, when they feel absolutely desperate, they take their first antidepressant. As the emotions improve, they attribute the longed–for change to the drug. Very often these individuals even become evangelists for their antidepressant, sharing their testimonial freely and encouraging their friends to try the drug themselves. It is possible, aside from any placebo effect, to become a believer in their power in this way. But now let's consider the amazing power of placebos—the other way "healing" may occur.

The Placebo Effect

For several years I introduced the placebo effect to my students by describing a study done at the University of Wisconsin.[74] Americans are well aware that alcohol is known to increase aggression, but Alan Lang and his colleagues suspected that drinkers often start acting out a role long before the alcohol could have significant physiological effects. To put that theory to the test the researchers used an alcoholic drink (vodka with tonic water) and a non–alcoholic placebo (tonic water only) that could not be told apart. They tasted the same, but only one actually contained alcohol. College men were then recruited and divided into four groups with half of all subjects being deceived as to what they would be drinking. In reality, half of the men who thought they were getting only tonic water actually got alcohol, and half of those who thought they were getting vodka and tonic water actually got just tonic water. The other half of the men were not deceived, being honestly told if they were getting vodka and tonic water or just tonic water.

When the results of the experiment were in, the researchers found that what each man drank was immaterial. The only factor which mattered was what he thought he was drinking. Those who thought they were getting alcohol (and did) became aggressive, but so did those who thought they were getting alcohol but consumed only water. On the other hand, for those who thought they were getting tonic water but actually got alcohol, there was no change in their behavior.

That study tells us something about placebo effects, but I stopped sharing it with students years ago as the finding is not too surprising. After all, we know what alcohol's end effect is, and in some circles it is considered "cool" to be drunk. Today I prefer to share studies that are sometimes old studies but speak more clearly to the amazing power of placebos. For example can a placebo (saline) help control pain? The answer is a strong "Yes," being up to 70% as effective as morphine.[75] Even more surprising, give patients with high cholesterol a "cholesterol–lowering" placebo, and their cholesterol levels will drop.[76] Or test asthma patients with an inhaler which they are told will cause bronchoconstriction or bronchodilation, and you will bring on bronchoconstriction or bronchodilation—even if the inhaler contains no active chemicals.[77]

BOX #8–5

A Flawed Study of Placebo Effects

The May 24, 2001, issue of the *New England Journal of Medicine* reported that an analysis of a total of 114 placebo studies "found little evidence in general that placebos had powerful clinical effects."[1] That conclusion reflects a very poor research study design, not reality. Instead of limiting the definition of placebo to pills or to pills and hypodermic injections, the authors included studies in which the placebos included "talking about daily events, family activities, football, vacation activities, pets, hobbies, books, movies and television shows."[2]

The *New England Journal of Medicine* study also failed to distinguish between those conditions which are highly influenced by placebo effects (anything evaluated subjectively—like depression—versus anything evaluated objectively—like a parasite count in a blood sample). Thus, conditions which cannot be easily influenced were combined with those which could be, lowering (in their study) the placebo effect's power.

Other problems have been discussed in some of the many immediate responses and subsequent articles which critiqued this now–fully–discredited *NEJM* article.[3] The article's greatest value has been to illustrate again how erroneous conclusions can be if a good study design is not employed.

Many other studies point to actual physiological changes resulting from a placebo. One such study used patients with limb ischemia. Ischemia is a condition in which there is a lack of blood flow to a leg typically caused by the blockage of an artery. If ischemia is left untreated, gangrene will set in. But injecting patients with a vasodilator to open up the blood vessels causes blood flow to increase, and systolic blood pressure rises. Inject patients with a placebo and essentially equivalent physiological changes take place.[78]

A study from the 1950s is even more dramatic. It involved a surgical procedure which became common for controlling the pain of angina (chest pain due to inadequate blood flow to the heart). The procedure was known as internal–mammary–artery ligation. By simply making small chest incisions, a cardiologist could reach down with some suture and tie off the two mammary arteries. It was assumed the procedure would lead to greater blood flow to the heart because it was well established that it provided a great deal of relief to patients. Then a Seattle cardiologist and some of his colleagues decided to see if any of the relief was due simply to a placebo effect. Patients suffering with angina were taken to surgery, had the incisions cut into their chests, but unknown to them, some never actually had the surgical procedure. It did not matter. They improved as much as all the other patients. The surgery had never worked as hoped (new blood vessel formation), but those who had the surgery had less need for nitroglycerin, could exercise longer without pain and had improved electrocardiograph results—whether or not they had the real operation.[79]

All of these studies point to actual physiological changes resulting from the innocent little placebo. Placebos can change one's heart rate, blood

---

BOX #8–6

Can Placebos Produce Endorphins?

"Endorphin" is a word made from two other words, *endogenous* (meaning "originating within"—in this case, originating within the brain) and *morphine*, a pain–killing drug. Endorphins are classified as opioid compounds as they resemble opium from which morphine, codeine and heroin are made.

Numerous studies have now shown endorphins are produced during exercise[1] or when someone is given a placebo which he or she expects to be of help.[2] Endorphins are natural painkillers, which may explain why I felt no pain for a time following the most serious bone break I ever had. Ask a gathering of adults how many have had similar experiences, and you may be surprised. The fact that endorphins are produced during exercise may also explain what many runners have called a "runner's high." Placebos can also cause dopamine to be released by the brain.[3] And then, once the painkilling chemicals are released by a placebo, "a complex cascade of events" follows which impacts other parts of the body.[4]

---

pressure, pupil size, blood sugar level and, more importantly as concerns depression, they can release endorphins and cause measurable brain (electroencephalogram and PET scan) changes.[80] And the desirable brain changes brought about by an antidepressant appear to be no different than those brought about by the humble placebo.[81]

The Placebo Effect Variables

The research on placebos is rich. About this powerful medicine we also know:

- A placebo shot works better than a placebo pill.[82]

- The more frequently a placebo is administered, the more quickly healing occurs.[83]

- Placebos which are given the most openly are more effective than those which are given less openly.[84]

- The greater the expectation of effect, the greater the effect.[85]

- Placebos work better when they involve a well–known brand name.[86]

- Larger pills and larger doses have a more powerful effect than do smaller pills and smaller doses.[87]

- Placebos given by doctors have a more powerful effect than placebos given by nurses.[88]

- If the person giving the placebo seems particularly warm, friendly, and genuinely interested in the well–being of the recipient, the placebo will have a greater effect.[89]

- Placebos given by doctors who act enthused about the effectiveness of the drug they are prescribing have a more powerful effect.[90]

If a doctor's enthusiasm matters, then we should expect that as doctors become convinced of the power of antidepressants, the effectiveness of anti-depressant placebos increases. That is exactly what has occurred in America. A *JAMA* article's title tells the story: "Placebo Response in Studies of Major Depression: Variable, Substantial, and Growing."[91]

Placebos are not always equivalent to real medicines. You will not cure malaria or heal an infection or correct poor vision with placebos. We still need antibiotics, athlete's foot medicines and glasses. But placebos are highly effective for anything that is more subjectively measured (depression) rather than more objectively measured (bacterial infections, athlete's foot infection or poor vision). And this is not a recent discovery. For example, Lowinger and Dobie conducted four double–blind studies between 1959 and 1962 to measure the placebo effect on sleep disturbance, thought disturbance, interpersonal relationships, depression and anxiety. These are all issues which are subjectively evaluated and consequently, placebo effects were dramatic, "healing" as many as 76% of the cases in one study and proving more effective than the mind drugs in two studies.[92] When a good double–blind design is used, such results have now been found for decades.

Do antidepressants work? They do, but not any better than do bright lights, St. John's wort, negative ion generators and acupuncture, assuming you and your doctor are both convinced your treatment will work. The question then becomes, so why did the FDA approve these drugs? That is addressed by the following chapter.

9

"How can a drug that is associated with higher rates of both renal dysfunction and death than placebo—and that costs 50 times as much as standard therapies and for which there are no meaningful data on relevant end points—be given to more than 600,000 patients and be promoted throughout the United States for serial outpatient use, an indication not listed on the label?"[1]
— Eric J. Topol, MD
New England Journal of Medicine, *2005*

THE FDA DRUG
APPROVAL PROCESS

Is there really a drug which has never been proven effective, is incredibly expensive and is known to sometimes cause death but is commonly prescribed in America? There is. The drug, Natrecor (nesiritide) is given for acute congestive heart failure. But how is that even possible? Dr. Topol writes that the answer to his question is in large measure a matter of imperfect drug studies and near perfect marketing.[2] Those are major factors, but perhaps even more significant is an FDA drug approval process that allows drugs to enter the market which would never have passed the test earlier in our nation's history.

Many younger Americans have no memory or knowledge of the thalidomide tragedy. It is a story that should be remembered. Thalidomide is a relatively safe drug—unless it is taken during pregnancy. Yet thalidomide was marketed primarily as a remedy for morning sickness, which is most commonly experienced during the first trimester of pregnancy. That is the very time the developing child is most susceptible to the effects of harmful drugs.

The Thalidomide Disaster

In 48 countries around the world[3] 8,000–12,000 thalidomide babies[4] were born during the late 1950s and early 1960s. Thousands were so damaged that they did not survive their first birthday.[5] Those who did often had most severe birth defects. One British mother took a single pill. When the BBC interviewed her son 40 years later, he reported that his handicaps included "very short arms, no right eye and 10 per cent vision in my left eye."[6] Eventually the documented effects of thalidomide included damaged hearts, gallbladders and brains; malformed bowels, narrowed or closed anuses, deformed hips, missing genitals, damaged eye muscles, deafness, missing ears, missing fingers, and thumbs with three rather than two joints.[7]

But the most common birth defect, and the one most remembered by those of us who saw the full–page photographs printed in the news magazines when the danger of thalidomide was finally realized, was phocomelia, in which a baby is born with defective or missing extremities. Some had shortened limbs with hands or feet at the end of short stubs protruding from the body. Others had only toes attached to their hips.

Thalidomide was first synthesized in 1953 by the Swiss pharmaceutical company CIBA. They conducted extensive tests, seeking to find a profitable use for their new drug. By 1954 CIBA was willing to sell development rights to a German firm, Chemie Gruenenthal, as they had found no use for thalidomide. Chemie Gruenenthal first tried to market thalidomide as an anticonvulsant for those with epilepsy. However, the drug proved to be essentially ineffective for this, so they sought other possible uses. Their tests had revealed that thalidomide tended to bring on drowsiness. Thus, it was that this drug was then seen as a possible sleeping aid or general sedative.

The first child to be damaged by thalidomide was born on Christmas Day 1956. The baby girl was born without ears. Her father was a Chemie Gruenenthal employee, and he had given his pregnant wife a sample of his company's new drug. It was years before he came to realize that it was thalidomide that was responsible for his daughter's birth defect.[8] Thalidomide was seen as such a safe drug when it was released to the West German public on October 1, 1957, that it did not even require a prescription.

The drug was at first sold as a "completely safe" sedative. Ads for the new sedative were placed in fifty medical journals and 250,000 letters were sent to physicians which declared Contergan (the German patent name) the safest sedative available, perfectly suited to reduce the growing number of accidental barbiturate deaths worldwide. Even children could be given thalidomide, and in Germany it became common to give fussy children a dose.[9]

Over the next few years, thalidomide became so popular that it proved to be the most profitable drug in the company's history.[10] Thalidomide's sedative effect, combined with its safety, led physicians to begin prescribing it for a growing list of ills—asthma, headaches, colds and sleeplessness. Then in 1958 when Chemie Gruenenthal sent out a letter encouraging use for morning sickness in pregnant women, a new potential market was added to that ever–growing list.

Though thalidomide was first sold in Germany, its manufacturer aggressively marketed it to other drug manufacturers around the world. It was soon being sold in other European countries: Australia, Canada, Asian and African nations, and various Latin American countries. Nevertheless, it was not until December 16, 1961, that the first suggestion that thalidomide was causing birth defects appeared in print. An Australian obstetrician, Dr. W. G. McBride, wrote a letter to the editor of the *Lancet* stating, "In recent months I have observed that the incidence of multiple severe abnormalities in babies delivered of women who were given the drug thalidomide . . . to be almost 20%."[11] He then asked, "Have any of your readers seen similar abnormalities in babies delivered of women who have taken this drug during pregnancy?"[12]

In Germany Dr. Widukind Lenz, a pediatrician and professor at Hamburg University, also became aware of the surprising number of babies being born with missing fingers or short arms or with feet attached to the hips. He had been approached by a man whose sister had given birth to a severely deformed baby. Six weeks later the man's wife gave birth to a baby with similar defects. Lenz began a historical investigation. How common had these birth defects been in previous years? He went through birth records for 212,000 births, virtually every Hamburg birth between 1930 and 1955. Among all those births only one involved defects such as he was seeing.[13] He placed advertisements in German newspapers asking parents to contact him if they had a child with these birth defects and then visited dozens of them.

By November 1961, Lenz was sure thalidomide was the culprit and contacted Chemie Gruenenthal, the manufacturer, to tell them of his discoveries. A personal conversation did no good. A formal letter was then sent stating, "Every month's delay in clarification means that fifty to one hundred horribly mutilated children will be born."[14] Lenz next shared those fears (publicly announcing the drug's name) at a pediatrician's association meeting. The following day Lenz found Chemie Gruenenthal representatives, including its lawyer, at his door. The company threatened him with a lawsuit and then immediately sent out 70,000 letters to German doctors who were now hearing of the thalidomide–birth defect link, telling them that thalidomide was completely safe to prescribe.[15]

In meetings with German health authorities, Lenz convinced them of thalidomide's dangers, and they asked Chemie Gruenenthal to voluntarily withdraw the drug. Gruenenthal refused. Either Lenz or someone aware of his first letter to Gruenenthal took the action which would bring the quickest possible change—they took the story to a major German newspaper. Lenz's declaration, "Every month's delay in clarification means fifty to one hundred horribly mutilated children will be born," was included in the article. It was sensational news, and it forced thalidomide off the German market.

Though thalidomide was removed from the German market, worldwide sales continued to be strong, and Chemie Gruenenthal was determined to keep it that way. They sent out letters to distributors around the world indicating their decision was only a temporary action and due only to the sensationalism of the German press. They also began a blistering attack on Lenz. "Idiots and clever people are both equally harmless," they declared. "Those halfwits and half–educated people [who] always recognize only half–truths alone are dangerous."[16]

Chemie Gruenenthal would not surrender, but soon it would not matter. McBride's *Lancet* letter was a warning to the rest of the world and within just five months, the first published report of the effect of thalidomide on the offspring of animals appeared. Once again, it was the *Lancet* that announced the findings:

> We have succeeded in producing deformities in rabbits remarkably similar to those seen in humans. . . . Our chief animal technician, Mr. R. E. Hughes, states that he has never seen anything like this during fifty years' experience of rabbit breeding.[17]

Balancing Benefits and Risks

There are always lessons to be learned from tragedies. In this case, it may be that we should recognize the potential disregard for objective data which may occur when profits are at stake. Chemie Gruenenthal acted to protect the public only when forced to do so. It is possible that corporations are more responsible today than in the past, but it will continue to be human nature to struggle with putting the interest of others ahead of our own. That is why we have a Food and Drug Administration. They are there to protect us, and they have done so by denying approval to thousands of drugs.

Even among those who have heard about thalidomide, many are not aware that, though it was prescribed in countries all around the world, it was never approved for use in the United States.[18] The FDA's approval process, though inadequate by today's standards, was more stringent than that found in most countries. Those more demanding standards saved countless babies from the terrible physical effects continuing to plague thousands of adults in countries all across the world.

The result of prescribing thalidomide to pregnant women[19] was truly a tragedy, but that tragedy also brought large amounts of funding to pregnancy research and changed the drug approval process. Many countries began demanding various animal studies that had not been required before thalidomide. The FDA further tightened its requirements. It was this very conservative approach that caused many to believe that if a drug was approved in America, it must be quite safe.

The problem with this very cautious and, hence, very slow process is that it also prevents newly discovered, life–saving drugs from getting to the market quickly. The person with a life–threatening disease might die long before the drug that could save his or her life is ever approved for use. There was a time when those Americans with cancer or other serious diseases, desperate to find a miraculous cure, knew that they could go to Mexico, Canada or a European nation to get the latest drugs—drugs which might not be approved in America for months or years, if ever.

This more cautious approach put the FDA on the front page of the nation's papers in October of 1988. The FDA headquarters in Rockville,

Maryland, was the site of a protest by AIDS activists. Over 1,000 protesters chanted, "Hey, hey, FDA, how many people have you killed today?" The activists did not want an explanation concerning why the FDA used a very deliberate approval process. They knew AIDS would likely take their lives before life–saving drugs were ever available to physicians. One AIDS victim from Chicago announced, "We are here for all the people with AIDS, but we are also here for all the other people with life–threatening illnesses who need drugs now."[20]

Drug manufacturers also wanted to speed up the approval of new drugs. In 1992 new drugs took, on average, 22 months to get approved.[21] The average person can barely conceive of how much potential revenue this costs the industry. In the year 2000 drug companies were making, on average, $1.3 million per day on their new drugs.[22] Thus, for popular drugs, each day of delay in getting a new drug to market could mean a loss of literally millions of dollars. The key fact here is that the patent laws start counting days whenever a new drug patent is approved by the patent office, not when it is approved by the FDA for use by the American people. So speeding up the FDA's approval process even a few weeks could mean hundreds of millions of dollars to the industry.[23]

The combined energy of activists and the drug industry led Congress to pass the Prescription Drug User Fee Act (PDUFA) of 1992. I believe few could imagine how dramatically the legislation would transform the FDA and the drug approval process in ways unforeseen by Congress or the FDA.

Money Influences Drug Research and Drug Approval

Merck's arthritis drug Vioxx made front page news in 2004 when Merck announced it was going to remove the drug from the market because of concerns over increased cardiovascular risks. Most of the public still believes that the Vioxx–heart problem link was only discovered in 2004. The 2004 edition of the *Physicians' Desk Reference*[24] (*PDR*), the compilation of

FDA–approved drug package inserts, makes it plain that the danger was known years before the drug was pulled from the market.

During the clinical trials comparing Vioxx with its logical competitor, the previously top–selling arthritis drug Naproxen, Vioxx came out looking terrible with more than twice as many serious cardiovascular events (45) during 10½ months of testing.[25] Those 45 "events" in 10½ months of use by 4,047 patients are just a little over a 1% chance of having a stroke or heart attack during less than one year of use. In small but legible print the *PDR* has been warning patients of this risk for years. "Serious cardiovascular events included: sudden death, myocardial infarction, unstable angina, ischemic stroke, transient ischemic attack, and peripheral venous and arterial thromboses."[26] In other words, this drug can kill you, a conclusion coming out of trial data submitted to the FDA in June 2000.[27]

It wasn't until a longer–term study was indicating years of use could jump that risk of death appreciably[28] that Merck decided it should act, stopping the study two months before its completion. After the drug's withdrawal I began to hear discussions concerning whether or not the withdrawal was really necessary. "All drugs have some danger, but the risks are so minimal I think we ought to be able to choose whether we take the drug or not." I doubt if anyone who made such comments was aware that Merck had cut the typical dosage in half for the clinical study in order to reduce adverse events—a common drug trial trick of the trade (at least when there is cause to suspect your drug might be killing people). I also doubt many of these individuals realized that at the higher 50 mg/day (the maximum recommended dose for pain), the risk of having a heart attack or stroke was more than 1 in 100 during just the first 42 weeks of use![29]

The Vioxx recall prompted the FDA to assemble an advisory panel during the third week of February 2005 to make a recommendation to the FDA about the entire group of Cox–2 inhibitors (Vioxx, Celebrex and Bextra). Then something very surprising happened. By a very close vote (17–15) the panel of experts voted to allow Vioxx back on the market. They also voted not to remove Celebrex and Bextra. The vote made headlines and seemed to say again that the safety concerns were overblown. The message seemed to be that, yes, there were risks, but they were so minimal even Merck was overreacting. That was undoubtedly a huge disappointment to the many law firms that had started national advertising campaigns to solicit potential lawsuit clients. (Anyone watching much television at that time likely saw numerous "Have you been hurt by Vioxx?" commercials.)[30]

There may never have been additional discussion of the FDA's panel of experts except for the work done by The Center for Science in the Public Interest. That organization had been keeping a list of scientists whom they identified as receiving financial contributions from drug manufacturers. During the fourth week of February, they released their findings to the *New York Times*.[31] The Center for Science in the Public Interest did not have records for all the members of the panel, but they had enough information to reveal why the committee voted in favor of the drugs.

Ten panel members had financial ties with either Pfizer (maker of Celebrex and Bextra) or Merck. Those ten experts voted 10–0 in favor of keeping Pfizer's two Cox–2 inhibitor drugs on the market and 9–1 in favor of allowing Vioxx to be made available again. No one can prove that the financial ties influenced the votes of these panel members, and all of those willing to discuss it claimed it had no influence on their votes. However, none of us is as objective as we think we are. Those ten experts should have simply said they had a conflict of interest and felt it improper to vote. But then Vioxx would have been rejected by a vote of 8 to 14.[32]

The big question concerning this story is why did the FDA allow those panel members to vote on these drugs? The FDA knew what financial ties each member had with various drug companies. (They are required to disclose this information.) The fact is, the FDA just did not see a problem. They acknowledged there were many ties but argued that most experts have ties to the drug industry, and it is not realistic to think a full panel of experts who do not have those ties can even be found. Of course, it would be helpful if the FDA would at least tell us which panel members have stock, stock options, research grants, consulting arrangements and so forth with the drug companies. The FDA refuses to do so.

The FDA grants both general and specific waivers for those with financial conflicts of interest. Several general waivers were granted to Vioxx advisory committee members. A statement of a general nature is read into the record at the beginning of a meeting. However, it usually requires a Freedom of Information Act request to discover what specific financial ties advisory committee members have with the pharmaceutical companies.[33]

Prior to 1992 the FDA relied on their own scientists to determine a drug's safety. The changes made during that year were not designed to allow drug companies to influence the FDA's decisions, but that is clearly what has occurred. The Vioxx committee was not unique. Most of the drugs Americans take today were approved by FDA committees whose make–up includes individuals who were paid large fees or given stock in the drug companies whose drugs they were asked to approve or disapprove. Today most drug trials are designed, not by independent researchers, but by the very companies which hope to market and profit from the new drugs. Most of those doing the research are even paid, not by our government, but by the drug companies themselves. The data coming out of these studies typically cannot be viewed by independent researchers. (Think of my experience when I sought to examine the Effexor ad studies discussed in Chapter 5.) The drug companies own and control the data.

The new FDA is so riddled with conflicts of interests that this has been an issue raised by the media every time there is a major blunder ever since the passage of the Prescription Drug User Fee Act (PDUFA) in 1992. Unfortunately, the result of this occasional media attention to a problem needing correction has not been a more open FDA. Instead, the FDA decided to stop releasing much of the information about committee members' financial ties with the drug companies. The FDA claims the decision was a matter of protecting the privacy of committee members.

Financial Conflict of Interest Rules

The rules for when a financial conflict of interest occurs fail to insure even some semblance of objectivity. Committee members can receive up to $50,000 per year from a drug company for any reason without it being considered a financial conflict of interest if the "work" is not directly tied to the drug the committee is evaluating.[34] Not until a committee member has stock holdings greater than $100,000 is exclusion expected to prevent participation in a drug's approval process.[35]

Despite the lack of openness concerning conflicts of interest, investigative reporters have been successful in gathering sufficient data to make it clear the system is extremely tainted today. *USA Today* reporters found that though, as already noted, federal law does not allow the experts who vote to approve a new drug to have a direct financial interest in the drug they are evaluating, more than half of the experts do have these conflicts of interest. But if the law does not allow this, how could this be possible? The answer is found in the fact that the experts are given waivers by the FDA. This is not a rare event. It occurs nearly 200 to 400 times per year.[36]

This problem is not limited to the FDA. The National Institutes of Health (NIH) is the world's leading biomedical research institution. Yet, since 1995 its policies have allowed incredible exchanges of cash and stock from the drug companies to NIH employees. (See Box #9–1, NIH Policies on Outside Financial Ties for Employees.) This "almost anything goes" policy has undoubtedly caused FDA officials to adopt softer attitudes toward industry ties.

Money's Dramatic Influence on Published Research

In a perfect world, money would not influence anyone's judgment. But a continuing stream of research studies makes it clear that money very much influences the judgment of both individual researchers and the entire system. A *JAMA* article entitled "Evaluation of Conflict of Interest in Economic

BOX #9–1
NIH Policies on Outside Financial Ties for Employees[1]

Before 1995	After 1995
Employees limited to no more than $25,000/yr from any single source and no more than $50,000/yr from all sources combined	No dollar limit on the amount of money employees can earn from outside activities
Employees limited to a maximum of 500 hr/yr of outside activities	No limitations on the amount of time employees can devote to outside work, as long as it does not interfere with their NIH work
Employees could accept only money for performing outside activities; payment in stock or stock options was banned	Employees can accept money as well as stock and stock options for their services

Used by permission of the *New England Journal of Medicine*

Analysis of New Drugs Used in Oncology" reported that "studies funded by pharmaceutical companies were nearly 8 times less likely to reach unfavorable qualitative conclusions than nonprofit studies."[37] They also discovered that "1 in 5 articles contained overstatements of quantitative results."[38]

We are not talking about bias in an area of research which would "do no harm" if results were not reported honestly. Oncology is the study of cancer. A less than objective study of new drugs would result in the deaths of many people, and this research team determined that the published oncology research is far from objective.

And even this study, which sought to determine how pharmaceutical money was influencing the conclusions found in the medical journals, had the following note concerning the study's funding. "The data collection efforts for this study were funded by an unrestricted grant from Amgen Inc., Thousand Oaks, California, as part of a larger, on–going study. The sponsor had a contractual right to review and comment on manuscripts and abstracts prior to submission."[39]

This is an unconscionable system. If a study were to find a pharmaceutical company's new drug had no positive benefit or had serious side effects or was less effective than a competitor's, they could simply refuse to allow the study to be published. Such potentially life–threatening acts have occurred often.[40] The American Society of Clinical Oncology published revised conflict of interest guidelines in June 2003[41] (which went into force for new research beginning June 2004). That policy is still in effect today. It requires disclosure of stock ownership, honoraria, gifts and other remuneration from pharmaceutical firms by authors who submit articles for publication by the society's journal. However it cannot force researchers to submit articles which find that the drug under study is harmful.[42]

A Canadian research team examined virtually all the research published in English language medical journals over a 19–month period, recording each author's position on one type of drug. The authors were then assigned to a favorable conclusions, a neutral conclusions or a critical conclusions group. They then contacted the authors of these published reports and made inquiries concerning any financial relationship they might have with the drug manufacturers. The results were dramatic. Ninety–six percent of authors with favorable conclusions had financial ties to the drug manufacturers compared with "only" 60% of those who had neutral conclusions and 37% of those with negative conclusions.[43]

Defending the System

The *New England Journal of Medicine* published three letters to the editor which were critical of the study. Some of the research design criticisms had merit; however it is interesting to note those who responded to the research did not deny the financial ties. The first letter argued that we should expect financial ties. "But those receiving the support were clinical researchers and would have been expected to require grants to perform these studies."[44] The second denied being influenced by the money. "I receive support from pharmaceutical companies that supplements basic grants from our medical research council. These funds go to university accounts with nothing going into my pocket. This support does not buy silence. I proposed to our ethics committee that all adverse drug reactions need publication, irrespective of company attitudes."[45]

My response to this last comment would be, "Do you mean to tell me that your ethics committee does not already *demand* that you publish adverse drug reactions, not just the positive drug results?" Add to this another fact of which few Americans are aware: not securing funding can keep a university researcher from getting tenure, being promoted or receiving a positive evaluation. Can you see how objectivity can clearly be compromised? Drug companies do not want to continue funding departments that publish reports which hurt their company's business. (And industry funding of academic institutions has now surpassed federal funding, so this is no minor issue.[46]) Conflicts of interest can either be very clear and manifest or very subtle and unspoken.[47]

To their credit the *Journal of the American Medical Association* and the *New England Journal of Medicine*, arguably two of America's most prestigious medical journals, have both published several studies in recent years which have revealed conflicts of interest in drug research. An example is the study by Justin Bekelman and his colleagues entitled "Scope and impact of financial conflicts of interest in biomedical research: A systematic review" which appeared in *JAMA*. In their study the authors looked at English language studies appearing between January 1980 and October 2002 which examined the financial relationship between drug companies, researchers and academic institutions. Their conclusions reveal how concerned we all should be:

Strong and consistent evidence shows that industry–sponsored research tends to draw pro–industry conclusions. . . . Consistent evidence also demonstrated that industry ties are associated with both publication delays and data withholding. These restrictions, often contractual in nature, serve to compound bias in biomedical research. Anecdotal reports suggest that industry may alter, obstruct, or even stop publication of negative studies.[48]

Why the FDA Doesn't Demand More Impartial Research

When the Prescription Drug User Fee Act went into effect, its declared purpose was to speed the approval process of new drugs aimed at treating life–threatening or serious diseases. "Life threatening diseases" was the focus of AIDS activists. But it was drug manufacturers who lobbied to include "serious diseases" in the act. This could speed the approval of drugs for "diseases" not seen as particularly life–threatening, including mental diseases. In order to speed up the process, the FDA had to hire additional reviewers. Congress chose to allow drug manufacturers to pay for these new positions by requiring fees to be submitted with new drug approval applications. The fee in 2005 was over $625,000.[49]

One result of PDUFA has been to force a closer relationship between drug manufacturers and the FDA, the agency which regulates the drug manufacturers. Kathleen Holcombe, a drug industry lobbyist who has previously worked in government, understands how different the relationship is today than it once was. "There has been a huge shift. FDA historically had an approach of 'Regulate, be tough, enforce the law, don't let one thing go wrong.' But now," she added, "the FDA sees itself in a much more cooperative role."[50] Today, close personal friendships are commonly seen among the FDA scientists and the drug company scientists assigned to getting a company's new drug approved. Informal contact occurs daily, and formal meetings with drug company representatives occur over one thousand times a year.[51]

FDA scientists and occasionally FDA administrators admit to the pressure they feel to approve drugs and to do so quickly. Janet Woodcock who once was the director of the FDA's Center for Drug Evaluation and Research (responsible for the approval of all new drugs) admitted her understanding of PDUFA was that "industry would pay fees to add to FDA's resources for reviewing new drug applications. In exchange, FDA made a commitment to meet certain goals for review times."[52] Her understanding is right. That's the way it works. But human nature is such that when a neighbor invites us over for a meal, we aren't apt to leave until we say, "Well, we will be sure and have you over soon." FDA scientists know who pays for their meals. That was evident when Dr. Woodcock noted the discomfort she feels when she considers rejecting a company's drug. As she noted, it might mean an immediate loss of $150 million or more in development costs.[53] Of course, $150 million is nothing compared to the potential loss to the industry that could result if the FDA declared antidepressants and antipsychotics unsafe.

The FDA and Mind Drugs

During 2005 the FDA testified before Congress about the creation of a new and independent Drug Safety Oversight Board (DSOB) "to oversee the management of drug safety issues."[54] The testimony stated that the new DSOB "will enhance the independence of internal deliberations and decisions regarding risk/benefit analyses and consumer safety."[55] The goals for the DSOB are commendable and needed, but I can assure you the new board will not look at how the antidepressant drug studies are designed (Chapter 7, Tricks of the Trade), the actual effectiveness of antidepressants (Chapter 8, Do Antidepressants Work?) or the side effects of these drugs (Chapters 10, 11 & 13). The controversy and costs would be too great.

At risk would be drug industry jobs, lawsuits against drug companies and physicians who have encouraged their use, and the anger of millions who genuinely believe they could not survive without their antidepressant. America has been thoroughly fooled, and pronouncements from the FDA could stir up a hornet's nest. Then add in the fact that many FDA jobs would be lost if the pharmaceutical industry seriously stumbled. The FDA expects to collect $260 million in PDUFA user fees in 2007.[56] That's an impressive number considering the FDA only spent $187 million in 2000 to run their Center for Drug Evaluation and Research (again, the department which approves new drugs).[57] With the increase in fees from the drug companies, the FDA plans to add 376 new drug review employees by 2007.[58] That many new employees should allow greater care to be given to examining new drug applications and considering important benefit–risk issues, but it will not likely make the agency more independent. The sense of obligation (although perhaps unconscious) will likely grow.

Changes May Be Coming

I discussed in the Tricks of the Trade chapter the lawsuit Eliot Spitzer brought against GlaxoSmithKline for hiding the results of studies which found their antidepressant to be associated with suicide. I did not mention that Mr. Spitzer was not just upset with GlaxoSmithKline. "Where has the FDA been all these years when clinical data has been hidden from public scrutiny? They have simply failed to confront the problem."[59]

It is truly remarkable what media attention can accomplish. As the media announced Spitzer's intention to sue other drug companies unless they provided public access to all clinical trials, the American Medical Association added its voice to the call for a public database of trial results.[60] Later that month the Association of American Medical Colleges voted to support a federal registry for all new clinical trials.[61]

Next came an announcement from the International Committee of Medical Journal Editors, an association of some of the most important medical journals in the world—*JAMA, New England Journal of Medicine,*

Lancet, Canadian Medical Association Journal and *Annals of Internal Medicine* among others. They announced that after July 1, 2005, only studies which have been registered would be considered for publication.[62] The World Health Organization also jumped on the bandwagon.[63] The deputy editor of *JAMA*,[64] a long–time proponent of registering trials, entitled his *JAMA* commentary, "Trial registration: A great idea switches from ignored to irresistible."[65] Congress decided it, too, should do something as a bill was introduced which could conceivably pass into law in 2006 or 2007, the Fair Access to Clinical Trials (FACT) Act.[66] I am delighted that the need for changing this aspect of the system has finally been recognized and accepted. If all trials (not just those with pro–drug outcomes) are registered, it will mean a harmful drug side effect will not be hidden away, a practice that for a single class of drugs once cost up to 75,000 American lives (25 times as many as died on 9/11)—our worst medical disaster ever.[67]

But I am also realistic. The journal editors and the World Health Organization's efforts are praiseworthy, but unless the FACT Act becomes law and is *enforced*[68] (see endnote comment), the changes will be inadequate.

The Unique Problem of Evaluating Mind Drugs

Now let's return to the FDA and the drug approval process, and let's imagine that every clinical trial was registered, that drug manufacturers did not provide any of the funding for FDA employees' salaries and did not give grants, honoraria and consulting fees to any of those sitting on FDA advisory panels. Could the FDA then make wholly objective judgments about the drugs they are asked to approve? The FDA and its expert committees make their decisions based primarily on the results of the research they examine. Consequently, the answer would be a resounding "no" until the drug manufacturers are no longer allowed to design the clinical studies.[69] Cutting doses in half (to reduce adverse events) or doubling doses (to achieve a measurable effect) and all the other tricks of the trade (Chapter 7) would never occur if the studies were designed by truly independent researchers.

Nowhere is drug research more susceptible to manipulation than in the area of mental health. Is our patient over his or her schizophrenia or just drugged up? Is our patient depressed or just blue? I have already emphasized that depression is so subjective that determining its severity and relative change from hour to hour, day to day, or week to week is a unique problem. It is not like the falciperum malaria discussed in Chapter 2. We could ask 100 labs if I had malaria, and all would have said "Yes." Ask 100 doctors if person "A" has depression, and you will not have agreement. Even for a mental problem like schizophrenia which should be easier to diagnose accurately (if they hear voices no one else hears or think they own France, it should not be too hard to determine what the diagnosis should be), we may not get it right 100% of the time like we would with malaria, but we should not miss too often.

Yet a famous study found incredible disagreement even here. The researchers showed some film footage of a 30–year–old bachelor who was moody and asked both U.S. and British psychiatrists for a diagnosis. Surprisingly, 69% of the U.S. psychiatrists diagnosed him as schizophrenic. Only 2% of British psychiatrists did so.[70] That is an older study, and today I am sure agreement would be much higher since we now use a checklist (which was developed because diagnosing mental problems was so inconsistent). But the point remains that measuring mental problems presents unique dilemmas. Without independent researchers designing clinical trials the FDA and its experts can continue to be fooled.

The Most Fundamental Flaw in the System—Efficacy

The FDA's mission statement reads, "The FDA is responsible for protecting the public health by assuring the safety, efficacy, and security" of drugs."[71] "Security" refers to the fact that drugs must contain the ingredients listed on the drug label. It is also a reference to the FDA's responsibility to be sure that drugs are not marketed out of someone's garage laboratory. The middle word "efficacy" in the FDA mission statement simply means effectiveness. All FDA–approved drugs are supposed to be effective, but I believe the most amazing fact of all when it comes to drug approval is this: to receive FDA approval, new drugs do not really have to work; they only need to be more effective than a placebo. That is not a contradiction.

BOX #9–2

What Gets Published?

Hans Melander and his colleagues published an article in the *British Medical Journal* entitled "Evidence Biased Medicine" (in contrast with "evidence based medicine").[1] Examining studies sponsored by drug companies and submitted to the Swedish government's "FDA," they discovered that drug companies can greatly influence our perceptions by

(1) publishing those studies with positive drug outcomes more than those with less positive drug outcomes,
(2) publishing positive outcome studies repeatedly in different journals and
(3) reporting their drug's more favorable aspects.

Such a biased handling of drug study results gives a distorted view of a drug's effectiveness and safety. Unfortunately, this study was typical of drug studies paid for by pharmaceutical companies. Many high quality evaluations of even the best research design for drug testing in humans (randomized, placebo–controlled trials) have found strong publication bias and more positive results when the study is paid for by a drug company.[2-10] In other words, (1) even RCTs can be manipulated and (2) studies that do not find that a drug has benefits may never get submitted for publication. The end result is a distortion in the research literature which favors drugs.

When the FDA votes to accept or reject a new drug, the most influential factor in making their decision is the published research. (They supposedly have access to all clinical trials, but published research still has significant influence. Amazingly, one analysis found only 1 of 37 clinical trials was ever published.[11]) You can see why the FDA's decisions must sometimes be reversed by means of national drug recalls.

If you now understand that any drug which has side effects is likely to be more effective than a placebo at treating depression, then you understand that this is a worthless standard. I could treat depressed patients with cancer–fighting drugs, blood pressure drugs or common antihistamines, and any of them would also work better than a placebo because they all have side effects. None of these actually works to cure depression but, because they have side effects, they will be "effective" compared with a no–side–effect–producing placebo.

This is exactly the standard that allowed Prozac, the first SSRI, to receive approval. In *The Creation of Psychopharmacology* David Healy gives the history of Prozac's development and notes that Prozac "could not be shown to be beneficial in treating patients hospitalized for depression . . . and indeed has never since . . . been shown to work."[72] In reality Tofranil (imipramine), with which it was compared, outperformed Prozac.[73] But the set of rules that guides the FDA does not care if there are better drugs. Drugs are never compared to the best drug available. That would be ideal, but that would mean many hugely profitable drugs would never have been approved. If we used that standard, the bar for getting a new drug approved would become "*How* effective is it?" not "Is it effective?" That is a night and day difference.

If that were the standard, we would have far fewer drugs available to treat arthritis and high blood pressure and the many other ills for which there are numerous "equivalent" drugs. By using the "better than placebo" standard, Prozac entered the market. After all, though it has minimal benefit for depression, Prozac does indeed have significant side effects, one of which is agitation. That side effect, in fact, is what prompted Eli Lilly researchers to give the subjects in the clinical trials a benzodiazepine tranquilizer at the same time they received Prozac.[74] How could the FDA know which drug was overcoming depression if those getting Prozac were also getting a tranquilizer? Such was the state of drug approval when the first SSRI was introduced to America.

Matching Antidepressants with Other Subjective "Diseases" to Increase Sales

When a more objective measure of change is used (white blood cell count, the presence or absence of parasites in the blood, or the increase or decrease in oral staph), the placebo cannot match the real drug over time. But depression is subjectively measured. (The Hamilton Rating Scale for Depression is the most commonly used measure of depression for drug studies, but it has been found to yield what appear to be very invalid scores.[75]) So researchers willing to deceive can "prove" that Prozac can cure depression—and all kinds of other subjectively measured mental "diseases."

Eli Lilly thus got FDA approval to add Obsessive–Compulsive Disorder (OCD) to Prozac's label after completing clinical trials that "proved" it could help solve that problem. Two years later they received approval to list bulimia. Next came approval to list geriatric depression. That was 1999. Prozac was nearing the end of its patent protection. Whenever this happens, drug companies seek to alter the ingredient in a minor way. It must be advertised as "new and improved" or "the same as but with better tolerance," and the revision will start receiving all the new advertising dollars. Sometimes changing the ingredients is not even necessary to create a new market or stimulate additional sales.

When Prozac went off patent in 2001, Lilly simply renamed it, changed its color (pink and purple) and began marketing it for treating Premenstrual Dysphoric Disorder.[76] (See Box #9–3 for definitions for these diseases.) How can the same drug change the various chemical imbalances that are supposedly responsible for depression, Obsessive–Compulsive Disorder, bulimia, geriatric depression and Premenstrual Dysphoric Disorder? It can't. Can Americans be fooled into believing such nonsense? They can. Billions of dollars in sales prove that they have been.

What Does the FDA Mean by "Safety"?

The FDA's mission statement reads as follows:

BOX #9-3

The "Diseases" Which Prozac is
FDA–Approved to Help Cure

Obsessive–Compulsive Disorder: Being unable to stop continuous, anxious thoughts (fear of germs, being harmed or losing control being commonly reported) and/or engaging in repetitious, abnormal behaviors (commonly handwashing, checking door locks, counting or hoarding).

Bulimia: Repeatedly engaging in binge eating followed by vomiting, fasting, the use of laxatives, enemas or some other means of food removal or weight control so binge eating can continue without weight gain.

Geriatric Depression: Depression in patients age 65 and older.[1]

Premenstrual Dysphoric Disorder: A disorder which typically emerges monthly for about a week prior to the menstrual period involving depression, anxiety, tension and disinterest in normal activities.

Personal Note: I acknowledge that individuals manifest the symptoms associated with each "disease," but I do not agree that any of these meet a traditional definition of "disease" or that any of these is caused by a chemical imbalance in the brain.

The FDA is responsible for protecting the public health by assuring the safety, efficacy, and security of human and veterinary drugs, biological products, medical devices, our nation's food supply, cosmetics, and products that emit radiation. The FDA is also responsible for advancing the public health by helping to speed innovations that make medicines and foods more effective, safer, and more affordable; and helping the public get the accurate science–based information they need to use medicines and foods to improve their health.[77]

I have no criticism of that statement. The words are excellent. The goals are excellent. But, realistically, the FDA falls far short in their supervision of mind drugs. The first task the FDA mission statement demands of the agency is to protect the public's safety. Yet there is a judgment call here.

The agency recognizes that all drugs carry some risks. Therefore, a risk–benefits analysis is used to determine if a drug can justifiably be marketed to the public. But if a drug's "efficacy" is no greater than a placebo, the risk–benefits analysis would demand that the drug not have harmful side effects. That reasoning should have kept antidepressants from ever getting approved since the benefits are marginal at best while the potential harm is real. The "risk" of the equation will be discussed in the next chapter.

10

"Man is becoming the primary guinea pig."[1]
— *Dr. Ross Baldessarini*
Psychopharmacologist
Harvard Medical School

PHYSICAL SIDE EFFECTS OF ANTIDEPRESSANTS

Following a lecture on the uncontrollable muscle movement which results from taking some mind drugs, June approached me about her mother. "Could long–term stimulant use also cause dyskinesias?" I did not know, but as June told me more, I became suspicious. I had known June's mother for at least a decade longer than I had known June. We attended the same church, and I had often witnessed the spurts of severe shaking that emerged every few minutes. But I was unaware that she had been on Ritalin and had been on it for over 30 years to control her tendency to fall asleep in the middle of the day. I decided to call Carolyn, June's mother, and learn more.

211

". . . And are you still on it, Carolyn?"

"No, I got off it a little over a year ago because my liver had been damaged by taking it for so long."

"What was your daily dosage?"

"When I started, I took between 8 and 10 20–mg pills a day." [Note: Ritalin comes in 5–mg, 10–mg and 20–mg tablets. The manufacturer states that taking more than 60 mg per day "is not recommended."[2]]

"Weren't you concerned about the dosage being so high?"

"That's what the neurologist put me on, and it was better than sleeping all the time. But when my local doctor learned how much I was on, he jumped up from his chair. He said he had taken half of a 10–mg tablet once while in medical school so he could stay awake and study for an important exam, but then he couldn't go to sleep for 24 hours."

"Has anyone ever suggested that the Ritalin may be responsible for your muscle spasms?"

"Oh, no. No one thinks it is something caused by the Ritalin. I even researched that myself, and it's not."

Carolyn and every doctor she ever consulted could not be more wrong. As soon as I got off the phone, I opened my *PDR* and there, under Ritalin, I saw "dyskinesia" as a potential side effect. I went to Medline and quickly found numerous studies which confirmed this. Large dosages[3] and long–term use[4] are especially significant risk factors. One case report of a Ritalin–induced movement disorder involved an elderly man with Parkinson's disease who, when given only two 2.5–mg doses of Ritalin, developed uncontrollable muscle movements.[5] Carolyn took 40 times that amount each day. Carolyn will live with her dyskinesia the rest of her life. There is no cure. But this should never have occurred. Even in the 1970s when Carolyn was first prescribed Ritalin several studies had already linked high doses of amphetamines to dyskinesias.[6]

There are two messages I hope you will reap from Carolyn's experience. First, there is too little awareness and concern about adverse drug effects among physicians. Today many physicians freely prescribe Ritalin or other stimulants without any awareness that 7.8% of children given them will develop tics, including those on low doses,[7] or that a smaller number will develop other movement disorders.[8] Second, I want you to recognize how little we know about long–term exposure to Ritalin or to antidepressants. Carolyn is the only person I know with over 30 years of stimulant exposure. No one in our world today has had that many years of SSRI–antidepressant exposure because the drugs only came to market in 1987. But if you are even a relatively long–term user, you are a guinea pig. That is not to say that we are unaware of harmful effects today. There is enough published research for you to make very informed decisions. Unfortunately, that research is in the medical journals where few in the public ever see it. That probably does not surprise you. What should surprise you is what that same medical research has found concerning how little those writing antidepressant prescriptions know about these drugs and their side effects.

What Do Doctors Really Know?

General practice physicians have very inadequate knowledge of antidepressant side effects.[9] Many physicians are unaware of antidepressant withdrawal effects.[10] Many feel uncertain that they are even prescribing the right mind drugs.[11] If the prescribed antidepressant causes unpleasant side effects, most psychiatrists simply experiment with another antidepressant.[12] Off–label antidepressant prescriptions (writing prescriptions for non–FDA approved reasons) is a common practice including off–label prescriptions for pregnant and breastfeeding women.[13] However, if the depressed patient does not have health insurance, the chances of receiving an antidepressant prescription drop dramatically.[14] As one psychiatrist pointed out, such haphazard treatment of patients is not tolerated in any other field of medicine.[15]

This is a situation that must change as it undoubtedly contributes to the casual overprescribing of antidepressants.[16] Of course, if antidepressants were not expensive or had no side effects, this would not matter greatly, but neither is true. The adverse side effects of antidepressants include movement disorders, agitation, sexual dysfunction, improper bone development, esophagus and stomach bleeding, and a host of other even lesser known problems. These are not rare events, but most real harm comes only after months or years of use, a fact which can lead to the false impression that antidepressants seem quite safe. "I've been on antidepressants for several years now, and I can't tell that they have hurt me" is sometimes voiced as I begin sharing the research. The same objection could be expressed even if we put all women on thalidomide, the drug that led to thousands of babies being born without ears, arms, hands or legs. Many drugs that are very dangerous cause no apparent harm unless taken long term or in combination with another drug or by someone with special circumstances. (In the case of thalidomide, the special circumstance was pregnancy.)

More than half of those beginning an antidepressant (whether an older tricyclic antidepressant or a newer SSRI antidepressant) have one of the more common side effects.[17] Examining the most popular antidepressant ever sold (Prozac) and what is currently the most popular antidepressant (Zoloft), we can get some idea about how often these mind drugs affect both the mind and the body.

Movement Disorders

My single greatest concern related to antidepressant use is brain damage that may result in parkinsonism, tardive dyskinesia and other movement disorders. The incidence of these adverse side effects is much lower with antidepressant use than with the use of antipsychotics, and they are not apt to show up as quickly. This contributes to a limited literature and may give a false sense of safety. In fact, my impression, based on my never having had a single student or client indicate that they were told about these risks, is that physicians are unaware that antidepressants (tricyclic, SSRI and SSNRI types) can cause movement disorders. Nevertheless, the risks are real,[18] though as with antipsychotics, the risk is greater in older people. (See Box #10–1, A Window Into the Future?)

I want you to know why I believe we will some day see large numbers of former antidepressant users developing movement disorders, but I first want to remind you of the conclusion which must be reached by examining the best of the double–blind studies on the effectiveness of antidepressants. That conclusion is simply that antidepressants do work, but they do not work any better (or just barely better in some studies) than a sugar pill placebo (see Chapter 8).

BOX #10–1

A Window Into the Future?

Zoloft is considered one of the better antidepressant choices for those who want to reduce the risk of developing the jerking and twitching symptoms of parkinsonism. However the research literature has many cases that should give us pause. For example, a woman in Spain who was on Zoloft developed parkinsonism after long–term treatment with the drug. The involuntary movements finally went away three months after she stopped taking the drug. Nevertheless her brain had been damaged. Though she stayed off Zoloft and other antidepressants, the jerking and twitching suddenly began again 14 months later—movements that will not likely ever go away again without additional medication.[1]

The fact that this woman was older means she was more likely to develop these symptoms than would a child or a young adult. But we have no longitudinal research that would assure us that years of antidepressant use early in life will not lead to movement disorders in old age.

The point that must be emphasized, though it may seem it should be obvious, is that if serious health risks are being accepted, major health benefits should be expected. Sometimes trade–offs have to be made. In 2005 *JAMA* reported that those on the heart drug Natrecor (nesiritide) were 80%

more likely to die during their first 30 days on the drug.[19] Yet, the drug (used for acute decompensated heart failure) *reportedly* brings so much comfort to patients struggling with shortness of breath that accepting an increased risk of sudden death *may* not be unreasonable. But the trade–off being made with antidepressants is unfair to patients. Most believe they are getting real help in the form of a pill, and most have never heard what health consequences may result.

If you examine the PI (package insert) for Prozac or Zoloft, you will not find "parkinsonism" or "tardive dyskinesia" included in the tables which list adverse events. However, you will find the term "tremor." In the case of Prozac you can see that the trials Eli Lilly conducted (and reported to the FDA to get their drug approved) examined Prozac's effects compared with a placebo for 5 or 6 weeks.[20] In only 5 or 6 weeks 10% of those put on Prozac developed tremors.[21] For Zoloft which used 6 and 8 week trials, 11% of those taking the drug developed tremors.[22] That concerns me.

It concerns me that when the Department of Biochemistry, Molecular Pharmacology and Anesthesiology at the Jefferson Medical College subjected the brains of rats to various antidepressants (including Prozac and Zoloft), they found it resulted in brain cells that were shriveled and twisted in five different regions of the brain.[23] We cannot subject humans to these same experiments, but there is no reason to believe these drugs are not damaging human brain cells as well. The doses given the rats were higher than recommended for humans, but the damage occurred after only four days on these drugs!

It concerns me that Parkinson's patients who take an antidepressant immediately develop more severe symptoms.[24] When those patients stop taking the antidepressant, the tremors and other Parkinson's disease symptoms also diminish. And it is, at least, suggestive that Parkinson's disease causes brain shrinkage,[25] and brain shrinkage also occurs in those on antidepressants.[26] Someone who is knowledgeable might object to these suggestions and point out that Parkinson's disease is associated with a loss of dopamine in the striatum part of the brain and that antidepressants are supposed to alter serotonin levels, not dopamine levels. They would be right. Antidepressants are only supposed to impact serotonin (and noradrenaline in the case of SSNRIs). However, what is supposed to happen and what actually occurs are two very different matters. Rat experiments have now proven that antidepressants do impact dopamine levels also.[27] (See Box #2–1, Is It Possible To Measure Serotonin and Dopamine Levels Or Not?)

Objection and Response

An objection to my concern is sometimes voiced. "But millions of people have been taking antidepressants for years." I have three responses. First, we have many cases of drugs being pulled from the market after years of use by millions of people. Think of Pondimin, discussed previously, which was approved for use in 1973 and was taken by millions despite the fact that Pondimin damages heart valves and can cause a life–threatening pulmonary disorder. Yet the drug stayed on the market until 1997. Other examples include Rezulin, Propulsid, Seldane, Hismanal and Posicor.

Second, tardive dyskinesia is unique. The very name means that symptoms are not supposed to show up until long after the damage begins. ("Tardive" is related to the word "tardy.")

Third, the law requires that drug companies conduct what are known as Phase 4 studies after their drugs come to market. These studies are required because the Phase 1 and Phase 2 studies required for receiving FDA approval are very short studies (4 to 8 weeks generally) and use very small numbers of people (20 to 80 individuals are typical).[28] Phase 3 studies (which involve giving the drug to a group of physicians who will prescribe it to their patients and then notify the drug manufacturer of any adverse events) still involve relatively short periods of time and only several hundred to near three thousand patients.

But once the drug is released to the entire nation, it may be taken by millions of people and be taken by many patients for years. Some kind of monitoring system is obviously needed after the drug is released, and this is the purpose of Phase 4 studies. Drug manufacturers are required to send Phase 4 reports to the FDA every three months for a year after a drug is released. Two reports must be submitted during the second year, and after the second year annual reports are required.[29] It is a good system, but there is a problem. Drug companies are not obeying the law, and the FDA claims it lacks the ability to enforce the law.

When this defiance made headlines for a short time in 2004, many astonishing facts were uncovered, including the fact that Forest Laboratories which manufactures the antidepressant Celexa had never submitted any Phase 4 studies information.[30] It was also reported that though for–profit drug companies fund over 80% of all drug trials, only 13% of all listed trials were submitted by for–profit companies.[31] Most of those willing to obey the law were government agencies and non–profits.

This situation will not last forever.[32] But, until compliance with the law becomes the norm, how are we to know about adverse drug effects that may not develop for years after drug exposure? We may not have any clear indication of how many antidepressant users will develop movement disorders for years.

Breast Cancer

Do antidepressants cause breast cancer? Here is another example of an issue about which we must not be dogmatic. The research is too contradictory. For example, Paxil has been reported to be associated with a breast cancer risk that is 7.2 times the "no use" risk, and use of tricyclic medication (such as amitriptyline) for two or more years more than doubles the risk.[33] But some studies find only a modest risk when various statistical adjustments are made for other factors associated with breast cancer.[34] And yet other research finds that, with adjustments for all these other risk factors, virtually all the antidepressant–breast cancer risk is either not significant or eliminated.[35]

What should a woman conclude? I think it is reasonable to assume that the risk is not great. However, this is where doing animal studies makes great sense. We can do experiments on animals which would not be possible on humans, and it is possible to control variables that may contribute to cancer risk in them, unlike human experiments. Many animal studies have found an antidepressant–cancer link.[36] Add to that the fact that we have little long–term research, and an argument for caution becomes necessary.

Sexual Dysfunction

Sexual dysfunction may impact a larger percentage of antidepressant users than any other symptom. Though the packaging inserts for Prozac and Zoloft report only 2% and 7% of those taking these drugs developing sexual problems, respectively, independent studies suggest much, much higher rates of problems.[37] A review of the research that included several randomized, controlled trials (the ideal design for investigating this subject) found that among those taking SSRI antidepressants (which include Prozac and Zoloft), between 30% and 60% experienced sexual dysfunction.[38]

I have no idea how Eli Lilly and Pfizer came up with such minimal numbers when every study I have read points to dramatic effects for large numbers of both men and women. (Actually, I do have some idea how they managed this since I understand some of the clinical trial tricks commonly used.[39]) What treatment options are available? One review of the research concluded that "few proposed treatment options, apart from avoidance, have proved effective for antidepressant–associated sexual dysfunction."[40] And the problem rarely improves on its own.[41] How many people who are given an antidepressant prescription are aware of this side effect before they take their first pill?

Esophageal and Stomach Bleeding

SSRI antidepressants have been found to cause upper gastrointestinal tract bleeding in many studies. The odds of developing this problem are over three times as high in SSRI users as non–users. The really significant increase, though, involves being on an anti–inflammatory drug as well, like aspirin, ibuprofen (Advil, Motrin, etc.), naproxen (Aleve) and celecoxib (Celebrex). This raises the chance of bleeding by a factor of over 15—much more than the SSRI or the anti–inflammatory drugs would by themselves.[42]

Many years ago my father almost died as a result of taking naproxen. Naproxen is still commonly given to those with arthritis, but a frequent side effect is an ulcer leading to internal bleeding. The occurrence of this side effect is so common that many physicians use the phrase "naproxen–induced ulcer."[43] That experience keeps him from taking aspirin which is really very similar to naproxen. (Both help control pain, but both can also cause ulcers and internal bleeding.)

Heart Attacks

It is commonly known, thanks to TV and magazine ads, that small doses of aspirin can actually help prevent heart attacks. Since SSRI antidepressants also thin one's blood, we should expect that, in addition to causing internal bleeding, SSRIs should lower the incidence of heart attacks, and this benefit has been reported.[44]

SSRI antidepressants are very different than the older tricyclic antidepressants. Today, partly because of concerns about SSRI side effects, some physicians are writing prescriptions for the tricyclics. However, they carry several risks of their own, one of which being a doubling of the risk of having a heart attack.[45]

However, the largest study ever conducted on this concern came to a very different conclusion. Looking at over 60,000 cases of myocardial infarction (heart attacks) and 360,000 randomly chosen matched controls, it was found that both the older tricyclics and the newer SSRIs could result in sudden death—even within days of starting an antidepressant.[46] For example, more than 2½ times as many patients taking Prozac had a first acute heart attack during the first seven days on the drug than did the matched controls.

Was this increased risk purely a drug effect, or was the stress of depression the primary culprit? I don't know, and I believe it may be several years before we are certain. For now, it is best to emphasize again that all drugs carry risks and with human research, unlike animal experiments, the variables are so many that we often arrive at very contradictory conclusions. When this occurs, we need to emphasize that if good alternatives are available (and they are in the case of depression), it is wise to avoid the drug.

Dental Cavities

There have been published reports of patients with excessive dental cavities related to antidepressant use for many years. In 1981 a Dutch article stated the case succinctly in its title "Antidepressive agents can cause dental damage in children and adults."[47] Because antidepressants cause the mouth to produce less saliva (xerostomia), the bacteria that cause tooth decay are not removed as well as needed. The result is that a higher number of dental patients are antidepressant users (21%) than is found in the general population.[48] (Of course, as always, we find it is possible to challenge the cause and effect assumption. For example, we could ask if depressed people are less likely to brush their teeth.) And we know that depression itself can reduce saliva production.[49] Nevertheless, the close proximity in time of antidepressant initiation and the high rate of tissue damage in the mouth (72% in 12 months or less) and new dental decay (55% in 12 months or less)[50] points to another harmful effect.

Children's Vulnerability to Proper Bone Development

Bones of mice exposed to antidepressants are narrower, have less bone mass and even have inferior mechanical characteristics.[51] The implications are most serious. Will children exposed to antidepressants today have skeletal problems and frequent bone fractures as they age? No research will exist for many years that will be able to document what the impact is.

Children's Vulnerability to Proper Brain Development

"The use of SSRI medications in pregnant mothers and young children may pose unsuspected risks of emotional disorders later in life."[52] That was the conclusion of a research team headed by Dr. Mark Ansorge at the Columbia University College of Physicians and Surgeons. The researchers gave newborn rats doses of Prozac comparable to what humans take or saline (salt water) which has no brain damaging effects for rats or humans. Nine weeks later they measured the willingness of these rats to explore their environments, to take risks to earn food and to quickly leave their environment when it was made unpleasant. What they found was frightening. Rats injected with saline handled the stressful environments as would be expected. However, rats given Prozac had apparently suffered abnormal brain development that caused them to become anxious and unable to properly respond to the experimental tests.

I am unfamiliar with anyone prescribing Prozac to preschoolers; however, the studies which have measured use by preschoolers have found that this is the group among whom we have seen the greatest increase in antidepressant use. The rate is still a small fraction of the rate for children over 5, with only 3.7 preschoolers per thousand on antidepressants.[53] But calculate that by the number of preschoolers in America, and we can assume that there are over 70,000 children under 5 who are having their developing brains harmed. (See Box #10–2, What Upsets Me.)

The Columbia University study is not alone in suggesting that we are doing irreparable harm to children with antidepressants. A subsequent study that came out of the laboratories of the National Institutes of Health began, "There is growing evidence that serotonin has major influences on brain development in mammals."[54] The NIH researchers performed a simple whisker stimulation procedure on the mice and measured their cerebral responses. It was a highly sophisticated experiment that boils down to one simple truth. Serotonin exposure in young mice impairs their brain's cerebral development. Again, there is no reason to assume the same would not occur in developing children.

One other point: brain development does not stop at age 5 as once believed. Today we know from both human and animal studies that the nervous system is rapidly growing from conception through pre–adulthood.[55] If the brain is changed during childhood or adolescence, antidepressant use may have results we have never considered and still won't realize for many years.

BOX #10–2

What Upsets Me

Prozac is approved by the FDA for use by children **age 8 and over**. So why is it being prescribed to preschoolers—and very large numbers of children ages 5–8? That upsets me. And why are many other antidepressants being prescribed to children when Prozac is the only FDA–approved antidepressant for children? That upsets me.

Anyone who prescribes drugs must be somewhat familiar with the fact that it typically takes several years before some of the drug's effects are discovered. They must also know that a developing child is more vulnerable than an adult. So why would anyone prescribe an antidepressant to a preschooler?

Children's Vulnerability to Other Health Effects

Most preterm and small–for–date babies will do fine. Yet, both of these are risk factors for many negative health effects. Therefore, our goal is always a full–term, full–weight baby. Unfortunately, babies who have been exposed to antidepressants before birth are at increased risk of premature birth, lower birth weight and a lower Apgar score, a measure of a newborn's health.[56] As would be expected, babies exposed to antidepressants before birth are between 62% and 121% more likely to experience respiratory distress, convulsions and hypoglycemia.[57] Subtle effects on newborns' motor development and motor control are also recognized today.[58] What additional health effects will impact the child as he or she grows? We simply will not know for many years. We know there is some small risk for liver damage for adults who have long–term exposure to antidepressants.[59] But there has never been even one study that has examined the long–term exposure effects on the liver for those who began taking antidepressants as children. You can see why I have concerns about not just what we know, but also about what we do not know.

Other Concerns

I have not discussed insomnia which is one of the more commonly reported adverse effects for many mind drugs.[60] I have not discussed akathisia which is one of the antidepressant side–effects that is the greatest concern for some psychiatrists.[61] I have not discussed problems with weight gain which is the complaint that has proved the most disturbing for many of my students.[62] Space does not allow for a discussion of all the antidepressant side effects or even a full discussion of those I have covered. That's okay. My real goal is to make you aware that these drugs carry real risks. Those risks should be known by patients before they ever take their first pill. That only rarely occurs.

11

"Adults being treated with antidepressant medications, particularly those being treated for depression, should be watched closely for worsening of depression and for increased suicidal thinking or behavior. Close watching may be especially important early in treatment, or when the dose is changed, either increased or decreased."[1]
— *FDA Public Health Advisory*
June 20, 2005

PSYCHOLOGICAL SIDE EFFECTS OF ANTIDEPRESSANTS

Debbie grew up in a traditional Mennonite home. Her life, even in her youngest days, involved daily prayers, listening to her father read from the Bible and helping prepare meals for her dairy farming family. There was no television or radio in the home, and vulgarities and lewd comments were never heard. During adolescence, following her baptism, she began wearing a head covering which, along with the modest homemade clothing and the absence of jewelry, lipstick or fashionable hairdos, helped make her easily recognizable as a member of the Mennonite church.

At 21 the shy and quiet Debbie was approached by one of the very quiet Mennonite men in her congregation about marriage. It was discussed by the families and, with their approval, they were soon married. When the wedding ceremony was over, the couple headed to St. Louis. Her husband John opened the door to their hotel room and immediately turned on the television. That was a startling surprise, but it would not be the last. The next came when he got angry over nothing. This was a side of her new husband she had not seen before. And when he seemed to have little interest in spiritual discussions, Debbie began to wonder if she had made a huge mistake.

Then came John's experiment. John had a fascination with psychology and had read a number of psychology books. And now he had a subject he could analyze. "What is your earliest memory?" "Did you feel competition with your mother when you were young?" "What kind of conflicts did you have?" When Debbie expressed her unhappiness, John had done enough reading to know the answer immediately. "You just need some Prozac."

Debbie knew she did not need Prozac, but she also wanted to please her husband. So only two months after her marriage began, she went to her local doctor, asked for Prozac and began the experiment with antidepressants. What occurred next must have shocked her hometown as much as it scandalized her church. Debbie went into the local corner store and purchased a six pack of beer and a *Playgirl* magazine. She had never tasted beer before, but she went home and consumed two cans while she looked at the *Playgirl*. She still finds it hard to believe. She did it. She knows she did it, but nothing could be more out of character.

I made notes as she shared that experience with me again. I recorded her saying, "I felt like I was floating. I just didn't care." Then she added with genuine embarrassment, "Can you imagine what the people at the Quick Stop thought when they saw me, this Mennonite woman with a head covering, buying beer and a *Playgirl* magazine?"

The Blunting Effect

Debbie's experience illustrates what I call the blunting effect. Antidepressants cannot cause a depressed person suddenly to become happy any more than alcohol can do so, but, just like alcohol, they do impact the mind. Either one of those drugs could cause a blunting effect. In studies conducted by the manufacturer of Remeron and submitted to the FDA it was reported that in six–week clinical trials over half (54%) of those taking Remeron had a problem with sleepiness. Unlike alcohol, Remeron is not a depressant. (Supposedly it is an antidepressant.) So why do most patients on this drug report a desire to sleep? That is the blunting effect. Seventeen percent of Remeron users reported an increased appetite—over eight times the rate of those on a placebo. Interesting, since most users feel sleepy. High energy activity should increase appetite, but low energy activity (like sleeping) should decrease it.

This is more evidence of the blunting effect. If we "just don't care," we won't control our eating as well and will likely eat more, and then report an increased appetite. The manufacturer's own study reports that 4% of users report abnormal dreams and 3% report abnormal thinking. Other nervous system effects which occurred *frequently* included apathy (the blunting effect) and agitation.[2] Again, these effects are those reported to the FDA by the maker of this antidepressant. And the results would have been even worse for Remeron except that 16% of those taking the drug dropped out of the study because of adverse experiences and are not included in the final analysis.

Similar statistics have been reported for all the major antidepressants—Zoloft, Luvox, Effexor, Paxil, Celexa, Lexapro, Wellbutrin—and even the one antidepressant the British still allow to be prescribed to children—Prozac. Take out the packaging insert for Prozac and, if you can read the fine print, you will learn that while on Prozac 16% of depressed subjects experienced insomnia, 12% experienced anxiety and 14% reported feeling nervous. How did a drug with those numbers become known as the happy pill? But read on.

When you get to the nervous system effects, it becomes apparent that we should not be surprised when a client or friend taking these drugs reports a bizarre experience. I have heard story after story from students and clients who were on these drugs which convince me that, though most of those on an antidepressant never have a bizarre experience, they do occur. The nervous system effects which occur frequently (again, this is as reported by Eli Lilly, the maker of Prozac) include

(1) agitation (Definition: extreme emotional disturbance[3]),

(2) amnesia (Definition: partial or total loss of memory),

(3) confusion (Definition: impaired orientation with respect to time, place or person) and

(4) emotional lability (Definition: not listed in my dictionary, so I tried the *Webster's New World Medical Dictionary* and found it defined as "susceptible to change, error or instability." It comes from the Latin word *labilis* which means "prone to slip.")

There you have it from Eli Lilly themselves. Those who take their drug may experience an "extreme emotional disturbance," "partial or total loss of memory," and "emotional instability." And that's the safest of the antidepressants?

How can a drug blunt the emotions and inhibitions? To answer that question we need to understand the function of the frontal lobes. The answer to that question will also help us understand a condition known as "amotivational syndrome."

Amotivational Syndrome

Scientific reports of indifference, apathy and loss of initiative associated with antidepressant use have appeared in the research literature ever since Prozac, the first SSRI antidepressant, was initially approved. This extreme reaction to SSRI drugs is rare; yet it is common enough to have a name—amotivational syndrome.[4] The earlier reports involved only adults, but that was before widespread use of antidepressants by children became common.

Amotivational syndrome is also known as frontal lobe syndrome. The frontal lobes located just behind our foreheads hold within their cells our personality, more than any other part of the brain. People who have damaged frontal lobes may still score well on intelligence tests and may not experience memory loss, but they are likely to suffer dramatic changes in their personalities.

The classic case involved Phineas Gage, a 25–year–old railroad foreman who survived a most horrendous accident in 1848. Gage's crew was blasting rock to level the ground in preparation for new track. The crew would bore the rock, fill the hole with gunpowder, cover the gunpowder with sand, tamp it down with a tamping iron and then ignite the powder. One day as he was tamping the powder, the explosive ignited prematurely and the 3½ foot tamping rod shot up through Gage's left cheek, his frontal lobes, and out through the top of his head. Incredibly, Gage not only survived, but before the day was over he was walking and speaking. Yet the accident was not without serious consequences.

Gage's memory and intellectual abilities seemed unaffected, but Gage lost control of his emotions and his inhibitions to some degree. Though reported to have been a dependable and responsible foreman before the accident, Gage became dishonest, temperamental and antisocial. His friends declared he just was not the same person.

Antidepressants do not destroy the frontal lobes, but they do affect them. Two Canadian physicians sought to determine if the impact of Prozac and Paxil on the frontal lobes was influenced by dosage. What they discovered was that their subjects experienced the same disinhibitions, impulsiveness, apathy and poor concentration found in earlier studies, but they also found a relationship between the dosage given and the degree of personality and mental changes.[5]

How many of those taking these drugs are aware that the brain is physically changed by SSRIs? Those of us who read the scientific literature in this area are keenly aware, but I'm not sure I have ever had a student or client tell me they had heard this. I can understand the average person not reading *Neuropsychopharmacology* or *Brain Research*. Journal research is often difficult to understand. But how can we excuse the constant marketing of mind drugs with messages that do not warn of the permanent brain damage which can occur or of the dangerous psychological effects which sometimes occur? One of those effects, now widely known, is an increase in agitation.

Agitation

When Yale University's Department of Psychiatry decided to analyze the admissions to their hospital's psychiatric unit, they found that 8.1% of the patients "were found to have been admitted owing to antidepressant–associated mania or psychosis."[6] Effects which the average patient has never associated with antidepressants are common and were known by drug manufacturers long before their antidepressants were ever released to the public. "Agitation" is one of the most common antidepressant side effects, something Pfizer learned in the 1980s when they began testing their new unnamed drug (which eventually was called Zoloft) on their own employees. They provided female volunteers either their antidepressant Zoloft or a placebo. These employees were not seeking medical help. These were healthy, typical employees who simply volunteered to participate in an early trial of a new drug (though a substantial financial gift was likely provided each volunteer). None of the participants was told if he/she were taking the sugar pill or the real drug, but 25% of the Zoloft takers reported "agitation."[7] Agitation was so common with the SSRI antidepressants that it was an adverse event that manufacturers sought to hide. But how can an agitation effect be hidden? Think back to Chapter 7, Tricks of the Trade, and perhaps you can come up with an answer.

If all Prozac or Zoloft or other antidepressant takers were also given a tranquilizer (a sleeping pill), perhaps it would keep the agitation from emerging. But again I ask as I did in Chapter 7, would it be fair to mask one of the very real effects of a drug by giving the subjects in your drug study a tranquilizer? I can tell you that every time I have shared with my classes that this was, in fact, exactly what was done in some of the trials used to get

Prozac and other antidepressants approved, most of my students have found it shocking.

The facts about Prozac's clinical development are no longer secret. Because of lawsuits brought against Eli Lilly & Company, makers of Prozac, Lilly's company files were opened. Following a 1995 lawsuit,[8] one of those able to inspect the Lilly documents and data was Dr. David Healy, noted earlier in this book to be one of the world's foremost authorities on mind drugs. Dr. Healy's numerous articles on mind drugs, many published in leading medical journals, brought him to the attention of the law firm suing Lilly.

Securing Dr. Healy as an expert witness was extremely valuable. Healy is a licensed psychiatrist, but more importantly he is a brilliant researcher who holds the equivalent of both an MD and a PhD and has the training and background which make him highly qualified to analyze drug trial data and documents. Many of the documents and data that were found in Lilly's files were never allowed to be shown in court. (See the small portion of pre–trial rulings concerning what could be used in evidence.[9]) But sufficient internal documents were admitted as evidence to prove that Lilly had long known that their drug could have dramatic effects on a small percentage of users. The Lilly files from 1978 and 1979 when the earliest tests were being conducted substantiated concerns about agitation effects. The committee minutes of the Prozac project team included the following comment: "Some patients have converted from severe depression to agitation within a few days; in one case the agitation was marked and the patient had to be taken off [the] drug. *In future studies the use of benzodiazepines to control agitation will be permitted* [emphasis mine]."[10]

There it was in Lilly's own documents. Agitation was one of the effects of Prozac's use, and it was discovered by Lilly in even their earliest trials. It was sufficiently common that in future studies they felt it important to give all drug trial subjects on Prozac benzodiazepines—that is, tranquilizers.

Lilly won the lawsuit, but having to release their internal documents to Dr. Healy for his inspection made it a hollow victory.

Dr. Healy who had often prescribed Prozac became so concerned about the unknown dangers that he wrote a book detailing the trial experience, the dangers of antidepressants, and the industry's promotional tactics of these drugs.[11] He also created a website where the court documents can be seen by anyone.[12] Other documents that came to light during the trial revealed that Lilly purposely excluded those from the Prozac group who had risk factors for violence or suicide—the divorced, unemployed or retired, an alcohol abuser, a person with an arrest record—the very kind of factors that might be associated with increased violence. The result? Increases in violence associated with Prozac would be reduced in these studies. These were not honest, objective studies of Prozac. These studies were designed to get the best possible responses and have the fewest possible negative events.

Other minutes revealed that the committee seeking to develop Prozac as an antidepressant could never have dreamed their chemical would some day be so successfully marketed that it would eventually be seen as a true miracle drug. Their own minutes declared Prozac did not appear to help depression but did result in several adverse effects. (Remember as you read the following minutes that fluoxetine is the generic name for Prozac.)

> None of the eight patients who completed the four–week treatment showed distinct drug–induced improvement. . . . There have been a fairly large number of reports of adverse reactions. These have been varied, and their relationship to fluoxetine is not clearly established. The first depressed patient to receive fluoxetine showed dystonia resembling an extrapyramidal reaction . . . [meaning the patient experienced involuntary muscle movement which likely included twitching and twisting, which ceased during sleep]. Another reported enlarged thyroid and liver . . . . One patient developed psychosis manifested by paranoid delusions . . . [meaning

the patient had lost touch with reality and had an extremely irrational fear that others were seeking to harm him in some way]. Akathisia [ceaseless, agitated movement that can be unnerving] and restlessness were reported in some patients.[13]

Antidepressants and Suicide

Another document emerged from an earlier lawsuit[14] from the German's drug licensing agency, the BGA. It noted the BGA's concerns about the suicide risk. It stated, "During the treatment with the preparation, 16 suicide attempts were made, two of these with success. As patients with a risk of suicide were excluded from the studies, it is probable that the high proportion can be attributed to an action of the preparation."[15] The "preparation" was, of course, Prozac.

So great was the BGA's concern, they told Lilly they could not approve Prozac for use in Germany. That was 1985. Prozac was approved in 1987 in the U.S., and the marketing was so effective that German psychiatrists were clamoring for "the safest and most effective antidepressant ever developed." The Germans finally licensed Prozac, but only with the following warning: "For his/her own safety, the patient must be sufficiently observed, until the antidepressive effect of [Prozac] sets in. Taking an additional sedative may be necessary."[16] Don't miss this point. The Germans were so concerned about how some of those taking Prozac would react to this drug that they asked physicians to consider giving Prozac patients a sedative. The hope, of course, was that the sedative would decrease the danger of suicidal disinhibition and agitation.

Legal proceedings also brought to light a document by Dr. John Heiligenstein, one of Lilly's own research scientists, written when Lilly decided to issue a statement saying that reports of suicide and aggressive behaviors were not related to Prozac usage. His response as found in a memo dated September 14, 1990, was "We feel caution should be exercised in a statement that 'suicidality and hostile acts in patients taking Prozac reflects the patient's disorder and not a causal relationship to Prozac.' Post–marketing reports are increasingly fuzzy, and we have assigned, 'Yes, reasonably related,' on several reports."[17] Do not miss this point either. As early as 1990 Eli Lilly's own employee was stating he believed Prozac was causing "suicidality and hostile acts."

Most Americans are very aware of the much reported FDA warnings concerning suicide risk for children on antidepressants. Based on 24 trials the FDA stated that they believed the risk was twice as great for children on antidepressants as compared with those on placebo.[18] It was unfortunate that the FDA did not issue a similar warning for adult use as the German drug regulators felt would be necessary if Prozac were ever to be approved in Germany. That was 1985, two years before Prozac began to be pre-scribed in our nation. The German regulators concluded that if Prozac were to be approved (as it was in 1990, 5 years after they had first rejected it), it would be "on the condition that physicians be warned of the risk of suicide."[19] Those should have been prescription–stifling warnings. But marketing can always trump science. The German warnings were ignored by our FDA as were the many research reports suggesting the suicide risk was very real.

Describing the situation that existed as of October 1993, Ann Blake Tracy wrote, "Prozac has been out only six years and the most severe emo-tional side effects did not even come to public or professional attention until February 1990 and yet there are 28,623 complaints registered [with the FDA], a figure higher than any other drug in the history of the FDA."[20] Of those registered complaints, 1,885 involved suicide attempts.[21]

David Kessler who was the FDA commissioner at that time estimated that only about 1% of serious drug side effects were/are ever reported to the FDA. If his estimate is even close to being accurate, then the number of sui-cide attempts (and actual suicides) related to just the first of the SSRI drugs is staggering.[22] As Tracy noted, it was in February of 1990 that the suicide concern came to "public and professional attention."

Specifically, she was referring to an *American Journal of Psychiatry* article published by Dr. Martin Teicher and his colleagues from the Department of Psychiatry at the Harvard Medical School which received much attention.[23] Their article provided six case reports in which "patients free of serious suicidal ideation developed intense, violent suicidal preoccupation." For each of the patients the persistent suicide thoughts started within 2–7 weeks after they began taking Prozac and eventually ended after they were taken off Prozac.[24]

Many letters to the editor followed, including one by fellow psychiatrists which said they had for some time given only one–fourth the lowest dose because the same phenomenon occurred so frequently in their own practice.[25] Several others responded with similar stories. One who expressed a differing view reported his patients were very pleased with Prozac in part because it "improved modulation of emotions."[26] What does "modulation of emotions" mean? That the emotions are blunted. It means a more neutral affect. Giddiness is blunted. Sadness is blunted. And the strong self–preservation instinct we all possess is blunted as well.

That article brought a debate that could not be fully resolved since there were no large randomized, placebo–controlled trials (RCTs) in existence. But media stories were suggesting Prozac could cause suicide or murder. Article titles such as "Wonder drug/killer drug" in the popular media forced the FDA to act.[27] In September of 1991 their Psychopharmacological Drugs Advisory Committee was asked to meet and hear testimony and examine the research. Eli Lilly called on their Psychopharmacology Division to get ready. They also prepared new articles for publication in the medical journals. Those publications found Prozac actually reduced the chance of suicidal thoughts as well as suicide.[28] The FDA committee voted unanimously in favor of Lilly's position.

BOX #11–1

A Tragic Lesson for Lilly's Chairman

Lilly knew Prozac could increase the risk of suicide, but Lilly's chief scientist and spokesman Leigh Thompson also knew that if they acknowledged the Prozac–suicide link, "Lilly could go down the tubes," to use Thompson's own words as found in a memo Thompson never dreamed would be seen by others.[1]

Those comments were made as stories about Prozac–induced suicides were being written in the popular media following the *American Journal of Psychiatry* article of February 1990 which identified the link. It took 19 months before the FDA hearings on this concern were held, but Lilly (rather than develop fair RCT studies which they already knew would destroy their miracle pill) plotted the strategy which would keep the public from knowing the truth and would influence the FDA committee members.

As revealed by other uncovered memos, the strategy was to promote three messages:

(1) Suicides are due to the "disease" of depression, not to Lilly's anti-depressant.
(2) Prozac was the most researched drug ever made.
(3) If Prozac were banned, Americans with the disease of depression would be denied the very treatment they most need.[2]

Lilly won the FDA vote, but Lilly's chairman, Randall Tobias, may someday admit that he wishes they had not. Only 3 years later his wife decided to take Prozac. She committed suicide shortly thereafter.[3]

2004, The FDA Gets It Partially Right

Fast forward 13 years. The date is September 13, 2004. The FDA's Dr. Robert Temple announced to the nation that an analysis of 15 studies found that antidepressants clearly increased suicidal behavior.[29] That conclusion was the polar opposite of the FDA's 1991 conclusion. The obvious question is how did the FDA go from agreeing there was no threat to the point where they announced that they would immediately begin requiring that makers of antidepressants place the dreaded "black–box warning" on their antidepressant drugs? The answer is not that new research studies uncovered a danger not seen before. Most of the data upon which the 2004 decision was made came from studies completed more than a decade earlier. (Recall the details of Dr. Andrew Mosholder's experience told on p. 144.) The more reasonable answer is that: (1) the FDA has many "true believers" who have been convinced depression is caused by a chemical imbalance, and they did not want to take drugs off the market that many undoubtedly believed might be saving lives; and (2) the analysis of research data by those outside the FDA, coupled with related media stories, forced a reevaluation of the FDA's position.

Dr. Peter Breggin, perhaps America's leading expert on the purposely hidden effects of stimulants, antidepressants and antipsychotics, had by 2004 published numerous books aimed at educating the nation about the dangers of mind drugs.[30] Ralph Nader's Public Citizen and other non–profit organizations took on the task of disseminating information which the drug companies sought to keep out of the public's eyes. Reports in the media began suggesting that antidepressants might be behind the horrific murders that shook the nation. These stories typically noted that Andrea Yates (Houston bathtub drownings), Kip Kinkel (Jonesboro, Arkansas, shootings), Eric Harris (Columbine school shootings) and Christopher Pittman (South Carolina grandparents murdered) were on or had been on antidepressants.[31] The relationship between violence against others and violence against self is apparent. Whether these suggestive stories had merit or not, they got attention. The British government announced in December 2003 that the only antidepressant which appeared not to increase the suicide rate among children was Prozac. Other European nations and Canada soon issued sim- ilar warnings. And then the Mosholder story broke. The FDA was forced to revisit the issue.

No one should imagine the antidepressant–suicide link applies only to children. Since the hearings which led to the "black boxes," we have heard over and over that these suicide warnings apply only to children. When the suicide concern was focused on by the media in 1990, the issue was adult antidepressant use and suicide. The blunting effect which is associated with antidepressant use impacts both children and adults. We have a strong innate desire to live, but if that self–preservation sense is blunted, we must expect a rise in suicide. (See Box #11–2, Alcohol Also Blunts [Disinhibits].)

When the FDA issued their public health advisory in June 2005 concerning antidepressant drug use and "increase suicidal thinking or behavior" (see epigraph, p. 225), they were nearly two decades late. The data has made the danger apparent since Prozac was first tested. Nevertheless, the FDA's June 2005 health advisory also noted the FDA was in the midst of a review of antidepressant use and suicidality, a review they announced "will take a year or longer to complete."[32] You can wait until the middle of 2006 or 2007 or later to hear their conclusion, but an unbiased reading of the research makes it clear right now what they should be forced to conclude.

BOX #11–2

Alcohol Also Blunts (Disinhibits)

Should we be surprised by the studies which show an increase in suicide or violence related to the use of mind drugs? Alcohol, though consumed in a liquid form rather than a pill, is also a drug that blunts. It is widely known that alcoholics have a suicide rate that is many times that of a matched group of non–alcoholics.[1] But alcoholics are also far more likely to be divorced, have lost their jobs and have major health problems—other suicide risk factors. So let us leave the research on alcoholics alone and simply ask if there is an increase in suicide among those who have simply had some alcohol to drink.

The results of this inquiry make it plain that the strong sense of self–preservation we all possess can be dramatically blunted by alcohol. For example, an American study found that a third of all persons committing suicide had been drinking.[2] A British study reported that 41% of those attempting suicide were intoxicated at the time.[3] And those states which have a minimum drinking age of 21 have lower rates of suicide among 18– to 20–year–olds.[4]

Alcohol can also lower our inhibitions to avoid violence. People who would not assault another person when sober may do so if they have been drinking.[5] Placebo–controlled studies find "expectation" is a primary factor in changed behavior (the Lang study reported on p. 182 being the classic example). Yet experimental designs have also found that alcohol itself does increase aggression "not by 'stepping on the gas' but rather by paralyzing the brakes," as one researcher put it.[6] Said in another way, alcohol, like antidepressants, disinhibits our inhibitions. Or, you could simply say, alcohol blunts.

Part Two

The Antipsychotic Story

12

"Biological psychiatry is a total fraud."[1]
—*Fred Baughman, MD, neurologist*

FOOLED, FOOLED AND FOOLED AGAIN: THE HISTORY OF TREATING MENTAL PROBLEMS

How should those who have become so disturbed that their thinking is confused be treated? Physical abuse has been seen as a necessary part of the cure throughout recorded history. And even when purposeful abuse was no longer seen as helpful, the abuse continued, albeit in the guise of modern medical treatment.

Beating Some Sense Into Them

Sir Thomas More, the great scholar, author and Lord Chancellor of England, was beheaded by Henry VIII for not submitting his own conscience to the will of his king. More, praised as "a man for all seasons," was known for his goodness, kindness and his ideals. His description of an ideal society he entitled *Utopia* and thereby added a new word to the English language. And yet in his book *A Dialog of Comfort Against Tribulation* (1553)[2] he advises treating the mentally unstable with "betynge and correccyon."

More describes his treatment of one unfortunate soul who came wandering to his door. Translating the English of his day into our vernacular, we read that the man was "taken by the constables and bound to a tree in the street before the whole town, and there they beat him with rods till he became weary. . . . It appeared that his memory was good enough, except that it wandered till it was beaten home."[3]

Sir More's advice was likely influenced by *De medicina*, a medical book from ancient Roman writer Aulus Cornelius Celsus, which declared, "It is necessary to oppress with very harsh, corrective measures" even those whose problems did not exceed confused speech, and for the more serious cases he advocated fetters.[4] *De medicina* was printed in 1478, less than three decades after Gutenberg invented the printing press. Ironically, many of the Greek and Roman writers came to have greater influence during that era than they did in the ancient world. Andrew Boorde, a contemporary of Sir Thomas More, was also apparently influenced by the ancient writers. He wrote that those afflicted with madness required "merry communication" but that they must also "be kept in fear of one man or another, and if need require he must be punished and beaten."[5]

In the 17th century Thomas Willis, considered the greatest doctor of his day, wrote, "Maniacs often recover much sooner if they are treated with torture and torments."[6] John Brown's tremendously influential *Elementa Medicinae* (1793) counseled "intimidation and frightening of patients to the point of arousing in them a state of desperation."[7] "Non–injurious torture" was the term chosen by German neurologist Johann Christian Reil to describe the ideal treatment for delusional mental patients. In his highly influential 1803 volume,[8] he expressed many enlightened views including providing socialization for those who had "turned inward," but he also advocated plunges into water, inflicting pain and arousing anger and fear as means of awakening a more healthy mind.

Mental hospitals did not provide a refuge from this abuse. True to the wisdom of that day, many asylum superintendents would see that their wards were beaten in hopes that the pain might help the lunatics overcome their madness by causing them to forget their delusions. However, it was even more typical for those who lost their minds but had no family willing to provide for their care to simply be chained and neglected. In cold cells the insane would sit in their own filth before eventually contracting tuberculosis or some other disease that would bring an end to their suffering.

Europe's oldest hospital, London's St. Mary's of Bethlehem (whose name evolved into the shorter "Bethlem" from which we get our word "bedlam"), even permitted those who sought entertainment to purchase a ticket which allowed them to gawk at the unfortunate souls who were confined there.[9] Yet Bethlem Hospital's administrators viewed their institution with pride. A poem written in 1744 which was sold to visitors praised the institution's governors for the quality of care provided its patients even as it revealed the true plight of those committed to "Bedlam"—drugs, vomits, bleedings, cold baths, and cold and dirty cells for those who had become the most wild.

> . . . to our Governors, due praise be giv'n
> Who, by just care, have changed our Hell to Heav'n . . .
> The Physic's mild, the Vomits are not such,
> But, thanks be prais'd, of these we have not much.
> Bleeding is wholesome, and as for the Cold Bath,
> All are agreed it many Virtues hath.
> The Beds and Bedding are both warm and clean,
> Which to each comer may be plainly seen,
> Except those rooms where the most Wild do lie . . .[10]

Even George III, King of England when America rebelled and declared its independence, was not immune from the abuse given those who became mentally ill. Five times during his reign King George lost the ability to think clearly, and each time he was placed in a straight jacket and mistreated or tortured. This could not have occurred if the best medical men of that era were not convinced that fear reduced the wanderings of the mind. "Sometimes it may be necessary to inspire [awe] even by blows and stripes," declared his doctor.[11]

BOX #12-1

"He's Gone Battie!"

William Battie (1703–1776) became the leading "mad doctor," as they were then known, of 18th century England. He first developed an interest in madness when he was elected a governor of London's Bethlehem Hospital. In time he devoted himself to the study and cure of madness and wrote *A Treatise on Madness* which argued that "madness, though a terrible and at present a very frequent calamity, is perhaps as little understood as any that ever afflicted mankind."[1]

Battie's treatise was the first by an eminent physician on this topic, and it had a great impact, making madness a respectable concern of medicine. Battie rejected what he termed the "general methods" for treating madness: "bleeding, blisters, caustics, rough cathartics, the gumms and faetid anti–hysterics, opium, mineral waters, cold bathing, and vomits."[2] The good doctor wrote that he knew it would seem almost heretical to reject these treatments, but, he argued, "Many a Lunatic who by repetition of vomits and other convulsive stimuli would have been strained into downright Idiotism, has, when given over as incurable, recovered his understanding."[3]

Bethlehem Hospital's physician John Monro published his own treatise condemning Battie's rejection of vomits, bleeding, purges and other physical treatments. But for those fortunate enough to have been admitted to the new St. Luke's Hospital for Lunaticks which Dr. Battie helped found, the physical treatments were replaced with kindness, private rooms, warm meals and, for many, a complete cure after several months, though it often required a whole year. Dr. Battie then opened his own private mad houses from which he grew very wealthy and from which we added another expression to our language.

When asylum reform began in Europe, reports of abuse—including the abuse suffered by King George—led Parliament to begin the investigations of 1815. Appearing before the Select Committee on Madhouses that year was Bethlem's physician Thomas Monro, son of the hospital's Dr. John

Monro. As evidence of their quality care, he testified that patients experienced "bleeding, purging, and vomit; those are the general remedies we apply. That has been the practice invariably for years, long before my time; it was handed down to me by my father, and I do not know any better practice."[12]

"Bleeding, purging and vomit" were widely practiced because it was believed that the origin of melancholia (abnormal depression), mania (abnormal excitement) and madness was a result of chemical imbalances. Though Hippocrates recognized that emotional stress could cause chemical imbalances to develop in the body,[13] it was, nevertheless, Hippocrates's belief that good mental health required the proper balance of four bodily substances (humors)—black bile, yellow bile, phlegm and blood.[14] (See Box #12–2, Hippocrates on the Origin of Madness.) The proper treatment of insanity and other serious mental problems was a matter of removing excesses of the bodily fluids.

A 17th century text, *The Anatomy of Melancholy* by Robert Burton, assumed the Hippocratic view. Its influence was dominant for nearly three centuries. When the 1821 edition was published 200 years after the first edition, the Hippocratic explanations remained.[15] Benjamin Rush, the father of American psychiatry, actively sought to reform the treatment provided the insane. He opposed abuse, but he also was influenced by Burton's classic work. He was convinced insanity was likely due to too much blood flow to the brain (Hippocrates's theory). Thus, he bled his patients.

BOX #12–2
Hippocrates on the Origin of Madness

"The corruption of the brain is caused not only by phlegm but by bile. You may distinguish them thus. Those who are mad through phlegm are quiet, and neither shout nor make a disturbance; those maddened through bile are noisy, evildoers, and restless, always doing something. These are the causes of continued madness."[1]

—Sacred Disease (25, XVII)
Hippocrates

Modern Medical Treatment: The Disease Model

The Cause of Mental Problems: Disease

The Renaissance brought a steady progression of new insights into human anatomy, physiology and disease, but it was not until the work of Louis Pasteur in the 1800s that the door to modern medicine was swung wide open. The application of Pasteur's discoveries was important to every branch of medicine. No one questioned that bacteria could cause disease following Pasteur. But what would be the application in psychiatry?

From Hippocrates on, medicine generally hoped to find simple cures for mental problems. If bleeding or a drug which induced "purging and vomit" could be administered and mental problems thus resolved, the medical profession's contribution would immediately be recognized as immense. Psychiatry began looking for disease, including unrecognized disease, that might be harming the brain. After Hippocrates was "rediscovered," many physicians looked for ways to reduce mental instability by treating the uterus or the ovaries. (See Box #12–3, Do Hysterical Women Need a Hysterectomy?) However, following Pasteur, psychiatry began looking for bodily disease in more than just the female organs. Since mental problems often arose unexpectedly, it was assumed that the responsible disease might be relatively hidden within the body.

Dr. Henry Cotton, the medical director of the New Jersey State Hospital at Trenton and a lecturer at Princeton University, began removing teeth from his mental patients on the assumption that infection of the teeth might be responsible for much insanity.[16]

> The removal of all infected teeth is imperative. This means the impacted and unerupted molars as well, especially in young people. From our experience, we consider that all impacted and unerupted teeth are infected. It is useless to quibble over this point.[17]

246

Unfortunately, he found that this procedure only helped about 25% of his patients, so he concluded that removal of other bacteria–harboring sites was clearly necessary.

> The tonsils are fully as important as the teeth, for among the psychotic group very few if any patients have had their tonsils removed in childhood. . . . We have found that many patients have been prevented from recovering by the fact that an error in the diagnosing of infected tonsils was made, thus allowing an infected tonsil to remain.[18]

When not every patient recovered, Cotton assumed infection must be present elsewhere in the body. "The infected cervix is frequently over-looked and if not attended to, in spite of the fact that infected teeth and tonsils have been removed, the patient's recovery will be hindered."[19] After careful study the good doctor reported the cervix was infected in about 80% of his cases.[20] And yet even then recovery often did not follow surgery, so other parts of the body needing surgical removal were sought. Out came sinsuses, appendixes, gall bladders, ovaries, fallopian tubes, seminal vesicles and entire colons. Amazingly, Dr. Cotton was unafraid to publish the results of these surgeries. Out of 281 full or partial colon removal operations completed over a two–year period, 27% of patients recovered, 37% did not recover and 36% died![21]

Dr. Cotton's work received high praise from many quarters. Adolf Meyer, one of the nation's most prominent psychiatrists, stated in the foreward to Dr. Cotton's book *The Defective, Delinquent, and Insane: The Relation of Focal Infection to Their Causation, Treatment, and Prevention* (1921) that Dr. Cotton's "evaluation of focal infections is an outstanding contribution of twentieth century medicine." He even suggested that Dr. Cotton had "results not attained by any previous or contemporary attack on the grave problem of mental disorder."[22]

How is it possible that such barbaric treatment was not more seriously challenged? Factors likely include elements that can always help bring

---

BOX #12-3

Do Hysterical Women Need a Hysterectomy?

Webster's Definition of Hysteria: (1) a psychiatric condition variously characterized by emotional excitability, excessive anxiety, sensory and motor disturbances, or the unconscious simulation of organic disorders, such as blindness, deafness, etc.; (2) any outbreak of wild, uncontrolled excitement or feeling, such as fits of laughing and crying.[1]

The term *hysteria* was once one of psychiatry's most common diagnoses, and it was a common diagnosis more than 2,000 years before psychiatry ever became a profession. The Greeks often described mental problems as hysteria, and as it appeared more in women than in men, it was assumed to have its origin in a female organ—specifically the uterus. Indeed the Greek word for uterus was *hystera*, and the origin of our word "hysteria" is the Greek word *hysterikos* which literally means "suffering in the hystera" (womb).

Old ideas can be slow to die no matter how silly they may be. Nineteenth and even twentieth century physicians would sometimes remove parts of the female anatomy in order to help the mind. Concerning insanity, one physician wrote in 1850, "Among the causes, females are alone exposed to those which grow out of the uterine and mammary structure and functions."[2] In 1866 another physician declared, "With woman it is but a step from extreme nervous susceptibility to downright hysteria, and from that to overt insanity."[3]

---

acceptance of error: (1) support from some of the profession's leaders, (2) excellent credentials, (3) working under the authority of a government institution, (4) presentation of research findings in reputable medical journals and (5) presenting optimistic reports to a psychiatric community that needed hope that psychiatry could have a brighter future.

Dr. Cotton concluded one review of his infection removal work by arguing that "the successful treatment of 1,412 cases during the last five years, must be accepted as evidence that our work has been efficient."[23] Other psychiatrists practicing infection removal to cure mental problems could not achieve Dr. Cotton's 80% success rate. This finally brought challenges to the statistics Dr. Cotton was reporting when the American Psychiatric

Hysterectomies and ovarianectomies (oophorectomies) would not be unreasonable if the female organs really were responsible for mental disorders. In fact, the link was so strongly associated in the minds of some that one popular nineteenth century book actually argued that if women engaged in excessive use of their minds by attending college, they could cause the uterus to atrophy![4] Such conclusions inevitably led to the surgical removal of female organs in order to improve mental health, an 1893 article arguing that the benefits were remarkable: "Patients are improved, some of them cured; . . . the moral sense of the patient elevated. . . . She becomes tractable, orderly, industrious and cleanly."[5]

By the beginning of the twentieth century many doctors could boast of having removed the ovaries from as many as 2,000 women.[6] The pace of ovary removals slowed (following 1910) only as the removal of the uterus became more popular. Such convictions were never held by a majority of physicians, but even the *Journal of the American Medical Association* published an article in 1907 with the title "To What Extent Can the Gynecologist Prevent and Cure Insanity in Women?"[7] upon which the journal's editor commented, "Finally by curing these pelvic irritations in women of unstable nervous organizations, before insanity occurs, its development may often be wholly prevented."[8]

The transition in the second half of the twentieth century was towards supplementing the hormones produced by the ovaries rather than removing the ovaries. (Think in terms of Dr. Robert A. Wilson, discussed in Chapter 1.) Nevertheless, for many, treatment of the mind still looked toward organs which were unique to the female sex.

Association met in 1922. One of the critics was Abraham Brill who as a member of the relatively new psychoanalytic profession could conceive of help without drugs or surgeries. He criticized "detoxification" (infection removal) as causing mental illness and death. He cited the case of a patient "whose depressive moods formerly lasted no longer than three weeks or a month and who, after all his upper teeth had been extracted, merged into a deep depression" and another case in which the lower intestine was removed resulting in sudden death.[24] But others present came to Dr. Cotton's rescue indicating that their results from gynecological removal procedures were also quite satisfactory. The critics were chastised for unjustified attacks on the march of science.

The next year, 1923, saw the publication of a controlled study comparing untreated patients with those who were operated on. No differences were found in outcome, a report that slowed down the march of science in this quarter anyway.[25]

Modern Medical Treatment: Insulin Shock

Dr. Manfred Sakel, a Viennese psychiatrist, discovered in 1927 that schizophrenics could be made tranquil if the patients received doses of insulin sufficiently large enough to put them into a coma and then were revived with the administration of glucose. To get the full beneficial effect of this treatment, Sakel learned that patients needed to undergo dozens of these near–death experiences.[26]

Like Cotton before him, Sakel reported wonderful results. For example, he described a patient who had lost his mind and had to be placed "for several weeks in a cage bed, under restraint." But then, "By treating him according to the method which I shall soon describe, it was possible to bring the patient back to a condition where he could resume his work and go his way again, free of psychotic symptoms."[27] Sakel's published comments led to the growth of insulin therapy across the nation. Both medical journals and the lay press declared insulin therapy a wonder cure.

I have witnessed the results of low blood sugar in my diabetic wife many times. On one occasion she was at the kitchen sink when she suddenly froze. She was trying to pour a glass of orange juice to counteract her dropping blood sugar but dropped the glass in her hands and lost awareness. Fortunately I was nearby and was able to carry her to the living room before she fell to the floor. In that condition she cannot speak or show any evidence that she is aware of the present circumstances. I always squirt sugar icing or something similar into her mouth so that the brain can once again begin getting the supply of sugar which allows it to function.

What Sakel did to his patients was far more harmful than what my wife has ever experienced as a result of her diabetes. He would inject massive doses of insulin into his patients. Adding insulin by injection lowers the amount of sugar available for use by the brain. Many diabetics have died by accidentally overdosing on insulin. Sakel put his patients on sufficient insulin to induce either an epileptic seizure or a coma that he would allow to last up to six hours. They would then be given carbohydrates when he was ready for them to come out of their coma. Sakel described the typical response as patients first began emerging from their trauma.

> As the patient awakens he first begins to mutter primitive sounds or to groan. He then starts to babble inarticulately and often expresses himself like a child. The ability to speak is the last function to return . . . . At a later stage of awakening, the patient is able to respond to simple and reit-erated commands. It appears that at first the patient is unable to understand the meaning of these commands. Only gradually does he comprehend them. But he is able to respond promptly and effectively as long as he is not required to express himself in speech. . . . When one attempts somewhat later to establish contact with the patient, one has the impression that he hears everything and wants to react, but that he is unable to grasp the meaning of the question put to him. . . . Finally, the patient will begin to understand the words he is hearing, but he continues to respond inappropriately or slowly at times despite his understanding.[28]

A single coma experience would tranquilize the undesirable outbursts and fantasies temporarily but did not bring permanent change. Sakel thus would put his patients through the experience again and again until the per-sonality was altered permanently. Sakel freely admitted that this essentially was a "lowering" of the personality but, nevertheless, psychotic experiences were reduced. The results were highly appreciated by most mental hospital staffs. Patients may have been somewhat "zombied," but they were clearly easier to manage.

The brains of autopsied patients who did not survive the treatment revealed what the mechanism was which reduced mental disorders and lowered the personality—brain damage. This was no real surprise. Experiments with dogs found that those which died during insulin coma or were put to death after several "insulin therapy" treatments experienced a shrinkage of nerve cells, microscopic hemorrhages and general destruction of brain tissue.[29] Sakel himself acknowledged that the mechanism by which the patient was "helped" was brain damage. He fearlessly described his insulin shock treatment as "a fine microscopic surgery to eliminate the cells diseased beyond repair."[30] (Note that the assumption that "the cells are diseased" persists.)

Various authors questioned the value of insulin therapy, but as late as 1953 Dr. Harold Bourne was able to write, "The widespread belief in the indispensable value of insulin treatment is a matter of general concern."[31] Bourne's article was a hard–hitting attack on insulin therapy. His article was entitled "The Insulin Myth," a title that reflected the data found in his analysis and critique of earlier reports which indicated insulin therapy to be highly effective in treating schizophrenia.

Despite such a scathing attack and despite the fact it appeared in the prestigious and widely read medical journal, *Lancet*, change came slowly. Writing in 1958, the director of the Psychiatric Clinic of Vienna argued that it was insulin therapy that first allowed "institutions of confinement" to become "true institutions of healing." He hailed Sakel's work as "a milestone in the advancement of psychiatry" and then declared,

> It is an eloquent testimony to the genius of its discoverer that throughout the period since its inception, the administrators of the Psychiatric Clinic of Vienna have not deemed it necessary to deviate from the classical procedure of insulin therapy as outlined by Dr. Sakel, in any essential.[32]

Modern Medical Treatment: Camphor and Metrazol Therapy

Long before Bourne's critique of insulin therapy appeared, many of America's asylums were looking for other approaches that might bring desirable results which were not as time intensive as insulin therapy. Insulin therapy patients had to be closely monitored. It has been suggested that at least 50–100 times as much attention and care had to be given insulin therapy patients compared with those not receiving insulin.[33] By definition, putting patients into a coma was dangerous. Vital signs had to be closely monitored. If breathing became too shallow or the heartbeat too slow, they would have to be given glucose quickly or death might result.

During the 1930s another shock treatment was developed which was much less time intensive. The treatment used metrazol, a synthetic form of camphor. Camphor is obtained from the camphor tree. Small branches are steamed until they "perspire" a clear liquid—camphor. It is a poisonous substance but in a minimal dose will cause delirium and convulsions in humans. It had long been believed that seizures and insanity were somewhat incompatible. It was an erroneous idea but one that led to various methods of inducing convulsions in hopes of curing schizophrenia, manic depression and other disorders.

In the 16th century a Swiss physician reportedly gave camphor by mouth "to cure lunacy."[34] During the 18th century Austrian physician Leopold von Auenbrugger administered small amounts of camphor every two hours to patients with mania to induce convulsions and overcome the manic disability. Other physicians experimented with camphor though it was never widely adopted despite an 1825 medical text reporting a case in which the camphor "produced a fit, and perfect cure followed."[35]

However, when Hungarian psychiatrist Ladislas von Meduna observed that the brains of epileptic patients had a huge number of glial cells whereas the brains of schizophrenic patients displayed a lack of those cells, he guessed that somehow epilepsy resulted in a biological change that might prevent schizophrenia. His colleague, Julius Nyirö who also had heard or observed that epilepsy and schizophrenia were incompatible, had sought to cure epilepsy by injecting blood from schizophrenics into epileptics. Of course, it was just a guess that causing epileptic seizures might benefit the insane, but it seemed to von Meduna worthy of pursuit.

He began testing the hypothesis using guinea pigs. The first experiments used camphor in an oil base which would then be injected into muscle tissue. After two months of testing von Meduna believed it was time to experiment on a human. He chose a schizophrenic patient whose body had been held in a frozen position for four years. The man had stopped eating and so was fed by a feeding tube. As he never moved, he had to be diapered and changed regularly. The camphor was administered. "After 45 minutes of anxious and fearful waiting the patient suddenly had a classical epileptic attack."[36] The result was miraculous. The man suddenly awoke from the seizures, sat up and asked how long he had been ill. Von Meduna reported he was thrilled beyond measure.

He began treating other schizophrenics and reported good though mixed results. He speculated results might be even better if a superior convulsion–inducing drug were used. Camphor was not highly reliable. A convulsion might not even occur or several convulsions might follow the injection. And it was never possible to know if the convulsions might begin in 15 minutes or not arrive for 3 hours.[37]

These problems led von Meduna to begin experimenting with a soluble synthetic form of camphor known as metrazol in the United States and cardiazol in Europe.[38] The metrazol would be injected into a vein and in 3 to 30 seconds the patient would experience a seizure of such violence that backs were broken and jaws dislocated.[39] In his review and appraisal of metrazol therapy Solomon Katzenelbogen, referring to the dislocation of patients' jaws, called it "a rather mild complication of frequent occurrence."[40] Whether or not the patient would consider this just "a rather mild complication" is debatable. A less debatable issue would be that the seizures produced by metrazol were incredibly violent. A New York State Psychiatric Institute study reported that out of 51 patients who had undergone metrazol therapy, 43% experienced an average of 3 to 4 vertebrae fractures.[41]

Metrazol therapy was always somewhat controversial. Though Katzenelbogen had often used metrazol convulsive therapy, he honestly reported patients' reaction to the treatment. "The most common and striking observation is the patient's facial expression of fright, of being tortured, of extreme anxiety. The descriptions by some of our patients of their feelings are in full harmony with their facial expressions."[42] But neither fractured vertebrae nor witnessing the terror felt by metrazol patients should have been as compelling as the reports of brain damage.

Katzenelbogen candidly stated, "The structural alterations found in the brains of animals . . . are of rather ominous significance."[43] Yet in 1940 when his review was published, Katzenelbogen reported that convulsive therapy had become "routine practice. Instead of being reserved for special, particularly ominous conditions, it is being used rather indiscriminately, without due regard for the nature and seriousness of the illness and without the circumspection such a procedure should command."[44] Nevertheless, that same year (1940) it was reported that some 70% of all American hospitals were using metrazol.[45] Many were using metrazol for manic depression while continuing the use of insulin therapy for schizophrenia.

Modern Medical Treatment: ECT

Few of my students have ever heard of insulin or metrazol therapy before they take their first psychology course. However, another shock therapy, electroconvulsive therapy (ECT), is more likely to be in their knowledge base. Insulin therapy's convulsions were believed to be so effective in restoring good mental health that any means of inducing convulsions was likely to be explored.

An Italian neuropathologist and psychiatrist, Ugo Cerletti, is generally credited with the development of electroconvulsive therapy.[46] Cerletti and his assistant, Lucio Bini, experimented with dogs to determine the voltage needed to induce convulsions. After many trials Cerletti found that passing 125 volts for just over one half a second (the electrodes being placed in the mouth and the rectum) brought the desired results.[47] Cerletti then learned that the Rome slaughter houses were using electricity and placing electrodes on the sides of the pigs' heads. Though this caused convulsions in the pigs, it did not kill them, a task which was still left to the butchers. This discovery greatly encouraged Cerletti and his assistant. They had lost many of their dogs to electrocution and hoped that passing current through the brain only and avoiding the heart might lower the rate of unwanted deaths.

Cerletti received permission from the slaughter house to carry out their next set of experiments on the business's pigs before they were handed over to the butcher.

> I carried out tests, not only subjecting the pigs to the current for ever–increasing periods of time, but also applying the current in various ways: across the head, across the neck, and across the chest. Various durations (20, 30, 60 or more seconds) were tried. It turned out that the more serious results (prolonged apnea sometimes lasting many minutes and, exceptionally, death) appeared when the current crossed the chest . . . ; and, finally, that passage of the current across the head, even for long durations, did not have serious consequences. It was found that pigs, even when treated in this last way several times, "came to" gradually, after a fairly long interval (5 to 6 minutes), then started moving, next made various attempts to get shakily to their feet, and finally ran rapidly to mix with their mates in the pen.[48]

Once the amount of electricity which would kill was clearly understood, Cerletti began looking for a human subject. It was over one year before a suitable candidate was found: a 39–year–old man without identification wandering around the train station. He had arrived from Milan but was lost and confused. As the authorities could not determine who he was, and he was incoherent and hallucinating, he fell into the hands of Cerletti, the local psychiatrist, and became the world's first ECT patient.

Electrodes were placed against the man's head, and 70 volts of electricity passed through his brain for a fraction of a second.[49] No convulsions (the desired effect) resulted. A second shock was attempted. The voltage remained the same, but the duration increased. After the second shock, the patient asked not to be shocked again. The experimenters, however, wanted to produce a convulsion and so continued, giving a third, even longer shock. Still the patient did not have a convulsion. Cerletti decided to end the experiment for that day but was determined to increase the voltage to whatever would be necessary the next time he brought his vagrant into the laboratory.

A few days later Cerletti assembled his assistants and some colleagues for what he hoped to be a historic event. Cerletti began with 70 volts and again did not achieve the convulsive seizure he sought. He then announced he would raise the voltage to 110 volts, but that immediately brought whispers of fear and even cries of protest from those who had been invited. Professor Brandon's history of these events states that "all of the staff objected to the further shock, protesting that the patient would probably die."[50] Cerletti later described the event himself.

> Upon closing the circuit, there was a sudden jump of the patient on his bed without loss of consciousness. The patient presently started to sing at the top of his voice, then fell silent. It was evident from our long experience with dogs that the voltage had been held too low.[51]

Those protests did not stop the experiment but actually hurried it up. Cerletti later admitted that he knew if he did not move quickly, the fear for the man's safety could bring an end to what he hoped would be an important medical triumph.

> The situation was such, weighted as it was with responsibility, that this warning, explicit and unequivocal, shook the persons present to the extent that some began to insist upon suspension of the proceedings. Anxiety lest something that amounted to superstition should interfere with my decision urged me on to action. I had the electrodes reapplied, and a 110–volt discharge was sent through for 0.5 second. The immediate, very brief cramping of all the muscles was again seen; after a slight pause, the most typical epileptic fit began to take place.[52]

That was the goal, and it was Cerletti who received great fame for bringing about the convulsion in a way that could be replicated everywhere. It cost little, was quick and, most importantly, amazingly effective. Cerletti wrote that after the electroshock, the convulsions and a period of comatose unconsciousness "to the immense relief of all concerned . . . the patient sat up of his own accord, looked about him calmly with a vague smile, as though asking what was expected of him. I asked him, 'What has been happening to you?' He answered with no more gibberish. 'I don't know; perhaps I have been asleep.'"[53] Eleven more ECT treatments followed after which Cerletti and Bini reported the man fully recovered.[54]

The relationship between convulsive fits and improved mental health was already widely accepted and widely pursued when Cerletti and Bini published their first paper on electroshock (Cerletti's term).[55] Cerletti did not become famous for discovering this link but for providing what quickly became the foremost means of inducing convulsions—one with numerous advantages over previous methods.

ECT was actually demonstrated at the American Psychiatric Association's annual meeting in 1940,[56] the same year muscle relaxants were introduced to the treatment so as to reduce the number of patients suffering broken vertebrae as a result of the violent convulsions.[57] During World War II ECT became so accepted that severely depressed soldiers were generally provided either psychoanalysis or ECT.[58] By the 1950s ECT had become a standard treatment in hospitals throughout the U.S. and Europe, which Edward Shorter, a professor of the history of medicine, calls "one of the discipline's great success stories."[59]

As I noted in the beginning of this section, many of my students have at least heard of ECT before I ever discuss it in class. Some are even aware that during the 1970s there were strong attacks on ECT, and that its use fell dramatically.[60] But most of my students are genuinely startled when they learn that ECT is still often performed and is continuing to increase in popularity today. The growth in the use of ECT began again after the National Institutes of Health (NIH) sponsored the NIH's Consensus Conference on Electroconvulsive Therapy in June of 1985. The praise for ECT was strong with their official report declaring, "Not a single controlled study has shown another form of treatment to be superior to ECT in the short–term management of severe depressions."[61] A summary of the consensus statement was then published in *JAMA* in October 1985. Several books followed which advocated increasing use of ECT.

In 1990 the American Psychiatric Association published *A Task Force Report on the Practice of Electroconvulsive Therapy* which strongly supported the use of ECT. The second edition was released in 2001, and again, it strongly encouraged its more widespread use.[62] This was followed by a *Journal of the American Medical Association* editorial which carried the title "Electroconvulsive Therapy: Time to Bring It Out of the Shadows."[63] Textbooks typically mimic the official recommendations of the professional associations which means that today students across the nation are being told that ECT works and that it should be more widely employed in treating major depression, dementia and various other mental problems. Whereas approximately 300,000 ECT treatments were administered in 1986, approximately 820,000 were done in 1995.[64] No figures are yet available to indicate how dramatic the increase may have been in the decade which followed the 1995 count, but it has likely increased significantly.

Modern Medical Treatment: Psychosurgery

> "It is probably like Rip Donderdunck's case," he exclaimed in a low, mumbling tone. "He fell from the top of Voppelploot's windmill. After the accident the man was stupid and finally became idiotic. In time he lay helpless, like yon fellow on the bed; moaned, too, like him, and kept constantly lifting his hand to his head. My learned friend Von Choppem performed an operation upon this Donderdunck and discovered under the skull a small dark sac, which pressed upon the brain. This had been the cause of the trouble. My friend Von Choppem removed it—a splendid operation! You see, according to Celsus . . ."[65]

The words are those of Dr. Boekman in Mary Mapes Dodge's *Hans Brinker or The Silver Skates* as he shares with his assistant his opinion concerning Hans's father, Raff Brinker, who had suffered a head injury. In the preface to her story published in 1865 Dodge tells us that "the story of Raff Brinker is founded strictly upon fact."[66] Since the beginning of time (long before Celsus) head injuries have been known to lead sometimes to coma and death, sometimes to loss of speech, sometimes to "stupidity" or "idiocy," and sometimes to personality change. It was this awareness that opened the door to modern psychosurgery.

In 1935 an international neurological conference was held in London at which Yale neurophysiologists John Fulton and Carlyle Jacobsen shared the results of experiments they had completed on Becky and Lucy, two laboratory chimpanzees. Fulton and Jacobsen had sought to determine the specific effect of removing the brain's frontal lobes on learning and problem solving.

They had devised a simple experiment in which the chimpanzee would enter a cage and then watch as food was concealed under one of two cups. The cups were then blocked from view for various lengths of time (from seconds to several minutes), and then the blind was removed. All the chimps had to do was to remember into which cup the food had been placed in order to receive the food as a reward. This simple test allowed the researchers to establish some standards for the chance of error to be expected after various time delays. The frontal lobes could then be removed and some indication of the importance of the frontal lobes for information processing and problem solving could be determined.[67]

If that was all that was shared at the conference, the prefrontal lobotomy would not have been born later that year, but the researchers also mentioned that one of the chimps had proved to be much more emotional and difficult than the other chimp.

> [Becky] was highly emotional and profoundly upset whenever she made an error. Violent temper tantrums after a mistake were not infrequent occurrences. She observed closely loading of the cup with food and often whimpered softly as the cup was placed over the food. If the experimenter lowered or started to lower the opaque door to exclude the animal's view of the cups, she immediately flew into a temper tantrum, rolled on the floor, defecated and urinated.[68]

Here was an animal who seemed to have real emotional problems, but then the lobotomy was performed and a most

> profound change occurred. . . . The usual procedure of baiting the cup and lowering the opaque screen was followed. But the chimpanzee did not show any excitement and sat quietly before the door or walked around the cage. Given an opportunity to choose between the cups, it did so with its customary eagerness and alacrity. However, if the animal made a mistake, it showed no evidence of emotional

disturbance but quietly awaited the loading of the cups for the next trial. . . . If the animal failed, it merely continued to play or to pick over its fur . . . it was quite impossible to evoke even a suggestion of an "experimental neurosis."[69]

Psychosurgery is generally considered to have been born on that day as the men whose names are most closely tied to prefrontal lobotomies, (António Egas Moniz and Walter Freeman) were both in attendance at the presentation. It was Egas Moniz who asked the now famous question, "If frontal–lobe removal prevents the development of experimental neuroses in animals and eliminates frustrational behaviour, why would it not be feasible to relieve anxiety states in man by surgical means?"[70]

In reality, it had long been known by others that the frontal lobes were central to personality and emotions. The countless number of soldiers who had suffered head wounds during the Great War (WWI) alone had taught that lesson to a large number of military doctors. Soldiers with damaged or destroyed frontal lobes had blunted emotions, little drive or will and a diminished maturity level.[71] Yet, intellectual effects would typically be rather minimal—unless problem–solving ability is considered a part of one's intellectual capacity.[72] Problem–solving ability could be dramatically affected as it was in the case of the Yale chimpanzees. Those facts did not overly concern Egas Moniz. He left the conference determined to conduct

---

BOX #12–4

Lucy—The Other Chimpanzee

Perhaps the most surprising aspect of Dr. Moniz's daring in performing lobotomies is the other chimpanzee, Lucy. Lucy was the calmer chimp who did not throw temper tantrums when she forgot which cup held the food. However, after she was lobotomized, her personality and behavior took a dramatic turn for the worse. Whereas the operation made Becky more apathetic, it resulted in less emotional control for Lucy. Suddenly she began having temper tantrums and acted emotionally distraught when she failed to correctly solve the "Which cup has the food?" problem.[1] If Dr. Moniz used Becky's greater apathy following frontal lobe damage as justification for damaging the frontal lobes of humans, the question becomes, "But how about Lucy?"

---

an experiment on a human. He would remove or destroy the frontal lobes of a schizophrenic and see if it did not cause the patient immediately to become less anxious and more manageable.

It was likely unknown to Egas Moniz, but he would not be the first psychiatrist to purposely damage a patient's brain in order to reduce a patient's symptoms.[73] In 1888 a Swiss psychiatrist Gottlieb Burckhardt guessed he might calm some of the patients in the mental hospital for which he was the director. Six of his schizophrenic patients had their skulls opened and had portions of their cerebral brain tissue removed. According to his biographer, "Most patients showed improvement and became easier to manage, although one died from the procedure and several had aphasia [a loss or impairment in the ability to speak or understand speech due to brain damage] or seizures."[74]

Dr. Burckhardt published the results of his experiments, but he was perhaps too honest for his efforts to be well received. (After all, "several had aphasia or seizures" would suggest a few of each, though only 5 of the 6 even survived the surgery.) Nevertheless, the patient's hallucinations were fewer, their anxieties calmed and their emotions blunted. On one level his experiment could be called a great success. Yet the medical community of his day did not receive his work with any enthusiasm, and it was soon forgotten.

António Caetano de Abreu Freire Egas Moniz was more fortunate. He was already one of Portugal's most famous and most respected senior physicians. He had held numerous prestigious positions for his nation including Minister for Foreign Affairs and president of Portugal's delegation to the Paris Peace Conference where he was a signer of the Treaty of Versailles which officially brought WWI to an end. He was celebrated by the medical community for developing the cerebral angiography, a most important medical advancement whereby blood vessels in the brain could be visualized on X–rays.[75] He had also already performed many experiments on patients' brains and was not likely to be challenged if the experiments were not successful.

Dr. Egas Moniz quickly located what he considered an excellent candidate. She was a 63–year–old schizophrenic woman with a long history of mental problems who was very disturbed at that time, evidenced by the following description:

> The woman had been diagnosed as an involutional melancholic with anxiety and well established paranoid ideas. . . . She believed she was being persecuted by her neighbors and the police and accused her pharmacist and physician of trying to poison her. She also had auditory hallucinations, strange bodily sensations, and episodes of severe anxiety, crying, restlessness, and insomnia. Before her second hospitalization she had secretly practiced prostitution in her apartment until the other female boarders forced her to leave.[76]

Dr. Egas Moniz drilled two holes to gain access to the brain's frontal lobes.[77] He then injected pure alcohol in order to destroy the tissue. The holes were covered and the hours of waiting began with hopes that the operation's effect would prove similar to the effect frontal lobe destruction had on Becky, the chimpanzee. Approximately five hours later the woman cried some, but the emotional intensity of her sadness was less. Dr. Egas Moniz declared her cured and quickly located 19 additional patients with which he could continue his experiment.

Results for the second patient were even more debatable than for the first. The third and fourth patients were schizophrenics who did not appear to improve following the operation. Egas Moniz decided it was time to increase the amount of damage the brain was to experience. He began drilling six holes in his patients and injecting even more brain–destroying alcohol. (Beginning with the eighth patient, he used a narrow instrument which was inserted into the drilled holes and used to cut the frontal lobe connections.[78])

The fifth patient was also a schizophrenic and, again, some of his symptoms continued after the operation. However, he had been a difficult patient who was often agitated. After the lobotomy the agitation was gone. He was calm and easy to control—both characteristics highly prized by asylum staff.

As Egas Moniz continued the experiment, it became apparent to him that emotions could be blunted more than delusional thinking could be eliminated. It may be that he used just whatever asylum patients were made available for the experiment. However, he may have chosen to focus on patients suffering depression rather than schizophrenia for it was those patients that began to dominate his experiments. When Egas Moniz summarized the results of his first 20 patients, he confessed that the benefit for schizophrenics was less than the benefit experienced by those displaying anxiety and depression. This is most ironic, for when Egas Moniz won the Nobel prize for medicine in 1949, the official statement declared it was "for his discovery of the therapeutic value of leucotomy [lobotomy] in *certain psychoses*" [emphasis mine].[79] (Again, a psychosis is a loss of contact with reality, of which schizophrenia is one type.)

Of course, even those Egas Moniz declared cured simply experienced the effects of brain damage. (Valenstein declared, "The evidence of 'cures' in Moniz's monograph could not have convinced a critical reader."[80]) When frontal lobes are damaged, the emotions are blunted. As evidence that a proper study and evaluation of the first 20 cases were not done, on March 3, 1936, only 3 months and 3 weeks after Egas Moniz's first patient was lobotomized, the results of all 20 cases were already written and at the publishers as Egas Moniz personally stood before an audience of his colleagues at a Paris conference and summarized the results.[81]

Dr. Egas Moniz was obviously anxious to be the first with a published report. Others were present at the London conference where the story of Becky and Lucy was shared. Someone else might be conducting the same experiment. Before the year was over he would publish five more articles on his lobotomy results—one of which used a new word he coined—psychosurgery.[82]

If credit and additional fame were what Egas Moniz sought, he need not have worried. He had in America at that very time a colleague who was to become his as well as his operation's greatest promoter. After Egas Moniz's book on his first 20 lobotomies appeared, Dr. Walter Freeman, an American neurologist, wrote the first book review. Freeman's review revealed his excitement—"Its importance can scarcely be overestimated"—and his willingness to accept Egas Moniz's report uncritically—"No case is reported in which there was any persistent disturbance of memory or intelligence."[83]

In evaluating Freeman's enthusiasm, it must be noted that surgery holds more prestige than general medicine even today. At that time psychiatry was becoming dominated by Freud's "talk therapy," and even Freud acknowledged his psychoanalysis was not suited to helping schizophrenics. ECT followed the first reports from Egas Moniz, but it was soon learned that the benefits of shocking the mind were very short lived. Additional ECT treatments were necessary for the blunting effects to continue. But lobotomies were quickly performed and could yield a permanent result.

We can only guess at other explanations for Freeman's enthusiasm, but upon reading one of Egas Moniz's papers, he immediately shared it with his friend and colleague James Watts. Freeman ordered a copy of Egas Moniz's "in press" book as well as his new lobotomy instrument. Freeman and Watts agreed they would perform their first lobotomy as soon as they returned from their summer vacations. By September 1936 Freeman and Watts were back on the campus of George Washington University in Washington, D.C., both eager to perform a lobotomy. They practiced on brains from the morgue before choosing their first patient.

The 60–year–old woman they selected was depressed and, more importantly, "agitated," the characteristic Egas Moniz indicated was most impacted by lobotomy. She agreed to surgery until she was told her hair would be shaved. With that news she balked until Freeman agreed to save her curls.

He didn't, but later, after the surgery, he noted, "She no longer cared."[84] After her recovery Freeman recorded his interview with the patient.

Freeman: "Are you happy?"
Patient: "Yes"
Freeman: "Do you remember being upset when you
                came here?"
Patient: "Yes, I was quite upset, wasn't I?"
Freeman: "What was it all about?"
Patient: "I don't know. I seem to have forgotten. It
                doesn't seem important now."[85]

Freeman's optimism and excitement were great. He and Watts quickly located other patients and completed several more operations during the following weeks. He also began writing papers on the procedure and seeking speaking opportunities at medical conferences. Medical articles must be written using temperate, even cautious language, but the Freeman–Watts articles did not always meet that obligation. The author announced that all their patients exhibited

> worry, apprehension, anxiety, insomnia and nervous tension, and in all of them these particular symptoms have been relieved to a greater or lesser extent. In some patients there has been amelioration or even disappearance of certain other symptoms such as disorientation, confusion, phobias, hallucinations, and delusions that were present before operation. The physical condition of our patients has also improved. . . . The condition of the patients after operation has been all that could be desired.[86]

> The symptomatic relief has been almost immediate, and has persisted to the present time. . . . In the patients operated upon up to the present, memory has not been obviously impaired and concentration has been improved, possibly on account of relief of the preoccupation. Judgment and

insight are apparently not diminished, and the ability to enjoy external events is certainly increased.[87]

The same article had photographs of patients taken before and after lobotomy. The despair and withdrawal seen in the "before" pictures turn into smiles and stability in the "after" pictures.[88] Freeman can fairly be called a promoter of lobotomies, including the procedure he eventually developed using an ice pick inserted under the eyelid and hit into the frontal lobes with a mallet.[89]

Opposition to Freeman's lobotomies began with the first medical convention at which he spoke about the procedure.[90] Destroying parts of the brain proved offensive to most neurologists, psychiatrists and related professionals. Such opposition may have conquered the average person's willingness to continue the experiment, but Walter Freeman had never been average. He was an MD, a PhD, and a fellow of the American College of Physicians. It was not unlikely that his own brilliance led him to assume that his hunches had to be right. He also received enthusiastic praise which may help explain the intensity of his efforts. "This is a startling paper. I believe it will go down in medical history as a noted example of therapeutic courage," declared the famous neurologist and psychiatrist Spafford Ackerly.[91] Freeman was able to win a number of converts as he continued writing and speaking, but the most enthusiastic support came during the 1940s as stories of transformed lives began appearing in newspapers and magazines.

Time magazine announced the publication of *Psychosurgery*, the new book on that subject by Freeman and Watts with a report which missed both facts and reality (thanks to Freeman, I presume), but it undoubtedly did much to promote an increasing number of lobotomies. Freeman's work was portrayed as pioneering, leading a movement and being amazingly successful. *Time* proclaimed that mental patients were having "their psychoses surgically removed. . . . A score of U.S. surgeons are now using the revolutionary new technique."[92] But how could damaging the brain heal the mind?

The article explained that the frontal lobes held the mental power which controlled the thalamus, that part of the brain containing "fear, rage, lust, sorrow, other purely animal instincts."[93] Readers learned that psychosurgery cut many of the frontal lobe–thalamus connections. "Not all the connections are severed, since a patient might then become a victim of his unrestrained thalamus."[94] The neurologist–neurosurgeon team acknowledged their patients had changed personalities but were quoted as declaring, "The freedom from painful self–consciousness, and also with preoccupation with former conflict, repressions, frustrations and the like, and the associated elevation in mood, renders life particularly agreeable to them and they enjoy it to the fullest."[95]

That was not the conclusion reached by more objective researchers. In 1955 Oxford University Press published *Personality Changes Following Frontal Leucotomy* by Macdonald Tow. Intelligence, vocabulary, tempo, persistence, creativity and many other performance variables were measured before the subjects were lobotomized and were then measured again after the operation. Chapter after chapter revealed that lobotomized patients did suffer some intellectual declines, but that other changes were even more worrisome.

> On the fluency test the responses of the 'frontal' subject are often vague or general. They become uncolourful and repetitive, where they had been interesting and varied.[96]

> The complete process of thinking out, initiating, and successfully pursuing the correct method seemed affected at all stages. This disability is no doubt associated with the blank, perplexed expression which frequently meets the examiner's instructions and encouragement. It is not necessarily that he misunderstands. But he fails to select and remember those particulars which are essential to a proper conduct of the task before him.[97]

He also has a different reaction to his own responses: he is not worried by failures; and he is not elated by success, for he does not seem really to appreciate it.[98]

There is, then, a greater tolerance of poor performance, less trouble to correct errors, and less care or worry as to whether his mistakes are noticed or not; and there is much less concern over the quality of his whole performance.[99]

These and a multitude of additional comments pointed to a blunting effect. Lobotomies blunted intelligence, motivation, foresight, reasoning, drive and emotions. But these effects had been discussed for decades. Studies from 1917, 1919 and 1926 reported patients with frontal lobe injuries to have "a loss of spontaneity and loss of memory,"[100] "a general loss of spontaneity and initiative"[101] and "disturbed attention and tempo; alterations of mood . . . loss of initiative; tactlessness and moral defects,"[102] respectively. The *Time* article of 1942 which praised Freeman and his surgery so strongly also noted, "After recovery a patient's emotional responses are vivid but somewhat superficial. He is indifferent to social amenities, may speak his mind and joke so tactlessly that he embarrasses his family and friends. . . . His foresight is impaired."[103]

How could it be that, despite this decades–old awareness that lobotomies blunted the personality, lobotomies continued and even increased in number throughout the 1940s and into the 1950s. The observation which is most important to note is the relative unimportance of the professional medical literature in determining actual practice. One can look, for example, at the weeks following the awarding of the Nobel prize to Egas Moniz in 1949 and find the medical literature had numerous articles reporting the blunting and personality changes caused by the lobotomy.[104] But those articles did nothing to change the number of such operations. Between 1948 and 1952 approximately 5,000 lobotomies were performed each year.[105]

The neurosurgeons and psychiatrists who had become committed to the procedure continued despite the knowledge that the lobotomy's harmful

The Lobotomy:
So Simple a Psychiatrist Can Do It

The lobotomy experienced a rapid evolution. The first seven patients had two holes drilled into their heads into which alcohol could be injected. Dr. Egas Moniz then conceived of an even simpler approach—using a "leucotome" which could be pushed into the brain and moved so as to cut the nerves connecting the frontal lobes to the rest of the brain. Both techniques effectively destroyed the part of the brain found immediately behind the forehead.

The first nerve–severing lobotomies (called leukotomies by the "inventor") still required drilling a small hole on either side of the forehead. Drs. Walter Freeman and James Watts together conducted their first lobotomy in 1936. However, Freeman sought an even easier and quicker means to lobotomize patients, and hence his famous "icepick lobotomy." His basic approach became the standard in the U.S. for the majority of the thousands of lobotomies performed annually during the 1940s and 1950s.[1] A medical textbook from the era, *Shock Treatments, Psychosurgery, and Other Somatic Treatments in Psychiatry*, 2nd ed.,[2] described it as such a simple procedure that psychiatrists could perform the operation without the help of a neurosurgeon. I have outlined for you their simple instructions (quoting freely from the textbook).

1. Lift the upper eyelid away from the eyeball.
2. Place the point of the icepick (leucotome) at the top of the eye socket about 3 cm from the face's midline.
3. With the icepick parallel to the nose, use a hammer to drive the icepick 5 cm from the upper eyelid into the brain.
4. Move the icepick as far to the left and to the right as possible. (This will sever the thalamofrontal fibers at the base of the brain.)
5. Move the icepick back to a position parallel to the nose.
6. Drive the icepick to a depth of 7 cm.
7. Move the icepick 20 degrees up and down and 30 degrees left and right. (This will sever the superior portion of the thalamo-frontal radiation.)

The textbook then notes, "To these two cuts Freeman later added a 'deep frontal cut,' which is now probably used by all who perform the operation."[3] Instructions are then given for that cut, and then we are also told that "sometimes it is difficult to withdraw the instrument when the bone is very thick. Therefore, Moore replaced Freeman's 'ice–pick–like' instrument with a 'transorbitoma' whose shaft is elliptical."[4] (Another step forward for psychiatry.)

effects were permanent. Why? Because the issue had been framed in such a way that many in the profession and the public were willing to accept that harm in order to prevent what was falsely called the inevitable alternative. As *Time* put it, "Some of these changes would be undesirable if the alternative—an unchanged psychotic personality leading to complete insanity—were not much worse."[106]

What did finally bring a dramatic reduction in lobotomies were two media (film and print) events which solidified the opinions of both physicians and the public: (1) mental hospitals began to be portrayed as snake pits and their more severe medical procedures (insulin therapy, ECT and lobotomies) as ghastly mistakes[107] and (2) the "miracle" of new antipsychotic mind drugs were declared "one of the most spectacular triumphs in the history of medicine."[108]

Behavior is influenced far more by the perception of what is true and right than by truth itself. That is a lesson for which evidence never seems to be lacking in psychiatry.

Modern Medical Treatment: The Drug Approach

The Greek physician Asclepiades (c. 124–40 B.C.) rejected Hippocrates's four humors theory of mental and physical health, insisting instead that disease, including mental disease, resulted from the particles that make up the body being either too constricted or too relaxed. He advocated releasing the insane from confinement and providing them hot baths, improved diets and body massages, as well as applying poultices, draining blood from their bodies and giving them opium.[109]

His goal was the reshuffling of the body's "atoms," but his means of doing so makes him one of the earliest advocates of using a psychotropic drug (a drug that influences the mind) to improve one's mental health. Yet it is not reasonable to tie the history of what we call antipsychotics or antidepressants to the ancient Greeks or Romans. Instead, the history of our modern mind drugs must reasonably be tied to the relatively recent discovery of Thorazine, a famous drug initially identified as RP4560.

In 1949 Dr. Henri Laborit, a surgeon in the French Navy, was actively experimenting with various drugs in hopes of preventing the shock which sometimes resulted from surgery. Shock causes blood vessels to dilate which, in effect, results in a progressive reduction in the volume of circulating blood. This, in turn, causes the heart to beat faster than normal, but it is unable to pump enough blood to maintain normal body functions and normal blood pressure. The skin becomes pale and clammy, and breathing may become shallow and difficult. Recognizing their own physical distress, patients typically become anxious and begin sweating profusely. If not aided, the patient will grow increasingly weak, enter a comatose state and die. Dr. Laborit sought to overcome this threat to life. When he experimented with antihistamines (commonly taken today by those with asthma or allergies), he found the class of drugs he needed.

Antihistamines block the effects of histamine, a chemical our bodies produce as an immune system response to any plant or substance to which we are allergic. When histamines are released, our nose runs, eyes water and sneezing and itching begin. These are discomforting effects, but they are not life–threatening. However, a surge of histamines is also released when a serious wound occurs or when the chest is opened during surgery. The histamines can cause the blood vessels to dilate—a reaction that can bring on shock. Antihistamines do not stop the release of histamines or inactivate histamine. Instead, they block receptor sites, thereby preventing absorption and the sometimes life–threatening physical effects of histamine release.

After many months of experimentation, Laborit decided the synthetic antihistamine promethazine was the most effective in reducing shock. It also had another characteristic. It seemed to have a "strong hypnogenic action" and an "appreciable analgesic action."[110] Laborit was delighted with this discovery. This new synthetic antihistamine allowed him to discard morphine with its many undesirable side effects. Promethazine so relaxed his patients that most lost their fear of having surgery, an effect Laborit recognized might prove useful to psychiatry.

The French pharmaceutical firm Rhône–Poulenc owned the drug which Dr. Laborit was so pleased to have found. Yet he hoped Rhône–Poulenc might have an even more effective drug or one in development. His inquiries led a company chemist to synthesize a new group of related compounds. One of these new compounds was RP4560. (During the pre-marketing phase of drug development, new drugs are assigned a number rather than a name.)[111] RP4560 was found to counteract the effects of adrenaline. Adrenaline puts the body into high gear; RP4560 put it into the lowest gear. Its benefits for surgery were obvious.

Laborit had reported promethazine to be a very effective anesthetic when combined with "barbiturates, morphine, curare, procaine, TEA, and synthetic antihistamines."[112] And it was as one ingredient in an analgesic cocktail that RP4560 was first marketed. However, Laborit believed RP4560 was a significant advance, especially in inducing the apathetic state which would be desirable for surgery.[113]

BOX #12–6

A Thorazine "Trip" Described

Toward the end of 1951 a psychiatrist who was a friend of Laborit agreed to participate in a brief experiment by taking Thorazine herself. At 11:00 a.m. on November 9, 1951, she received an injection of RP4560 while Laborit and 3 colleagues stood by as witnesses. A week after the injection the psychiatrist recorded notes on her experience.

No subjective change was felt until 12:00, when I began to have the impression that I was becoming weaker, that I was dying. It was very painful and agonizing. At 12:55 . . . I experienced an illness more pronounced than depression. . . . At 1:00, an intense affective change appeared that the group noticed immediately: the painful feeling of imminent death disappeared to make room for a euphoric relaxation. I had felt all along that I was going to die, but this new state left me indifferent. . . . Although very much in touch with my surroundings, I was more and more overcome by an extreme feeling of detachment from myself and from others."[1]

A commonly used experiment with rats called the rope–climbing test confirmed that RP4560 was a very effective compound for blunting the emotions. Using Pavlov's classical conditioning principles, a Rhône–Poulenc team taught rats to climb a rope and reach a platform to avoid receiving an electrical shock. By simply ringing a bell immediately before passing an electrical current through the floor of the rats' cage, the rats quickly learned that whenever the bell rang, they had to jump to the rope to avoid being shocked. However, when rats were given large doses of RP4560, they became indifferent to the bell. Their activity level and muscular strength were not affected, but they simply didn't care that they were about to be shocked.[114] Clearly RP4560 had a powerful blunting effect on the emotions.

Rhône–Poulenc was ready to begin more widespread clinical testing. In 1951 clinical testing was an amazingly uncontrolled stab in the dark. New drugs were sent out to researchers, physicians and institutions in hopes that new, unknown uses could be found. As stated by Rhône–Poulenc scientist Pierre Koetschet, it was felt RP4560 might be "useful once the best areas of its use were discovered through clinical trials."[115]

Samples of the drug were sent to numerous physicians, especially in Paris. Samples were also provided to Rhône–Poulenc researchers, one of whom was Dr. J. Schneider who was associated with the Broussais Hospital in Paris. Dr. Schneider treated a woman who was severely agitated with mania with a sedative, but it calmed her for only 30 minutes. He then gave her the same sedative in combination with RP4560, and the woman went into a calm, ten–hour sleep.[116] Not only was the new drug able to blunt the emotions, it had a powerful sedative effect as well.

Not long after this experience the Saint Anne's Hospital (Hôpital Sainte–Anne), the largest psychiatric hospital in France, also received samples of RP4560. The samples were sent upon the request of Dr. Pierre Deniker, the University of Paris psychiatrist who was over the hospital's male wards. He had learned of the new drug from his brother–in–law, an anesthesiologist, and Deniker was eager to try it on the more difficult patients.[117] The results were dramatic.

Patients whom the staff had tried to control but had no hope of helping were suddenly calmed. Dr. Jean Thuillier, a physician at Saint Anne's and a colleague of Dr. Deniker, was an eye–witness to the miraculous effects. He described the patients before and then after Deniker gave them the new drug. Those admitted to the closed men's ward "cried, shrieked . . . had to be tied up, supported or put in a straitjacket."[118] Some of the patients had to be strapped to their beds and could be made to eat and were kept clean only with difficulty. But he writes that after RP4560 began to be used,

> Delirious patients admitted to the department a short time previously, who could not give the day, the month or even the year of their hospitalization, or know where they were or the circumstances that had led to their arrival at the hospital, regained their orientation, remembered the beginning of their illness, and began to discuss their case. . . . And if the fury and violence had given way to calmness and peace, the most evident sign of this extraordinary therapeutic result could be appreciated even from the outside of the building of the men's clinic—there was silence.[119]

Deniker shared his discovery with Jean Delay, the head of the University of Paris Department of Psychiatry, and he expressed considerable excitement. Together they began experimenting with agitated patients with schizophrenia or mania, and by the spring of 1952 had written a series of papers on their experiences with what is generally considered the drug which gave birth to the modern mind–drug era.[120]

To encourage use of its drug, Rhône–Poulenc organized numerous seminars at university centers and brought psychiatrists from other countries to Paris to see for themselves the effect of RP4560 at Saint Anne's. However at the beginning of 1953, they still had not tapped into the massive U.S. market. They had approached a number of U.S. pharmaceutical firms, but none seemed to have any interest. Psychiatry in America was so dominated by Freudian psychoanalysis by that time that there was a natural resistance to using a drug to treat mental problems. Yet it is nevertheless somewhat surprising that no pharmaceutical company was interested since RP4560 had so many possible uses.

In addition to its sedative effects, its ability to control pain and its value as a potentiate (drug–effect multiplier), the drug was found to be a highly effective anti–vomiting compound. In fact, it was this quality that prompted the pharmaceutical company SmithKline & French to enter into a licensing agreement with Rhône–Poulenc to manufacture and market the drug in America. The drug's ability to control nausea and vomiting prompted the initial interest, but it was the reports from Europe of RP4560's ability to help schizophrenics and those with agitated mania which led SmithKline & French to ask several psychiatrists to experiment with the drug. The results and reports were generally positive but not glowing. Numerous side effects were noted.

It was then that Heinz Lehmann and Gorman Hanrahan, two Canadian psychiatrists from Montreal, learned about chlorpromazine (the generic name assigned the drug once the testing period's "RP4560" label came to an end) and administered it to 71 psychiatric patients. The results were remarkable. Among those patients with acute mania (the most difficult and unpleasant patients found in mental hospitals), 19 out of 19 who completed treatment improved or recovered. Among chronic maniacs the same miraculous result was found for 8 out of 9 patients. Though not all those with schizophrenia improved, most did. The two psychiatrists reported, "Manic patients often will not object to bed rest, and patients who present management problems become tractable. Assaultive and interfering behavior ceases almost entirely."[121] They also wrote, "Feeding problems disappear rapidly, and the patient soon becomes cooperative to nursing care. The psychiatrist is surprised to find his manic patients amenable to reason."[122]

BOX #12–7

Dramatic Effect of Thorazine

One psychologist who was in training in 1955, when Thorazine first began to be used in America, described the dramatic effect at the institution where he worked:

> The ward patients fulfilled the oft–heard stereotypes of individuals "gone mad." Bizarreness, nudity, wild screaming, and an ever–present threat of violence pervaded the atmosphere. Fearfulness and a near–total preoccupation with the maintenance of control characterized the attitudes of the staff. Such staff attitudes were not unrealistic in terms of the frequency of occurrence of serious physical assaults by patients, but they were hardly conducive to the development or maintenance of an effective therapeutic program. Then, quite suddenly—within a period of perhaps a month—all this dramatically changed. The patients were receiving antipsychotic medication. The ward became a place in which one could seriously get to know one's patients on a personal level.[1]

One must only imagine the stress on hospital professionals and staff caused by working in an environment where many patients often screamed, cried, and acted hostile and violent to see why such a report helped bring rapid acceptance of this new mind drug. Imagine an entire ward going from bedlam to stability and reason! That article appeared in 1954, the same year the FDA approved the drug.[123]

Psychiatrist and mind–drug historian David Healy described the clamor and the unexpected profits SmithKline & French received from their "antivomiting" drug in 1955.

> State mental hospital doctors were so eager to use the drug that when chlorpromazine was finally launched as Thorazine, in 1955, even though the license application had been for an anti–emetic, the take–up in psychiatry was astonishing—SmithKline & French reportedly took in $75 million the first year the drug was sold.[124]

That was an astounding sum for 1955—a year in which the annual earnings for a full–time employee averaged only $3,924.[125] That success spurred other pharmaceutical companies to recognize the tremendous profits that could be made from mind drugs.[126] As SmithKline & French's marketing campaign went into high gear, sales began to soar. Almost every mental institution in America began to administer Thorazine to patients.

BOX #12–8

SmithKline & French's "Research"

As SmithKline & French began to recognize the potential profit to be made with Thorazine, the marketing efforts entered the realm of medical research. Research studies which discovered their new drug could treat a whole host of mental problems were paid for by the drug company. The research was sloppy and self–serving. It did not matter. Far fewer psychiatrists would ever analyze and critique the research design and methods than would be impressed by the studies' widely circulated conclusions—that Thorazine "is especially remarkable in that it can reduce severe anxiety, diminish phobias and obsessions, reverse or modify a paranoid psychosis, quiet manic or extremely agitated patients, and change the hostile, agitated, senile patient into a quiet, easily managed patient."[1]

SmithKline & French then established a speaker's bureau and published promotional materials which showed how much money states could save if patients were given Thorazine. Broken window costs would drop, staff turnover would decline and the number of staff needed would be less. With patients in a lethargic condition, the states could save money in many ways.[2]

As patients were given Thorazine, many of them were released from their institutions. Dramatic drops in the number of patients in state and county mental hospitals followed. The graph on the next page reveals what a revolutionary change occurred at public mental hospitals.

In fact "revolutionary" is the word most commonly associated with this period of psychiatry's history. Drugs changed the role of psychiatrist, the treatment of the insane and soon thereafter, as drugs were developed for mental problems, the treatment of anxiety, depression, OCD and other common disorders. Even today treatment for mental problems is primarily

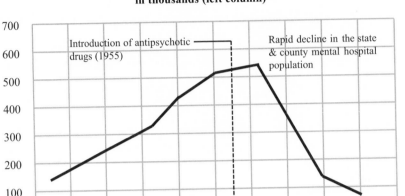

State and county mental hospital residents,
in thousands (left column)[127]

focused on choosing the best drug and the best dosage. Whether or not mind drugs should be given is hardly ever questioned by the psychiatrist. The issue has been settled. It should not be. In fact, this section on the history of Thorazine will leave you fooled unless you read "The Rest of the Story" which follows.

The Rest of the Story

It is understandable that so many are strong defenders of mind drugs. The history I just shared points to a far better world than experienced by the mentally ill before the advent of these drugs. Yet I am strongly opposed to their common use. "But why?" is the reasonable question. I am primarily opposed to these drugs because of the harm they do, but part of my opposition is also tied to the fact that most people believe mind drugs have benefits they do not have. They believe they have these benefits because they have been told repeatedly that they do. (It is also understandable that there were so many strong defenders of treating mental problems with torture, insulin shock therapy, metrazol convulsive therapy, ECT and even lobotomies. Families were desperate for cures, and each treatment did have some success. These treatments often boasted—whether true or not—of miraculous cures in cases that seemed hopeless.)

Praise and testimonials for antidepressants and antipsychotics are still found in almost any psychology text, in magazine articles, on "Oprah," in the literature found in doctors' offices and in advertisements on TV and elsewhere. But the truth is, the story I was taught about Thorazine when I took my first psychology course, the story that continues to be repeated over and over, is distorted. That story was the story I just shared with you. I, in fact, purposely presented a distorted story. I did not misquote anyone or falsify any facts myself. I chose, instead, to present the comments found in the textbooks I used as a student and the textbooks I have adopted as a professor, comments which contribute to America being fooled. These textbooks (and, again, the doctors' office literature, magazine articles, "Oprah" and advertisements as well) share "facts" that are nearly always unbalanced, distorted or simply myth.

BOX #12–9

The "Miracle" of Antipsychotics:
What Students Learn (Textbook Quotes)

"After the widespread introduction of antipsychotic drugs, starting in about 1955, the number of residents in state and county mental hospitals declined steeply."[1]

"Thanks to clozapine, Daphne Moss went 'from hating the sunshine in the morning to loving it.' No longer suffering from the paranoid delusion that her parents were witches, Moss began teaching school and living independently."[2]

"Drugs have shortened hospital stays and have greatly improved the chances that people will recover from major psychological disorders. Drug therapy has also made it possible for many people to return to the community, where they can be treated on an outpatient basis."[3]

"Where schizophrenia and major mood disorders are concerned, drugs will undoubtedly remain the primary mode of treatment."[4]

The chart on page 280 (the drop in the number of mental patients) is commonly found in popular psychology textbooks, but it is misleading. The earlier quote on the dramatic effect of Thorazine (Box #12–7) came from the abnormal psychology textbook I used in graduate school, but it is misleading. The quotes in Box #12–9, The "Miracle of Antipsychotics," came from two of the nation's most–used psychology textbooks—but these quotes are misleading. That story (more fairly called a myth) would lead us to believe that Thorazine and other mind drugs somehow repair broken brains. The textbooks fail to explain the real reason why loud patients became quiet. They do not discuss the permanent brain damage and missed opportunity for restored health that result from taking these drugs. They fail to note the "zombie" effect on patients who were given Thorazine, suggesting instead that Thorazine gave them back their lives. They fail to discuss any of the health consequences which result from taking antipsychotics. Neither do they explain the real reason the number of mental patients in state mental hospitals declined after 1955. It is time you knew the rest of the story. In the following pages I want to contrast the myth that is still taught and widely believed with facts that you have likely never heard before, even if you have been a psychology professor for decades.

Fact: Thorazine quieted mental patients with a "chemical lobotomy" effect.

Let's start with the 1954 article written by the two Canadian psychiatrists which reported such miraculous benefits for mental patients. Again, I reported the statistics and quoted from the article accurately. However, a careful reading of all their comments also points to the fact that Thorazine was, in effect, a "chemical lobotomy"—something never mentioned by any textbook. Thorazine researchers who considered Thorazine's psychiatric uses recognized this fact and actually used the word *lobotomy* to describe its effect.[128] So did the French naval surgeon Henri Laborit, who played such an important role in the development of Thorazine. He noted his colleague's view that Thorazine produces "a veritable medicinal lobotomy."[129]

Here are nine comments from Lehmann & Hanrahan's article that point out the sedation as well as the blunting of the emotions which characterize a patient who has been "chemically lobotomized."[130] To insure you see the real effect of this "miracle drug," the key drug–effect words are in bold type.

- Thorazine "produced a **type of depression** in animals which increased progressively with the dose." (p. 228)

- "Patients receiving large doses of [Thorazine] exhibit definite **motor retardation**, with an unsteady gait, while the **facial expression becomes rather wooden** and the general appearance resembles that of Parkinsonism." (p. 228)

- "There is usually **marked drowsiness**, which may increase to the point of [deep sleep]." (p. 228)

- "Tolerance develops rapidly and requires an increase in dosage after a few days to maintain a constant level of **sedation**." (p. 228)

- "After the first week of treatment the patients **remain retarded** but less sleepy." (p. 229)

- "Patients receiving the drug became **lethargic**." (p. 230)

- Patients "tend to **remain silent and immobile** when left alone and to reply to questions in a **slow monotone**."(p. 230)

- "Some state that they **feel 'washed out'** as after an exhausting illness, a complaint which is indeed in keeping with their appearance." (p.230)

- "Although a patient under the influence of [Thorazine] at first glance presents the aspect of a **heavily drugged person**, one is surprised at the absence of clouding of consciousness." (p. 231)

Drs. Lehmann and Hanrahan then noted that at that time there were only two therapies known to be effective in treating patients who were loud, aggressive and uncontrollable—electroconvulsive therapy (ECT) and sedation "including prolonged sleep therapy." They observed that "ECT provides excellent and immediate control of symptoms if administered intensively," but it had some unpleasant side effects. Thorazine accomplished the same effect (quieted loud patients), but was far easier to administer. No, Thorazine was not providing a missing chemical; it was getting the patient under control the same way ECT and lobotomies did—by powerfully drugging (and damaging) the brain, especially the frontal lobes. We should thus expect a "zombie" effect. (See Box #12–10, The Frontal Lobes.)

BOX #12–10

The Frontal Lobes

The frontal lobes of the brain contain much of what makes us human. Therein is found the seat of our own self–awareness, curiosity, drive, will, maturity, aspirations, emotions and foresight, as the following quotes make plain.

As human beings have the largest and most fully developed frontal lobes of all animals, these are considered "the organ of civilization" or "the seat of abstract intelligence." The frontal lobes are also important to insight, one of the primary capacities that separate us from the apes.[1]

There is no question that the area of the brain that contributes to your sense of self more than any other is the frontal lobe.[2]

The frontal lobes are concerned with understanding social and behavioral rules and using these rules to plan and anticipate the consequences of one's actions.[3]

The person with frontal lobe damage inhabits a robotic world. It would not be an exaggeration to say he is deprived of his humanity.[4]

As well as being the place where the will is generated, the frontal lobes play a role in the way we link our perceptions and our awareness of ourselves into a coherent experience. In other words, this is the area where we attach meaning to life.[5]

Fact: **Thorazine and other mind drugs were not responsible for a dramatic decline in the number of patients in the nation's mental hospitals after 1955.**

Look again at the textbook graph (p. 280) which reveals that the number of mental hospital patients dropped dramatically after Thorazine was introduced. Now, let's consider some facts. First, there was a decline, but there was not a dramatic decline in the number of patients in mental hospitals after the mind drugs were introduced. The table below shows the number of patients in state and county mental hospitals at the end of each of several years surrounding the 1955 peak. None of the annual declines following 1955 exceeded 1.35%. And the five–year decline (1955–1960) was only 4.19%.

Year	Patients	Decline
1951	520,326	--
1952	531,981	--
1953	545,045	--
1954	553,979	--
1955	558,922[1]	--
1956	551,390[1]	1.35%
1957	548,626[2]	.51%
1958	545,182[2]	.63%
1959	541,883[2]	.61%
1960	535,540[2]	1.18%

1. *Statistical Abstract of the United States*, 1960, Table 94, p. 78
2. *Statistical Abstract of the United States*, 1965, Table 96, p. 77

Germany, which also gave schizophrenics Thorazine and the other early antipsychotic (Reserpine), did not see a decline in the number of patients in its mental hospitals. Neither did Austria.[131] And Norway found that during "the important part of hospital stay between 2 and 6 months," providing patients mind drugs actually resulted in slightly longer hospital stays.[132]

Objection: "But look at that graph (p.280). Thorazine was approved in 1955, and the number of patients did immediately begin dropping. Thorazine must have been, at least, a major factor in that drop."

Response: Clearly that is the impression that both the textbooks' comments and the graph want to convey. But the reality is that this illustrates the kind of errors which we can find in most textbooks. That graph, if closely examined, has three major errors.

(1) The number of patients in state and county mental hospitals did begin dropping after 1955. However the graph shows that the decline did not begin until after 1962. The graph misses when the drop began by seven years!

(2) The introduction of Thorazine is shown to have been in 1955. But, the fact is, Thorazine began to be distributed in 1953[133] and then obtained FDA approval in March of 1954.

(3) The graph ties together the introduction of mind drugs and a "rapid decline in state and county mental hospital population." As I have already noted, there was no rapid decline beginning in the 1950s when the mind drugs became so widely prescribed. The rapid decline actually began in the 1960s. I have explained the real reason for the decline in Appendix 3 beginning on page 393.

A Better Alternative: Moral Treatment

Absent from this history on how mental problems have been treated is what became known as the "moral treatment" movement. It is the one approach that may honestly be termed a success. Evidence of its effectiveness is found in two facts I shared in the preface. (1) Those who develop schizophrenia in many third world countries (India, Nigeria, Columbia) which have little access to antipsychotic drugs have much higher recovery rates (where family members commonly care for the mentally disturbed) than do those in the United States and other wealthy nations who are prescribed those drugs.[134] (2) Two hundred years ago, long before antipsychotics were invented, when someone lost his or her mind and was sent to a moral treatment center or state hospital practicing moral therapy, he or she was much more likely to recover than are Americans who lose their minds today.[135]

Such statistics are hard to believe and, of course, strongly suggest that our nation has taken the wrong road. However if it were simply understood that drugs reduce the brain's ability to perform properly, then these facts should not be at all surprising. How can a brain that is not fully functional, that has been "blunted," be expected to return to normal functioning even when an ideal treatment is provided the person who has lost his or her mind? Yet psychiatry has so adopted the biochemical approach to "fixing" the brain that it is hard for most psychiatrists to accept these two condemning statistics.[136] Obviously, such studies make the Western world's psychiatrists look not just ineffective but dangerous.

As already noted, following the rise of the mental hospital, those placed in these institutions were commonly treated like wild animals. Many believed that insanity was incurable. Virtually all others were convinced that insanity could only be overcome if treatments were applied that in most cases could be described as nothing less than torture. Many were chained and consequently, forced to sit in their own filth. Most admitted to these asylums would not survive more than three years.[137] However another approach developed during the late 1700s that challenged the traditional methods. The name which is most often remembered as a leader of a more humane and moral approach is Philippe Pinel.

Pinel had been appointed as the director of a Paris asylum by the French Revolutionary government. The acting director had instituted humanitarian reforms which resulted in the impossible—some victims improved or recovered. Pinel was most impressed and proposed to continue the reforms. Despite opposition and abuse, he unchained the captives, occupied their time with meaningful activity, and soon witnessed the return to sanity for many patients. Pinel's efforts were very important and influential, but it is the work of a lesser known reformer, William Tuke, that advanced "moral treatment" to a new height.

It was only a few years after Pinel unchained asylum victims that William Tuke, an English Quaker, established "The Retreat," a home for Quakers who had developed mental problems. In 1791 a Quaker woman lost her mind and was placed in an asylum near Tuke's home in York, England. Her family lived a considerable distance from York, so they requested that Quakers living in the asylum's vicinity visit the woman. But the Quakers were not allowed to see the woman, the asylum claiming that the woman was not in a state suitable for a visit. Within a few weeks of her admission, she was dead.

The result of this sad conclusion was that at the close of the Quarterly Meeting of the Society of Friends at York in March of 1792, William Tuke proposed that the Society of Friends establish an asylum for the care of their fellow Quakers who might develop insanity. He hoped to establish an asylum in which the insane were treated with kindness rather than abuse. Some objected on the grounds that the insane could not be helped. Others felt that the severe treatment the insane generally received was necessary.[138] Tuke believed it was mental stress that caused insanity and that the abuse, insults and chaining of the asylums were both inhumane and not likely to help bring any healing to the mind.

He and his fellow Quakers did establish a home where patients were to be given adequate amounts of food; would take walks, exercise, read and take warm baths; and would be kept busy by engaging in labor or, if women, would be employed in sewing, knitting or other domestic work. Keeping the patient occupied "is perhaps the most generally efficacious."[139] Tuke observed that even the insane desired to be esteemed, and meeting that need "is found to have great influence, even over the conduct of the insane."[140] The superintendent would thus introduce topics which would allow the patients to display their knowledge.[141]

The superintendent and staff also sought to encourage a reflection on religious principles and participation in religious meetings. "A profound silence generally ensues; during which, as well as at the time of [Bible] reading, it is very gratifying to observe their orderly conduct, and the degree in which those, who are much disposed to action, restrain their different propensities."[142]

Tea parties would be held by The Retreat where patients were to dress up and vie with one another showing politeness and proper behavior. "The evening generally passes in the greatest harmony and enjoyment."[143] And what were the results of The Retreat's kind and common sense approach? Careful records were kept concerning every person admitted to The Retreat beginning with its founding in 1796. Examining their records we find that during its first 15 years, 66% of those who had been insane for no more than one year when admitted fully recovered their sanity within 12 months and another 6% recovered the state of mental health present before afflicted with insanity.[144]

The work of Pinel and Tuke became known as "moral treatment." The basic assumption of those who favored moral treatment was that life's stresses could rob one of his senses. The stresses to the mind were known to arise from both psychological causes ("the disappointments and tragedies of life") and physical causes. It was believed that treating these victims morally (with respect, dignity and kindness) and encouraging moral behavior (dressing properly, spending time in productive pursuits, engaging in social interaction) could restore their sanity if the brain was not organically damaged. They were observant of each patient, engaging each in regular conversation and giving compliments whenever improvements were noticed. Patients were treated as much as possible as though their minds were healthy. They were given the freedom to roam the grounds and enjoy the fresh air.[145]

John Butler, MD, the superintendent of the Connecticut Retreat for the Insane, put moral therapy into action at his asylum and was so impressed with the results that he published a book entitled *The Curability of Insanity*. In it he wrote that the "greatest evil" of asylums is monotony.[146] What is needed for cures to occur is the theme of his entire book, but even one sentence indicates how very different moral therapy asylums were when compared with today's monotonous mental hospitals.

> Music, games, all social or intellectual gatherings and recreations, excursions, changes of scene and localities, art, in its various forms of beauty, pictures, engravings, statuary, and above all other things, flowers—they are ever most welcome.[147]

We are fortunate that in the United States virtually all state–supported mental hospitals are required to submit reports to state legislatures each year. As these reports have been compiled and analyzed, a disturbing picture is painted. Worcester State Hospital began as an institution committed to moral treatment. As the years passed, the standards of treatment began to fall. Patient to caregiver ratios increased, and moral therapists were replaced by professional psychiatrists who focused on diagnosis. Most were trained to think in terms of brain pathology. J. Sanbourne Bockoven, author of *Moral Treatment in Community Mental Health*, compiled data from 120 years of Worcester's annual reports. Looking at the percentage of admissions discharged from that institution for having mentally recovered, he found it fell from 45% to 4%.[148]

When only those who had been mentally ill for less than one year were considered, the early recovery rate was even more impressive. Of the 734 patients admitted during Worcester State Hospital's first ten years, 72.8% recovered and another 7.2% improved.[149] This is a more rational approach to determining effectiveness, since organic cases (those who could not recover as their brains were permanently damaged by disease, alcohol or trauma) made up a larger proportion of the hospital's population each year.

Why is moral treatment essentially not used today? After all, recovery rates today are far below those reported by Dr. Pinel[150] or Samuel Tuke[151] 200 years ago. Tuke provided details on each patient admitted between 1796 and 1811, and from this data it is possible to document the truth of Tuke's assessment of York Retreat's effectiveness. Nevertheless their approach was criticized by some. Thomas Dunston, superintendent of St. Luke's Hospital for Lunaticks in London observed, "You carry kind treatment at the Retreat too far," and expressed his belief that fear was "the most effectual principle by which to reduce the insane to orderly conduct."[152]

But moral treatment has not been abandoned today because it fails to instill fear in patients. No, moral treatment has essentially disappeared because biological psychiatry has come to dominate the profession. Insanity is no longer seen as a response to tremendous stress or to fear or rejection or to an aimless life. It is now seen as a genetically influenced, biological problem that can only be successfully treated by drugs. How unfortunate that psychiatry has departed from the conclusions recorded by Philippe Pinel in 1806 in his "Treatise on Insanity":

> Desirous of better information, I resolved to examine for myself the facts that were presented to my attention. . . . I viewed the scene that was opened to me with the eyes of common sense and unprejudiced observation. . . . I then discovered, that insanity was curable in many instances, by mildness of treatment and attention to the mind exclusively. . . . My faith in pharmaceutic preparations was gradually lessened, and my skepticism went at length so far, as to induce me never to have recourse to them until moral remedies had completely failed. . . . Successful application of moral regimen exclusively gives great weight to the supposition, that, in the majority of instances, there is no organic lesion of the brain nor of the cranium.[153]

13

SIDE EFFECTS
OF ANTIPSYCHOTICS

Allen's schizophrenia developed over a two–year period following his graduation from high school. At first the behaviors were worrisome but not illegal or immoral. Allen claimed that he was Superman. He became convinced that the government was plotting against him. He called various family members regularly and talked on and on about fantastic facts which they all knew were proof that Allen was "going crazy." When he began ringing his neighbor's doorbell claiming they were living in his house, the police, courts and state mental hospital got involved. Allen was given antipsychotics and, after a few weeks, was released back to his family.

Allen returned home, maintaining his irrational ideas, but the drugs kept him so tame that everyone was relieved by the change. It was not until he stopped taking his antipsychotics that Allen became very troublesome again. His family had some concerns about the drugs he was on, but they would much prefer he be on drugs than continue the behaviors and "crazy thinking" that occurred before he was given those drugs.

Allen's case is typical. Not knowing what else to do and desperate for some way to end the crazy behavior, parents and other family members are often highly committed to mind drugs. They are almost never aware that taking antipsychotics will almost certainly keep their loved one from ever recovering. They are told the "disease" will likely require that the antipsychotics be taken for life. Since the drugs do blunt the mind and, hence, help control the behavior, this is a commitment they readily accept. I doubt they would be so willing to accept permanent drugging if they knew that though drugging keeps their loved one under control it also prevents his or her recovery and the opportunity to have a normal life. That is what most concerns me about antipsychotics, but that is just one of the several side effects that most family members have never heard about—permanent brain damage, shortened lifespan, tardive dyskinesia, akathisia and vacuous chewing movements just to name a few.

Permanent Brain Damage

If it were not for animal research, we would not know how damaging antipsychotics are to the brain. (See Box #13–1, Using Animals for Drug Research.) CT scans and PET scans and other imaging techniques each yield information, but some facts can only be discovered by methods that cannot be used with humans. The research studies that have done the most to shed light on the effects of antipsychotics on the brain are those involving macaque monkeys.

A research team at the University of Pittsburgh gave groups of macaque monkeys (consisting of six monkeys each) either one of two popular antipsychotics or a placebo for 17–27 months. The dosages were comparable to what are typically given to humans as determined by measuring the

Using Animals for Drug Research

Many Americans believe it is unethical to use animals in doing research. They may not be aware that no drug receives FDA approval until it has been used in animals. It would be unethical to give 50 premature newborns a new drug which might strengthen their immune systems but might also cause cancer or permanent brain damage. Of course, we never know for sure what harmful side effects a drug may have until it has been tested (and often discover unseen and unsuspected consequences years after approval for use in humans). To reduce the number of human tragedies, we use animals—approximately 85% of which are rats, mice and guinea pigs bred for use in laboratory research.[1]

Virtually every great medical advancement utilized animals in the early stages of the research program. Animals were used in developing insulin for diabetics, chemotherapy drugs for cancer patients and antibiotics for all of us. Animals were immunized for rabies, polio, measles, mumps and hepatitis before any humans ever received any vaccinations. Without the use of animals, we would never have developed the ability to perform coronary bypasses; heart, lung, kidney or liver transplants; arthroscopic surgery and hip replacements to name but a few examples.[2]

The other animal research question that arises is "Are animals enough like humans to make them valid experimental subjects?" The list I just noted of benefits we have already received from animal research should make the answer apparent. Other mammals may be very different from us in many ways, but they also have brains, hearts, lungs, kidneys, livers, a circulatory system, a nervous system, glands, hormones and neurotransmitters. Drugs that harm animals are likely to harm humans in the same way. Drugs that benefit animals are likely to benefit humans in the same way. Because of these facts scientists and governments throughout the world demand animal experiments be performed before experimental studies using humans are allowed.[3]

amount of the drugs in the monkey's blood. The results were dramatic. The monkeys receiving the placebo had no ill effects. The monkeys receiving either of the antipsychotics experienced brain shrinkage of approximately 20%![2] Humans tend to stay on these drugs much longer than just 17–27 months. Most are told they will need these drugs the rest of their lives.

It has been known for many years that the brains of schizophrenics are smaller at autopsy than the brains of healthy subjects.[3] It has been argued that this is proof that schizophrenia is a brain disease that damages the brain thus causing schizophrenia. But, once again, the cause and effect issues have been mixed up. Thanks to the macaque monkey experiments, we have proof that brain shrinkage results from taking these drugs.

If the monkeys were sufficiently stressed, the chemical changes caused by the stress would also damage and shrink their brains. There is an abundance of research on seriously stressed individuals (and rats) experiencing a decrease in brain size.[4] Is it not apparent why Americans who develop schizophrenia never get over it and eventually die with it while those in third world countries, if cared for by family when they lose their mind, are often free of schizophrenia symptoms within months or a year or two?

Shortened Lives and Sudden Death

Being diagnosed with schizophrenia is, to some degree, akin to a death sentence. Death rates for schizophrenics are much higher than healthy individuals. We have assumed that this was due to all the additional stress factors (see pp. 309–310 for risk factors associated with schizophrenia) as well as the several unhealthy behaviors and health problems more commonly found among schizophrenics—smoking, obesity, diabetes, HIV and hepatitis infection, and hypertriglyceridemia.[5] However, in 2005 the FDA issued a public health advisory which warned that these drugs can cause death.[6] The advisory was targeted at discouraging physicians from prescribing antipsychotics for elderly patients who have dementia. Some elderly people become more difficult to deal with as their minds begin to fail, and some physicians prescribe antipsychotics to help control their behavior.

However, the FDA has determined that the drugs themselves increase death rates by 60 to 70 percent. The most common causes of death are heart failure and infections (especially pneumonia) which indicate that when the mind is weakened, the entire body is weakened. Though the FDA's 2005 public health advisory was concerned with the elderly, we have had research for years that indicates that at least some antipsychotics can cause sudden cardiac death even in young adults. A study of 481,744 Medicaid patients in Tennessee found that those taking Haldol, Mellaril or some other older antipsychotics were more than twice as likely to die suddenly of heart failure even if they had never had heart problems before.[7] Newer (atypical) antipsychotics appear to have similar risks.[8]

In more recent years the study designs have improved and the antipsychotic–sudden death relationship is now firmly established with those taking antipsychotics having about three times the risk of sudden death. One study concluded, "Current use of antipsychotics in a general population is associated with an increased risk of sudden cardiac death, even at low doses," and then added, "Risk of sudden cardiac death was highest among recent users but remained elevated during long–term use."[9] How many patients on these drugs have ever heard such facts? I don't believe I have ever met even one who was familiar with this information.

Movement Disorders

Antipsychotic drugs cause several different kinds of movement disorders, more technically called extrapyramidal symptoms (EPS). The FDA fails miserably in requiring exact estimates of how many patients treated with antipsychotics will develop movement disorders over a length of time comparable to how long (many years) patients are actually on these drugs. The FDA's approved statement for Zyprexa, America's best–selling antipsychotic drug, in discussing one type of movement disorder known as tardive dyskinesia reads, "Whether antipsychotic drug products differ in their potential to cause tardive dyskinesia is unknown."[10]

Isn't it amazing that the FDA has routinely approved new antipsychotics though they claim to have no idea if one is any safer than another? It is even more amazing that this same statement has been included in the drug insert sheet for Zyprexa and several other antipsychotics for many years. What could be more important in prescribing these drugs than knowing exactly how much risk is involved? These drugs have been taken by millions of

Americans for years now. Claiming not to know how much risk is involved is inexcusable. (Remember, as noted in Chapter 9, in reality the FDA hates to compare one drug with other similar drugs. Doing so could cause a company receiving a "bad comparison" to lose business and employees. So the FDA speaks in general terms and claims it just does not know which drugs are the safest.)

More helpful are the results of the short six–week study Eli Lilly submitted to the FDA in seeking approval for Zyprexa. That study, available for viewing in the *Physicians' Desk Reference* (a copy of which can be found in any public library), reports that among patients taking 15 mg of Zyprexa per day, 20% developed "parkinsonism events" which also included tremors, a shuffling walk, slowed movements and a relatively expressionless face. (Many patients receive prescriptions for doses of 30–40 mg per day.)[11] Even at the lower 10 mg per day dose, 14% develop some kind of parkinsonism events.

Those numbers are higher than they should be. Why? The answer is simply that the shaking, twitching and other involuntary movements associated with taking antipsychotics are so well known that many patients actually fake some of these symptoms. (Proof of this is seen when some patients, given a placebo, develop these symptoms also.) But parkinsonism, like the slower to develop but similar tardive dyskinesia, is no minor event. Just a brief description of tardive dyskinesia will allow you to agree.

Tardive Dyskinesia

Tardive dyskinesia (TD) is a condition involving repetitive and involuntary muscle spasms or tics of the face, tongue, shoulders, arms, hands and/or feet. It is not a condition that is easily ignored. The victim has no control over the shaking movements, and one suspects they have Parkinson's disease. (In fact, TD is also termed "neuroleptic–induced parkinsonism," neuroleptic being another term for an antipsychotic drug.) Most commonly the symptoms include chewing, tongue protrusion, lip smacking, grimacing, blinking and foot tapping.

Conventional antipsychotics caused severe TD, and the search for drugs with less dramatic side effects brought us what are now called atypical antipsychotics.[12] However the atypical antipsychotics also cause movement disorders. (We have assumed they cause tardive dyskinesia at lower rates than the older antipsychotic drugs, but some research is suggesting that the superiority of atypicals to the conventional antipsychotics is debatable.[13]) And the atypicals are also known to carry weight gain and diabetes mellitus risks as noted in Chapter 3, How Psychiatrists and Doctors Are Fooled.

Symptoms can start immediately, but they usually begin several months or years after drug treatment begins. The longer patients have been on a drug, the higher their drug dosage and the older they are, the greater the chance of developing TD. It can even begin years after being off the mind drugs. There is no cure for this disorder, and it only rarely goes away. Remission, when it does occur, is typically in younger patients who have not been taking antipsychotic drugs for several years.[14]

A study of older patients (who are more prone to develop TD than younger patients) found that the condition emerged in 53% of the subjects within three years of drug exposure.[15] A study of younger patients that examined the first five years of drug exposure found that 20% had TD within that time period.[16]

I have already noted that TD is generally irreversible, but what will your psychiatrist do for you if you develop the shaking and twitching symptoms of TD? Believe it or not, the most prominent routine today is to treat these symptoms with a larger dose of the very antipsychotic drug that causes the brain damage to begin with. No one claims this will heal the problem. We know that it won't. But these patients will be treated again with antipsychotics. It will damage the brain further and shorten their lives, but it does help keep the shaking under control.[17]

The *Physicians' Desk Reference*
and Tardive Dyskinesia

The *Physicians' Desk Reference* (*PDR*) is the Bible of drugs. It is considered the authoritative work because all the drug information found in the *PDR* has been generated by the drug manufacturers, submitted to the Food and Drug Administration (FDA), rewritten and approved by the FDA and then sent back to the manufacturers for use as drug package inserts and inclusion in the *PDR*.

Concerning antipsychotics the official FDA warning reads as follows:

Tardive Dyskinesia

A syndrome of potentially irreversible, involuntary movements may develop in patients treated with antipsychotic drugs. Although the prevalence of the syndrome appears to be highest among the elderly, especially elderly women, it is impossible to rely upon prevalence estimates to predict, at the inception of antipsychotic treatment, which patients are likely to develop the syndrome. Whether antipsychotic drug products differ in their potential to cause tardive dyskinesia is unknown.

The risk of developing tardive dyskinesia and the likelihood that it will become irreversible are believed to increase as the duration of treatment and the total cumulative dose of antipsychotic drugs administered to the patient increase. However, the syndrome can develop, although much less commonly, after relatively brief treatment periods at low doses.[1]

Are patients routinely told that taking an antipsychotic even for a month may lead to permanent, irreversible, involuntary tics, tongue and lip–smacking, a gaited walk and other potential effects? It may seem unreasonable to believe that any physician would not explain this risk to the patient and his or her family, but my own experience has repeatedly found that those on these drugs are unaware of these risks.

Now, let's return to the FDA–approved package insert sheet for Zyprexa. and read what it says about tardive dyskinesia. (It is identical to the FDA–approved warning for all antipsychotics. See Box #13–2.)

Tardive Dyskinesia — A syndrome of potentially irreversible, involuntary, dyskinetic movements may develop in patients treated with antipsychotic drugs. Although the prevalence of the syndrome appears to be highest among the elderly, especially elderly women, it is impossible to rely on prevalence estimates to predict at the inception of antipsychotic treatment, which patients are likely to develop a syndrome. . . . The risk of developing tardive dyskinesia and the likelihood that it will become irreversible are believed to increase as the duration of treatment and the total cumulative dose of antipsychotic drugs administered to the patient increase. However, the syndrome can develop, although much less commonly, after relatively brief treatment periods at low doses.[18]

Most patients probably either do not read those warnings, do not appreciate the full implications of what these warnings are saying or perhaps discount the warning based on the assumption that their doctor wouldn't prescribe a drug that was not wise to take. My experience tells me that few patients who go to a psychiatrist (for any reason) leave without a mind drug prescription. For those who report hearing voices or have disturbed thinking, there is only the smallest chance that they will not be prescribed an antipsychotic.

Akathisia

Akathisia is another well–known side effect of taking antipsychotics. If we once again use Zyprexa as an example (we should assume that, as the nation's most popular antipsychotic, it has fewer side effects than would other drugs in this group), we learn that 11% of those on Zyprexa (10 mg/day) experienced "akathisia events" in a six–week trial developed by the drug's manufacturer.[19] To understand the nature of akathisia, consider the experiment conducted by the drug authority and researcher David Healy.

Using normal, healthy volunteers from among the students, nurses and other medical staff at a British university, Dr. Healy asked participants to drink some orange juice which contained low doses of an antipsychotic, a tranquilizer or a placebo. Obviously, none of the study's participants knew which of the three their own juice contained. The purpose of the experiment was to see if the effects of different drugs could be measured using computerized tasks. However, the purpose of the experiment was quickly overshadowed by the powerful drug effect on those given the antipsychotic.

> This was not akathisia with obviously restless feet; it was a restlessness whose sufferers might opt to move around without being fully able to explain why. Unlike foot–tapping restlessness, which can sometimes happen without the person being upset by it, these volunteers were uncomfortable. . . . We later convened a focus group for those who had been on [the antipsychotic] to get a better idea of what had happened to them. To a person, they felt [depressed and unwell], unsettled, and disturbed even while telling me they felt fine. They found it difficult to put their unexpected experiences into words. It was not like anything that had happened to them before. Some had said nothing because they didn't want to make fools of themselves, assuming they might be on placebo, and worried that complaints might simply demonstrate their suggestibility. Others felt awful but couldn't believe the drug was causing this. They had begun to think about some of the worst moments in their life. Highly personal memories of previous unhappy times—broken relationships or loneliness—seemed to be flooding back.[20]

Healy's account goes on to relate how a professor of clinical psychology who received the antipsychotic began crying within an hour of drinking his orange juice. Another colleague "became irritable and belligerent." A psychiatrist who also received the antipsychotic was transformed. She swung between feelings of restlessness and paralysis and became suicidal before the week was out—all from one pill! It is hard to believe that a single pill can cause such major disturbances as well as such different reactions. (See Box #13–3, Drug Reactions Are Not Always Predictable.)

BOX #13-3

Drug Reactions Are Not Always Predictable
"Benadryl Will Help You Sleep Well"

When I fly overseas I take two small Benadryl pills to guarantee hours of good sleep. A few years ago my father said he wasn't sleeping as well as he once did. When you are in your 80s, you are not supposed to sleep like a baby, but nevertheless, I thought I could help by suggesting he take a couple of Benadryl pills. He had never tried Benadryl, but I was sure it would give him a good night's sleep. The next morning when he came in he exclaimed, "Those pills! I've never had an experience like that in all my life. My legs were restless and I shook all night. I'm still just jittery."

I checked the warning label and, sure enough, listed as common reactions were drowsiness (my reaction) and insomnia, nervousness and restlessness (my father's reaction). Isn't it amazing that a drug that can give me a night of sound sleep would make my father nervous and sleepless? That difference may be due to the difference in our ages, but since that incident, I have had others who are younger than myself tell me their experience with Benadryl was similar to my father's.

Benadryl is generally considered one of the safest drugs a person can take because it has a long track record and has been taken daily by large numbers of people. Yet even Benadryl can cause unpredictable reactions, which should remind us that we must approach the decision to consume drugs with the knowledge that not all of us will react in the same way.

Endometrial Cancer

Because funding for and publication of studies that run counter to the interests of the pharmaceutical industry are suppressed (see Box #9–2, What Gets Published?) and because those that do get published always risk harsh professional responses[21] (remember that much of the published research on mind drugs is done by pharmaceutical company scientists and professors who are partially supported or receive extra income from drug companies), the number of studies examining the harmful effects of antipsychotics is only a small fraction of the total literature on these drugs.

Dr. Koji Yamazawa and his research team designed a high–quality research study (3 matched controls for every study subject) looking at a possible increased risk of endometrial cancer for those taking antipsychotics. They had good reason to suspect an increase since studies for more than three decades have been reporting that antipsychotics increase levels of the hormone prolactin,[22] and elevated prolactin has been known to cause the growth of tumors for nearly as long.[23] As anticipated, what they found was that antipsychotics put women at a 5.4 times increased risk of getting endometrial cancer.[24]

I was not surprised by this finding. However I could not find any other antipsychotic–endometrial cancer studies. That did surprise me, and it did not make sense because, as Dr. Yamazawa correctly realized, we should expect more endometrial cancer in those taking antipsychotics. I asked Dr. Yamazawa what his thinking was as to why other studies had not been done in this area. He was also surprised but found it difficult to explain.[25]

Being located in Japan, it is very likely he is not familiar with the extent of drug company sponsorship of research in the U.S., the publication bias of findings, the failure of drug companies to do Phase 4 studies and the pharmaceutical industry–FDA relationship. Drug companies have little incentive to investigate any adverse effects which the FDA does not insist they explore. Those side effects which do not show up for many years are not too difficult to ignore. Add to this the fact that we have forgotten how to help the schizophrenic recover and have been convinced it is a disease which only drugs can control.

If we believe there are no other options, then we are more prone to accept "what has to be done." Even many family members would likely prefer taking a chance on cancer than having to cope with the ongoing burden of a difficult, out–of–control person in their home who disrupts and complicates their lives. I am not unsympathetic, but I also know there is a better option.

14

WHAT REALLY CAUSES SEVERE MENTAL PROBLEMS (SCHIZOPHRENIA)?

Diane was typical of those students who come to see me as class ends whenever I lecture on schizophrenia. I had shared the Genain quadruplet hoax and the research on the lack of long–term recovery in America compared with those countries that do not use drugs to treat mental disorders. I had also shared how schizophrenia can develop in a mind that has been perfectly normal.

At that point in time, Diane's brother had been a schizophrenic for years, but she had never heard that schizophrenia could be caused by anything other than a chemical imbalance in the brain. I said, "Let's see how well the risk factors fit in your brother's case. How old was your brother when he developed schizophrenia?"

Diane: "20 years old."

"Are your parents married?"

Diane: "No, they divorced when he was 5."

"How was high school for him?"

Diane: "Awful. My father moved out of the country when my brother was 14. When they came back, he hated school. In fact, he stopped going and no matter what my dad tried, he couldn't make him go to school. In the end he got his GED."

I asked her to tell me more. After the divorce, Diane's mom got the kids, but she was always drunk or on drugs. They had been with her for just under two months when she exploded one day, called the police and said, "Get rid of them. I don't want them."

> The police took us with them right then, and we were placed in foster care for the next couple of months. Finally my dad took custody of us. Life with Dad involved a series of live–ins. One of them had a little boy, and she didn't want us around herself or her boy, so we could never come into the house until my dad got home. So we sat on the front porch a lot whenever she lived with us. Finally, one of his girl friends kicked me out, though my brother was allowed to stay. But he was hanging out with a bunch of guys who smoked marijuana and did drugs and were nothing but trouble. My brother was about 15 then, and he, of course, started doing whatever his friends were doing. But after he began taking those drugs, he would blow up over nothing.

Diane said the conflict at home became intense. Her brother and her father would argue constantly. Finally, the brother was forced to leave. He was working and was making it until he lost his job and became homeless. By the time he turned 20 he was hearing voices. His father brought him home and took him to counseling, but he grew worse and soon was getting SSI (Social Security Insurance). Diane wanted to assure me that she knew her dad didn't always make the best choices for herself and her brother as they grew up, but he did love and care about them both.

My dad really wants to help him now. He says he thinks the drugs the psychiatrist put him on are doing my brother more harm than good—my brother can't even engage in a coherent conversation now—but the psychiatrist won't even talk to him about it. Dad asked the psychiatrist if he could meet with him at his office, but all the bills are paid by SSI, so the psychiatrist can just ignore my dad. He won't even talk to him on the phone. Dad says my brother is just getting progressively worse, but he doesn't know what to do. He has debated taking the medications from him, but he just doesn't know but what my brother needs those drugs. Do you think there is any hope my brother will ever be able to be normal again?

I responded by saying it was very possible that if he had structure, goals and purpose in life; got a job, stopped doing drugs and so forth—he could maintain a job, marry, have children, be a responsible citizen, be happy and look back on these five years as a waste and a tragedy. When Diane heard that message of hope, she immediately had a rush of tears. No one had ever suggested that her brother could ever be truly normal again. Diane had never been told recovery was possible because today, despite recovery being very common in countries that do not prescribe antipsychotics,[2] in America it is "officially" assumed full recovery occurs only rarely if ever.

The APA's Position: There's Not Much Hope

The American Psychiatric Association's *DSM* (*Diagnostic and Statistical Manual of Mental Disorders*) at one time asserted that "a complete return to premorbid functioning is unusual—so rare, in fact, that some clinicians would question the diagnosis."[3] The current *DSM* modifies that gloomy statement with words that still offer little hope. "An accurate summary of the long–term outcome of schizophrenia is not possible. Complete remission (i.e., a return to full premorbid functioning) is probably not common in this disorder. Of those who remain ill, some appear to have a relatively stable course, whereas others show a progressive worsening associated with severe disability."[4]

How could it be otherwise? Do these patients and their doctors not know that 17 to 27 months of antipsychotic drug use will shrink the brain by approximately 20%?[5] Do they not know that even the more mild antidepressants can also cause shrinkage of brain tissue?[6] Are they not aware of the permanent brain damage that can result from both antidepressant and antipsychotic use?[7] My experience over and over has been to discover that neither patients nor their doctors are aware that such dangers come with the use of mind drugs.

BOX #14–1

Psychiatry Today—Ignoring the Research

It is distressing that in psychiatry, so unlike other specialties, research is ignored in favor of blind faith. An example of this is found in an article entitled "Can we find the genes that predispose to schizophrenia?" The authors declare,

> It is well known from genetic epidemiological studies that schizophrenia runs in families. Moreover, an impressive body of evidence from twin and adoption studies shows that individual differences in liability are largely genetic with heritability estimates close to 0.8.[1]

They give no citation supporting the notion that if your parents are schizophrenic then you have an 80% chance of developing it as well. In reality, nothing could be more false. Even true believers don't suggest such numbers today. How can they get away with this? Could I declare that the Jewish Holocaust never happened and not be challenged? Their article does not take issue with the works of Richard Lewontin, Don Jackson or Jay Joseph. No, they don't even mention the important research done by any of these authorities. This could only happen in psychiatry.

There is a better option, but it requires that we understand what causes the mind to break down. In order to see what does matter, I have provided a sampling of factors related to mental instability. I believe each factor can contribute to depression, but the studies I have cited all deal with the even more serious condition we call schizophrenia (see Box #P–3, Schizophrenia

Defined, p. 16). Each is well–documented, but I can assure you that my even sharing such a list will cause the few biological psychiatrists who read this book to get more than upset. They have been convinced that "you did not do anything to cause your illness, and it's not your fault that you have it," as Eli Lilly's marketing department put it. But you be the judge. Is losing your mind just like getting asthma (genetic fate—something you cannot do anything to avoid), or can you and your parents make choices that will help you avoid schizophrenia? Examine the research and see if you do not agree with me that modern psychiatry often destroys lives by excusing bad choices and by prescribing mind–shrinking, mind–destroying drugs. See if you do not agree that there is good reason to get more than upset with biological psychiatrists.

A Sampling of Risk Factors for Schizophrenia

(1) Being a young adult[8]

(2) Having parents divorce[9]

(3) Having a dysfunctional parent[10]

(4) Experiencing household tension or hostile family interaction[11]

(5) Having lower than average intelligence[12]

(6) Having low occupational status (or unemployment)[13]

(7) Having lower social class status[14]

(8) Living in a larger city[15]

(9) Smoking[16]

(10) Abusing alcohol and drugs[17]

(11) Using certain legal, prescription drugs[18]

(12) Having behavioral problems at school and at home as a child[19]

(13) Having fewer friends (most social interaction is with relatives— more contact with them than even the general population has)[20]

(14) Being socially isolated[21]

(15) Being a victim of child abuse[22]

(16) Being institutionalized as a baby[23]

(17) Being emotionally neglected as a child[24]

(18) Being deaf or hearing impaired[25]

(19) Having a drug–abusing parent[26]

(20) Having an older father[27]

(21) Being slightly brain damaged at birth (oxygen deprivation)[28]

(22) Having very low birth weight[29]

(23) Having unstable living arrangements (whether moving out of the parents' residence, becoming homeless or emigrating)[30]

(24) Experiencing life–threatening stress[31]

(25) Experiencing divorce[32]

(26) Being imprisoned[33]

(27) Having a child die—especially for mothers and especially during the first year after the child died[34]

(28) Not having a clear life plan[35]

(29) Spending much more time in bed sleeping and resting than the average person[36]

(30) Being an easily offended or a more self–centered person[37]

The Truth: Learned by Even the First Modern "Psychiatrists"

I have always been amazed that the causes of schizophrenia and depression are so often denied by those in the mental health professions. If they were not educated into adopting a belief in the "disease" model, I have no doubt most would come to the same conclusions that Philippe Pinel, the great reformer of France's mental institutions, discovered over 200 years ago. What causes desperate, hopeless depression? What leads to insanity? What is behind the development of the mental hyperactivity and giddiness we call mania? Through careful scientific observation and documentation, Pinel correctly saw each of these arising not from causes specific to any disorder (to suppose so "would be to fall into a very great error," he declared[38]), but from various types and severities of mental problems arising from the stress and trials of life. Most people overcome their difficulties, rejections and disappointments. But if the stress is particularly great and the individuals' social supports, purpose in life, personal desires and characteristics are not protective of good mental health, then they become vulnerable.

Though some of the terminology has changed, the most common causes of madness (schizophrenia) and melancholy (depression) during Pinel's era differ little from those that afflict us today. Pinel argued that the threats to good mental health included not fully employing one's faculties (not having a meaningful, challenging life), unsatisfied ambition (social, financial and occupational failure), domestic distress (family and marital conflict), lack of moral sensibility (guilt arising from violation of one's values) and drunkenness (alcohol abuse) among others.[39]

The Directional Problem

Such factors continue to be found by countless research studies, but they have been downplayed or even ignored ever since the chemical imbalance doctrine began its reign. The standard argument by biological psychiatrists is that the problems (e.g., alcohol abuse) are not what cause mental disorders, but rather it is the mental disorders that cause a person to turn to alcohol "to deal with the pain of mental illness." This "directional problem" is used to discredit each of the dozens of risk factors found by researchers. The argument is always the same.

Yet the honest observer would judge that the weight of the evidence is hugely in favor of the risk factors actually causing depression and anxiety and schizophrenia. This evidence is tied to using prospective designs, finding dose–response relationships, doing true experiments using animals (including experiments that find stress can quickly change body and brain chemistry) and examining quasi–experimental events among humans which occur naturally in the real world. Diane's brother had numerous risk factors before he ever developed any mental problems. Consider just his marijuana use for a moment.

Several studies, including some using prospective designs,[40] have found that marijuana use puts an individual at great risk of developing schizophrenia. Sven Andreasson, a professor of social medicine at the Karolinska Institute, one of Europe's largest medical universities, examined over 50,000 Swedish military conscripts from 1969 and found that those who had used marijuana 50 or more times by age 18 were six times more likely to develop schizophrenia over the next 15 years.[41] Dr. Andreasson and another research team then examined the group again 27 years later (after the risk for schizophrenia had greatly diminished due to the conscripts' ages).[42] In the newer analysis the researchers found the risk of developing schizophrenia for heavy (50+ times ever), early (by age 18) users was 6.7 times that of non–users. But even more significant, there was a dose–response relationship. In other words, the more marijuana a person smoked, the greater the chance of his becoming a schizophrenic. As the Swedish researchers observed, the results were "consistent with a causal relation."[43]

The relationship between marijuana use and schizophrenia was first reported nearly two centuries ago (more than 60 years before the word schizophrenia was even coined[44]), and that relationship has been reported by numerous studies.[45] Again, the biologically oriented disciples protest that this is because schizophrenics are drawn to marijuana to help mask their suffering, but the prospective research designs and the dose–response findings have now overcome this argument. No, marijuana stresses the brain and makes it more susceptible to losing touch with reality.

Experimental Studies Using Animals

That experimental animal studies have found stress can lead to severe mental collapse gives great weight to a stress model as well. The experimental designs have proven (only experimental designs allow us to use the word "proven") that it is the stress that causes hormonal, immunological and neurotransmitter changes.[46] Physical and psychiatric illness follows. These experiments have been done with rats[47] as well as monkeys.[48]

Saul Schanberg made his discovery of how dramatically stress in newborns can change their entire body chemistry quite by accident. He was studying brain development using the brains of rat pups. He would separate the mothers from the pups as he conducted the experiments but then began getting readings that were totally unexpected and seemed impossible. He even decided his means of measurement (assay procedures) must not be functioning properly. What was going on?

The answer was that separation from their mothers so stressed the newborns that within only two hours of being apart, all kinds of chemical changes were occurring—something Dr. Schanberg never considered until the strange readings were proven not to be due to incorrect data. ("It always amazes me how long it takes scientists to recognize the obvious," he later said about his experience.[49]) You don't need to be a chemist or even be able to pronounce the names of stress chemicals to understand that the stress of separation for pups is real and dramatic. (See Box #14–2, Some Effects of 2 Hours of Mother–Pup Separation.)

It is critical to understand that though thousands of studies like Saul Schanberg's have now documented a change in body and brain chemistry following stress, no study has *ever* found that an unexplained change in

---

BOX #14–2

Some Effects of 2 Hours of Mother–Pup Separation[1]

- Marked Decrease in Organ/Tissue ODC Activity and Polyamine Metabolism
- Suppression of Growth Hormone, Prolactin, and Insulin Action on ODC Expression
- Reduction in DNA Synthesis in Most Organ Tissues
- Slowing of Insulin Catabolism
- Increased Corticosterone Secretion
- Decreased Growth Hormone Secretion

brain chemistry *precedes* mental problems. In other words, no study has ever documented that the "direction" of cause and effect supports the theory that now dominates the mental health field!

Experimental Studies Using Babies

Human babies born prematurely have provided us with another opportunity for experimental research. Dozens of studies have found that receiving massage impacts the neurological development, endocrine system, enzymatic function and even weight gain of premies.[50] Tiffany Field, director of the Touch Research Institute at the University of Miami School of Medicine, has for many years been the leader in this field. I have been sharing one of her studies for 20 years.

Using 40 preterm babies, she randomly assigned half to an experimental massage group and half to a control group. The massage group was to receive 15 minutes of massage three times each day for 10 days. The results were astounding. Despite taking in the same number of calories, the massaged babies gained 47% more weight than did the non–massaged controls.[51]

The power of a less stressful environment (touch reduces stress for adults as well) changes us chemically. But, note again, it is the environment that changes the body's chemistry. Again, direction is everything in this debate. Though we cannot conduct some of the experiments on humans that we do with animals, we have an abundance of research that has found those who have been functioning quite well can very suddenly develop severe depression, schizophrenia or other mental problems following a severe stressor.[52] Of course, those who hold the chemical imbalance doctrine want to believe it is a chemical imbalance that causes maladjustment which consequently results in more life stresses. To address this objection, some studies have been designed just to get closer to the causation question.[53]

Extreme Stress Studies

This type of research has found certain very stressful events do indeed "trigger" depression and schizophrenia. Two British researchers found that approximately half of all the schizophrenics in their study had experienced extremely stressful events in the months prior to the onset of schizophrenic symptoms. The average member of the general population was hugely less likely to have had mental breakdowns during the same period of time.[54]

The same researchers later investigated the reoccurrence of schizophrenia in those who had regained their mental health and found that in these individuals as well, the clear pattern was that a crisis of some type preceded the mental collapse.[55] Again, we cannot generally use true experimental designs with humans, but there is an unlimited number of quasi–experimental events occurring in the natural world every day. By examining responses to unexpected and unplanned events—a natural disaster, a terrorist attack, the tragic accidental death of a child or being drafted and sent to a battlefield's front lines—we can get a picture of how humans respond to stressful crises. What we find is that most handle these events quite well. The National Opinion Research Center investigated numerous tragedies including an air show accident in which an airplane crashed into a crowd killing 20 and injuring 30, a coal mine explosion which killed 119 miners and an earthquake that did significant damage throughout a city. They found that only 1% to 3% of males displayed a "highly agitated state involving uncontrolled behavior."[56] Yet, the research is clear that a small number of individuals who have never shown signs of mental problems lose their minds in response to such trials. Victims generally move from mental distress to simple hallucinations to more severe hallucinations, but the pattern typically appears only in those who are in the most life–threatening situation. Life–threatening situations are more stressful than having survived a natural disaster, so they are even greater threats to good psychological health.[57]

The Extreme Stress of War

Following World War I so many Frenchmen were found to have amnesia from being shell–shocked that a rally was held in Paris. Thousands came. One veteran mounted the platform and anxiously called out, "Please, please, can somebody tell me who I am?"[58] The term "shell shock" comes to us from a British psychiatrist, C. S. Meyers, who coined the term after witnessing numerous cases of British soldiers who shared the same fate as some of their French allies.

During World War II, the battle at Dunkirk saw British troops trapped on the French coast opposite England with no way of escape. As Germany's much larger force moved toward the British troops and began the shelling, the Navy sent every available ship to rescue its men and called upon the nation to do the same. Commercial fishing boats, recreational craft and naval vessels made the dangerous dash across the English Channel to Dunkirk. Every ship and every boat were filled to the brim. Except for the wounded, it was standing room only for those put on ships.

Crossing the channel was also a frightful experience. Everyone knew they might not make it. German planes attacked from the air; E–boats and mines threatened from the sea. Two British psychiatrists reported that of the first 1,000 admissions at the Sutton Emergency Hospital which was set up to receive the evacuees, 144 had amnesia to the degree that they could not recall the event (and some had even more severe memory loss).[59]

Why Some Can Handle More Stress, Some Less

But why could most handle the strain while others fell apart mentally? The simple answer is that some went into battle with greater mental strength. They were better prepared to handle stress. That is what one researcher found when he examined the records of 1,500 WWII veterans who lost touch with reality. It was those with the most chaotic and stressful childhoods that were most apt to lose their minds under wartime conditions.

316

He also found that this occurred under conditions that were not extremely stressful for this group of men. For men with better backgrounds, these psychotic breakdowns nearly always came only under the most stressful battlefield experiences.[60] Some people have always been more prone to collapse under stressful conditions. These tend to be those whose upbringing was less than ideal and who are more likely to lack the social skills needed for handling difficulties.

A very enlightening study of men in the military looked at schizophrenia and length of service before the onset of symptoms. What the researchers found was that the mental breakdowns during the very first month of service occurred at rates that were six times higher than the rate for the entire second year of service.[61]

All of us are vulnerable under the most stressful situations. Another study of Normandy survivors found that once approximately 75% of a unit's troops had been "killed, wounded, captured, or otherwise made casualties," mental collapse to one degree or another became universal.[62] Universal means everyone. The implications of this are very significant. Every one of the few survivors of a decimated unit would begin to collapse mentally. Okay, biological psychiatrists, are we to conclude that all the survivors in a unit are genetically predisposed to a mental breakdown?

Variables — Important But Difficult to Measure

The true believers in biological psychiatry, presented with enough studies, will concede that stress does often push someone into mental instability. But they will continue to maintain that some are simply normal people who, even without any major stressors in their lives, developed schizophrenia. I have never seen such a case. I do, however, believe that in addition to the many risk factors which are objectively measured, there are many that are far harder to quantify but may be even more significantly related to mental health—dwelling on past difficulties or traumas, for example. The power of these subtle, internal conflicts or subjective interpretations to damage the mind is great.

In 1918 the *Lancet*[63] published the dramatic account of a British officer who had been buried alive when a shell exploded near him. He clawed his way out from under the mound of soil with only a severe headache, vomiting and some evidence of a concussion. Despite his experience, he was able to remain on duty for over two months. However, he collapsed suddenly when he went to find a fellow officer and discovered his body on the battlefield with the head, arms and legs all separated from the trunk. Duty demanded he gather any personal belongings from the body parts and clothing for the family, a duty he fulfilled. The experience was one he might have been able to handle if his own mind had not been so greatly stressed already.

In the days which followed he obsessed about his friend's dismembered body. He dreaded sleep as visions of the mutilated body haunted him. Before long he was relieved of duty and placed in the Craiglockhart War Hospital. At the hospital he was advised to avoid any thought or memory of the horror. His success during his waking hours was partial, but he found repression during sleep impossible. It was then that Dr. W. H. R. Rivers saw the patient and, instead of also advising repression, sat down and pointed out that his friend's mutilated body was absolute proof that he "had been spared the long and lingering illness and suffering which is too often the fate of those who sustain mortal wounds."[64] The patient "brightened at once"[65] and acknowledged he had never considered this before. The nightmares immediately ceased. He still had dreams of seeing his friend's dismembered body, but that sight no longer tortured him. He was released from the hospital very soon with no more indications of mental instability.

I think Captain River's case illustrates the degree to which stress can be very subjective. The same event can be handled well or can lead to a complete mental breakdown, depending on the person, the circumstance and, in this case, the intepretation of events. One's life view (Is my life in God's hands or happenstance?), view of self (Am I loved by family and friends or just tolerated?), view of right and wrong (Should I forgive my mother or hold a grudge?)—all influence one's stress level and thus one's mental health.

There are, of course, other important factors which influence our minds. Some of these will be discussed in Part 3 of this book, which deals with avoiding and overcoming depression. However, it must be recognized that the factors which allow us to avoid depression are related to mental health generally and thus to schizophrenia. It never has been anyone's unavoidable destiny to lose his or her mind.

Part Three

Good Mental Health Without Drugs

15

*"No medical forethought can prevent the occurrence of
insanity from accidental causes, but a vast proportion of
the insane become so in consequence of physical conditions of life and modes of living, which lead to the result
as certainly as unsanitary conditions of physical life lead
to typhoid fever or tuberculosis."*[1]

— *Dr. Samuel Tuke, c. 1813*

THE CONTINUUM MODEL

Over the last two decades I have told literally thousands of psychology
students that, contrary to what they may have always heard, depression is
not something which must plague persons all of their lives. In fact, depression can be overcome very quickly. I then add something else I fully
believe: any student can help someone who is depressed if the depressed
person can be motivated to change and the student possesses three qualities:
(1) common sense, (2) values compatible with good mental health and (3)
some understanding of depression.

But how about other serious mental problems: panic attacks, obsessive–
compulsive disorder, anorexia nervosa, schizophrenia and so forth? By
understanding what causes mental problems and encouraging good mental
practices, students or anyone can help prevent these problems from developing.

This is not the traditional view. The traditional view states that only those who have had many years of psychological training should even try to assist those who are mentally disturbed. The traditional view assumes a degree in psychology or psychiatry is needed or else the "helper" might "really mess up the mind" of the one they want to help. The problem with the traditional view is that it is simply not supported by the research.[2]

The Continuum Model is very simple. It argues that (1) we can make choices (mental health problems are not the end result of unavoidable bad luck, i.e., bad genes), (2) we can avoid poor mental health by choosing to follow good mental health practices, (3) good mental health principles can be applied to all of us and (4) foolishness can be avoided since this model is based on a massive foundation of research.

The Continuum Model: You Can Choose

The Continuum Model states that our emotional status *can* be influenced. Our emotional well–being must be seen as operating on a continuum—somewhere between very depressed and very joyful. Though being joyful is always the goal, we will never be without difficult and sad times in this life. But if we focus on our sorrows, if we do what leads to even more stress and depression, it will weaken us emotionally.

Depressed  **Joyful**

Mary Todd Lincoln provides a good example of this principle. Abraham and Mary Lincoln had four sons. The second son, Eddie, died in 1846 at 4 years of age. Mary's reaction was extreme. Three years after his death she continued to grieve.[3] But it was her reaction to Willie's death in 1862 when the Lincolns were in the White House which is most famous. As the First Lady, one might hope she would be a model for a nation filled with parents losing children to disease and war. But instead of accepting a natural period of grief for 11–year–old Willie, she chose to focus on her loss intensely. She ended all White House entertainment and ordered stationery with wide black borders.[4] The White House itself was filled with black crepe.[5] Mary Lincoln wanted everyone to know that her grief was especially great.

Months later a reporter came for an interview and had a surprising experience. "She entered the room where I awaited her, evidently striving for some composure of manner; but as I took the hand which she extended to me, she burst into a passion of tears and gave up all effort at self–control. . . . I put my arm around her and led her to a seat, saying everything I could think of to calm her; but she could neither think nor talk of anything but Willie."[6] Over a year after Willie's death the famous poet Walt Whitman who lived in Washington, D. C., during the war reported seeing Mary in her carriage still wearing a black mourning dress and a long, dark veil.[7]

The black slave who served Mrs. Lincoln later wrote a book which described some of what only her eyes and ears witnessed. One scene reveals that Abraham Lincoln understood that the mind can grow progressively weaker.

> The President kindly bent over his wife, took her by the arm, and gently led her to the window. With a stately, solemn gesture, he pointed to the lunatic asylum. "Mother, do you see that large white building on the hill yonder? Try and control your grief or it will drive you mad, and we may have to send you there."[8]

The literature placed in doctors' offices by drug reps typically stresses that depression is not something which you can *choose* to overcome. The rationale is that depression is a medical disease, just like diabetes or arthritis, and therefore it is impossible to make a decision to "just get over it" any more than one can decide to "just get over" diabetes or arthritis. In some circles it is considered heretical to disagree with this view, but not only do

I disagree, I believe those who accept this conventional view are robbed of the ability to provide the best quality of help to others.

About 1980 I had a woman come see me whom I have used ever since to illustrate the importance of *choosing* good mental health. Eleven months before she came to me her husband had died of leukemia. Because she was well off financially, she had the ability to stay at home and grieve over the loss of her husband as long as she wanted. As I visited with her I learned that she had essentially cut herself off from the rest of the world. For eleven months she had begun the day with tears and ended it with tears. She would sit on the couch and look at her husband's photograph and dwell on how much she missed him and how unhappy she now was. And then her health began to fail. She went to her physician who then referred her to me.

Did she need someone to write her a prescription for an antidepressant? Did she need someone to listen to how sad she felt? No, she needed someone who would emphasize values (the best of all motivators). I tell my students that what I said to her, I said with kindness but with firmness and conviction. I always suspect someone might perceive what I say as uncaring or harsh, but depressed people need someone willing to be more firm and directive than do those who are not depressed.

I emphasized that she did not have the right to take her own life—whether she did so suddenly by suicide or more slowly through daily grief. I emphasized that it was selfish to waste the rest of her life with daily grieving when she could help so many if she would choose to. We talked about her volunteering to hold premature babies at the hospital or volunteering at a local school to help children who needed one–on–one tutoring. She indicated no resentment. She agreed with my thoughts, and before she left she was committed to getting out of her house, socializing again and focusing more on helping and serving others rather than on herself. She committed to ending the daily ritual of sitting on the couch, looking at her husband's photograph and crying. If I had the opportunity to counsel Mary Todd Lincoln, I would have shared several of those same thoughts with her.

Is there a relationship between our experiences (and how we react to those experiences) and whether or not we become depressed (or even become insane in time)? To deny that relationship (which many advocates of the biological chemical imbalance theory do) is to deny the obvious. If your best friend were to accuse you falsely and declare the friendship over, would that move you toward depression or joy? If you were to find out your spouse was having an affair, would that move you toward depression or joy? If your alcoholic mother called and said your rebellious attitude 12 years earlier when you were 16 was what ended her marriage and she never wanted to see you again, would that move you toward depression or joy? To deny that life events play an active role in influencing our emotions and our mental health reveals a lack of knowledge (which generally results from too much "education" within a narrow point of view).

Today throughout America and throughout more and more of our world, even those who have experienced tremendously difficult life events such as these are routinely given antidepressant prescriptions by physicians after only a few minutes together. No careful analysis is made as to why the patient may be depressed. The marketing of antidepressants has been so successful that physicians sincerely believe a pill can help their patients be just fine again emotionally. These prescriptions are written despite the research which reveals the ineffectiveness (beyond the placebo effect) of antidepressants and the potential of antidepressants to cause physical harm. There is a far more reasonable approach.

The Continuum Model: Good Mental Health Practices Lead to Good Mental Health

The Continuum Model recognizes what the research proclaims over and over: that having good mental health is parallel to having good physical health. Failing to eat a healthy diet, exercise and get adequate sleep will not lead to just a single disease; it can lead to any one of many different diseases. In one person it may be high blood pressure followed by a heart attack. In another it might produce diabetes. In yet another it may result in cancer. The point is that poor health practices put a person at risk for not just one disease but for poor physical health generally and for diseases of many kinds.

Poor Mental Health 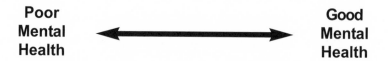 **Good Mental Health**

So it is with poor mental health practices. In one person it may lead to anxiety. Another person may become depressed. Someone else may begin to hear voices. And not following good mental health practices puts an individual at greater risk for all these problems. That is why we see so much comorbidity (more than one "sickness" at a time) among people with mental problems. Enter "comorbidity" into our government's National Library of Medicine PubMed search engine, and you will bring up over 27,000 research studies, about half of which deal with mental disorder comorbidity.[9]

Those with major depression are also more likely to have panic attacks, develop obsessive–compulsive behaviors, have agoraphobia (fear of public places) and become hypochondriacs (those who believe they are ill or will become ill even when medical examination indicates no problems).[10] Depression is also strongly associated with schizophrenia,[11] the relationship being strongest when the schizophrenia symptoms are most active.[12] Schizophrenics are more likely to have a diagnosis of antisocial personality disorder,[13] and they are more likely to be anxious, have panic attacks and have an obsessive–compulsive disorder.[14]

Those who have a personality disorder (what used to be called a psychopath or sociopath) are also more commonly found to be anxious,[15] depressed[16] and schizophrenic.[17] Anorexia nervosa and bulimia nervosa are likely to be accompanied by low self–esteem,[18] depression and anxiety.[19]

On and on we could go with the various relationships and interrelationships. The point is that all kinds of "comorbidity" relationships exist because not following good mental health practices puts us at risk for every kind of mental problem ever known. In other words, if you do not control your temper, pursue good relationships and have meaningful work, not only are you at increased risk of depression, you are also at increased risk of anxiety, eating disorders, personality disorders, schizophrenia and many other manifestations of poor mental health practices.

Not understanding this principle of the Continuum Model causes psychiatrists to see great difficulties and problems if a mental patient has more than just one mental problem. "Mood and anxiety disorders comorbidity is complex and presents a continuing challenge for both clinicians and researchers," concluded one team of psychiatrists.[20] That is a silly statement. That a person who is depressed should also be anxious should not even surprise us. Do what reduces anxiety, and you will reduce your chances of becoming depressed. Do what lessens depression, and you will decrease your chances of becoming anxious.

The Continuum Model, therefore, does not encourage more disciplined behavior for depression, responsible financial planning for anxiety, good social relationships for schizophrenia and exercise for an obsessive–compulsive disorder. The Continuum Model encourages good mental health practices no matter what kind of mental problems are seen.

Most of us trained in psychological therapy were taught that each disorder is unique and must be thoroughly understood before a treatment plan should be considered. Obviously, some adjustment should always be made to provide the most help for each individual. But the research makes it clear that we should not think in terms of nearly 400 different mental disorders (the number of mental disorders identified by the American Psychiatric Association's *Diagnostic and Statistical Manual*), but rather we should think in terms of a continuum. Do what leads to good mental health, and you will improve your mental health. Do what leads to poor mental health, and you will move toward the poor mental health end of the continuum.

The Continuum Model: People Are More Alike Than Different

It is almost a "law" in psychology that each person is so unique that much time must be devoted to learning a client's background, characteristics and personality. Intake forms generally ask about a client's family of origin, educational level, income and relationships, and include something akin to a personality test ("Are you an introvert or extrovert?", "Do you tend to be a saver or a spender?", and so forth). Of course, we are all unique, and I do not wish to imply that anyone's background is unimportant. However, what I have come to learn is that we are fundamentally far more alike than different. We all want to be loved. We all want close relationships. We all feel pain when rejected. We all need sleep, exercise and a healthy diet. We are all profited by being responsible and disciplined, and we are all hurt by being irresponsible and lazy. We are all stressed when we violate our values. We all have a tendency to be selfish.

This principle is important because it means that when we discover what leads to good mental health, we can apply it to ourselves and to all our friends and family. For example, we learned in Chapter 8 that exercise by itself is more effective than antidepressants, even though antidepressants have placebo benefits. But why? I shared in Chapter 8 some of the speculation of researchers who have studied this. However, I did not analyze the specific benefits of exercise that would push exercisers away from depression and towards joyfulness. I always ask students to suggest these mental health–related benefits, and with a class of 30 students they can generally build a list of 6 to 8 benefits. It would be profitable for you to write down as many as you can on your own. When you have done so, examine your list and see an interesting fact: each benefit moves you away from depression and towards joy. So do the benefits found on my list. My list includes the following:

(1) Exercise raises the body's metabolic rate. (Depression lowers the body's metabolic rate.)

(2) Exercise increases one's energy level. (Depression lowers one's energy level.)

(3) Exercise brings about better sleep. (Depression hinders sleep.)

(4) Exercise often involves a person with other exercisers. (Depression tends to result in more isolation and less socialization.)

(5) Exercise tends to release stress and tension. (Depression increases stress and tension.)

(6) Exercise gets your mind off the problem. (Depression involves an intense focus on the problem.)

(7) Exercise has physical health benefits. (Depression harms physical health.)

(8) Exercise often involves goals: improving strength, weight loss, etc. (Depression typically avoids goals, focusing on present problems and the past.)

(9) Group exercise requires you to get out of the house and, therefore, out of your rut. (Depression tends to keep you home and in a rut.)

(10) Exercise keeps the body from getting constipated, a major stressor for older people. (Depression reduces physical activity and, thus, "regularity.")

As you look back over your list (or mine), you can again see another truth. Those exercise benefits apply to all people everywhere. And that is because, despite our differences, we are all very much alike.

The Continuum Model: Foolishness Avoided

I believe common sense can be overcome with sufficient education ("indoctrination" is actually the better word). I have seen it happen to many good men and women. The dangerous tendency is to accept what we have been told simply because it comes from the "experts."

Thanks to Sigmund Freud many highly educated professors learned and then taught that babies put things in their mouths because it is sexually stimulating, and that if an adult chews gum, smokes, overeats or becomes an alcoholic, it is all related to that first year of life. Even becoming a sarcastic adult is supposed to tie back to one's oral stage of life.[21]

Thanks to Freud, many of us were also taught that all girls really desire to be boys and feel insecure because they are not.[22] These and a hundred other foolish Freudian teachings were not just accepted by two or three psychiatrists in some obscure locale. These ideas dominated psychiatry and psychology for decades. Writing in 1970 William Dember and James Jenkins described the dominance of Freud's psychoanalytic ideas in their general psychology textbook thus:

> With some exceptions, psychiatric theory today is virtually synonymous with Freud's psychoanalytic theory, or modifications thereof. The exceptions, while of interest to the psychiatrist, need not concern us here, since none has had an effect on psychology comparable to that of Freudian theory.[23]

What this psychology textbook is saying is that almost everyone in the profession had come to accept foolishness. But Freudian psychoanalysis is just one example.

Thanks to the behaviorist B. F. Skinner, I was informed that once we learned to fully control the human environment (which he said in 1948 we would soon accomplish), no one would commit crime or fail to live a good life.[24] This not–so–insightful sage became one of the most important names in American psychology (although the "utopian" communes he inspired have generally vanished, and we now have far more crime than we did in 1948).

Thanks to the evolutionary psychologists, I learned that men prefer young, attractive women for wives, not because they are young and attractive, but because men have an unconscious desire to produce as many children as possible to perpetuate their genes, and the most fertile women (according to the "experts") are young and attractive.[25] These and a host of other examples confirm that not only is it easy to be fooled (common sense can be quickly overcome), but "education" has not always been based on high–quality research.

Yes, common sense has its uses. As an example, consider a passage from the classic book *Swiss Family Robinson* which describes the father's effort to keep his family busy.

> When the great affairs were settled, we still found in all directions work to be done. Shelves, tables, benches, movable steps, cupboards, pegs, door handles, and bolts—there seemed no end to our requirements, and we often thought of the enormous amount of work necessary to maintain the comforts and conveniences of life which at home we had received as matters of course.
>
> But in reality, the more there was to do the better; and I never ceased contriving fresh improvements, being fully aware of the importance of constant employment as a means of strengthening and maintaining the health of mind and body. This, indeed, with a consciousness of continual progress towards a desirable end, is found to constitute the main element of happiness.[26]

Was the father wise to keep the family busy? Was he correct in assuming that having a goal ("a desirable end") and working to meet that goal brought happiness? I believe most people will recognize the wisdom of this view regardless of their educational status. That passage contains what I would call common sense.

But can either common sense or what we were taught by our teachers and professors be our guide? Believing so is what allowed foolish ideas (treating mental problems with beatings, purges, chemical–induced convulsions, ECT, prefrontal lobotomies, etc.) to grow and become widely practiced among highly educated people. Also note that I am not saying that until we saw the development of research published in scientific journals, we never took the right road. Tuke's Retreat was the right road. But we know it was the right path because they kept careful records on every patient that was admitted (and those records reveal their approach was very successful).

In other words, research was conducted, and their research found moral treatment far more effective than Bedlam's vomits and purges. The research also reveals it was far more effective than today's mind drugs. (See Box #15–1, Moral Treatment—1954).

BOX #15–1

Moral Treatment—1954

Though a number of mental hospitals practiced moral treatment during the 1800s,[1] the advent of "modern medicine" with its insulin, ECT and lobotomies, combined with inadequate funding for these institutions, resulted in the virtual disappearance of moral treatment from American asylums early in the 20th century. However, there was a remarkable resurgence in Kansas in the middle of the last century. Surprisingly that resurgence of moral treatment arose quite independently of Tuke's work—perhaps without any knowledge of moral treatment at all.

The Topeka State Hospital was typical of state mental hospitals in 1948. Only 1 of every 3 patients who was admitted ever left.[2] Patients would be housed for years, and most died there. They spent their days in absolute boredom. Patients were given rocking chairs and compelled to sit and rock quietly day after day, year in and year out. Those who disobeyed were put in straightjackets or strapped to their beds. "At all times at least 100 patients were in 'restraint,' screaming, tearing at their bonds."[3] These deplorable conditions became the focus of a 10–part exposé in a Kansas newspaper.

That attention resulted in the firing of the superintendent and the organization of a group called SHARE (State Hospital Aids in Recreation and Entertainment), made up entirely of volunteers from the community. A beauty shop was opened, and the standard "bowl" haircuts which identified patients as insane disappeared. Volunteers developed relationships with patients. Games began to be played. The legislature appropriated funds for social workers who sought to reestablish patient–family ties. The result was that a miracle occurred. By 1953 approximately 80% of those admitted were discharged as well.[4]

The *Reader's Digest* picked up the story under the title "They Go Home Again in Kansas" and reported, "Even more astonishing is the number of patients released who had for years been looked upon as hopelessly incurable: in 1949–1950, for instance, 112 of those who returned home had been at Topeka State for an average of nine years; one had been there 40 years."[5]

The article appeared in 1954. It should have marked the beginning of the resurgence of moral treatment nationally. But it didn't. For 1954 was also the year Thorazine (the first "miracle" mind drug) began to be marketed across America. The drug companies have won the last half century. They have made their money, but only at the cost of an incredible human tragedy.

Or consider John Butler's 1887 description of the causes and cures for mental illness. (Dr. Butler was a mental hospital superintendent for many decades.) He also used moral treatment with the thousands of patients he helped and also kept careful records which document his institution's success.

> A sensual and selfish, or idle and aimless life, must inevitably act as a predisposing cause to the development of one or more of these causes. In a large proportion of the cases which have come into my care insanity might have been prevented by the use of well–known measures, or natural and right development of body and mind, wise aims in life, and a reasonable exercise of self–control.[27]

Was Dr. Butler right? I know he was, but my confidence is not based on it fitting what I consider common sense. No, my confidence is based on the fact that it is supported by quality research and right values (values given us by God and supported by the research as superior—a purposeful life being better than an aimless life; a busy, occupied life being better than an idle life; unselfishness being better than selfishness, etc.).

Who would most disagree with those words? The answer is the men and women who have been trained in biological psychiatry—especially psychiatrists who spend years being indoctrinated by a drug–industry–promoted philosophy (as opposed to honest research) which teaches (1) "You didn't do anything to cause your illness, and it's not your fault that you have it";[28] (2) "Schizophrenia is not caused by bad parenting or personal weakness";[29] (3) "Schizophrenia is usually a life–long disease, like diabetes or high blood pressure. Most people with schizophrenia will probably need special medical care and medication for the rest of their lives"[30] (see Box #15–2, A Survivor's Close Call With Disaster) and (4) "Two key neurotransmitters that are needed for brain function are dopamine and serotonin, which play a crucial role in emotional health. . . . When the levels of these neurotransmitters aren't quite right, it may result in the symptoms of schizophrenia. For

---

BOX #15–2

A Survivor's Close Call With Disaster

Americans given antipsychotics immediately begin experiencing the brain damage that keeps most of them from ever having a normal life. It almost happened to Ronald Bassman. Today Dr. Bassman, a psychologist and survivor of a mental hospitalization, remembers his close call with a life of blunted emotions.

I couldn't see the nurse when she came in and said, "Get him ready." They quickly pulled my pants and underwear down to my knees. I winced at the violent thrust of the needle. I tried to prepare myself to fight the onslaught of the thought–dulling, body–numbing Thorazine. They waited for the drug to take effect before they stripped me of my clothes. I was left naked in the seclusion room, and no explanations were given. They did not tell me how long I would stay there.

Three decades have passed since I've had any kind of psychotic treatment, yet the memories remain. When I was discharged from the hospital I was told I had an incurable disease called schizophrenia. The doctor told my family that my chances of being rehospitalized were very high. His medical orders were directed at my parents, not me, and stated with an absolute authority that discouraged any challenge. He predicted a lifetime in the back ward of a state hospital if his orders were not followed.

"He will need to take medication for the rest of his life. For now, you need to bring him to the hospital weekly for outpatient treatment and he must not see any of his old friends."[1]

---

instance, too much dopamine in certain parts of the brain can cause symptoms such as hallucinations and delusions. . . . Too little dopamine in other parts of the brain can cause symptoms such as a lack of emotion, lack of energy, and lack of motivation."[31]

I pity the psychiatrist who has come to believe the biological chemical imbalance view. It makes the psychiatrist little more than a placebo pill pusher. And for those willing to research the literature who discover that depressed individuals given antidepressants are *more* likely to relapse and have more depression over time[32] or that schizophrenia is *less* likely to disappear if a person is given antipsychotics,[33] that discovery must be an emotional bombshell since it destroys the foundation on which their whole medical education was built.

Today, despite the dominance of the chemical imbalance view in psychiatry, there is an abundance of honest, well–designed studies supporting the Continuum Model which can guide us in helping others find good mental health. I will examine this research in the final chapter.

Note: The fact that "I will examine this research in the final chapter" does not mean to imply that I will address all the techniques, methods or issues which I cover when counseling the depressed or unstable individual. The research indicates there is much that can be done to help those in need, and many of my colleagues have developed specific techniques supported by sound research which should be widely adopted. The final chapter will focus instead on eight issues that can have a major impact on mental health which are often ignored or not adequately addressed. Each of the eight illustrates the truth that we are capable of making choices that can improve or worsen mental health. This is a much more positive message than today's conventional "It's not your fault, and there is nothing you can do about it."

16

What I've got they used to call the blues.
Nothin' is really wrong; feelin' like I don't belong;
Walkin' around, some kind of lonely clown.
Rainy days and Mondays always get me down.

What I feel has come and gone before.
No need to talk it out; we know what it's all about;
Hangin' around, nothing to do but frown.
Rainy days and Mondays always get me down.
              — *Sung by The Carpenters, 1971*[1]

AN EFFECTIVE GUIDE FOR AVOIDING AND OVERCOMING DEPRESSION

Using the Continuum Model, let us address how to avoid and overcome depression without drugs. Again, think of what we do as moving us toward depression or joy. As noted in the box on page 337, the "Eight Questions" which follow are not comprehensive, but the research as well as common sense support this model. Ignoring it only increases the risk of developing depression and other mental problems.

Depressed ⟵——————————⟶ **Joyful**

Eight Questions

(1) Are you getting adequate sleep?

Would lack of sleep move you toward "depressed" or "joyful"? Just as a baby who misses his or her nap is more apt to throw a fit over even a minor frustration, the adult who is not getting adequate sleep is emotionally weaker, not stronger. Randy Gardiner who holds the record for staying awake (11 days) found that in addition to experiencing speech difficulties and minor losses in physical coordination, by the third day he had also begun to have some significant mood changes.[2] Gardiner's story is anecdotal, but numerous scientific studies find that sleep loss adversely affects cognitive function and mood.[3] We should expect this as too little sleep impacts the mind in other ways as well. Inadequate sleep has been found to lower concentration, planning ability and the ability to employ high–level intellectual skills,[4] all of which are frontal lobe tasks.

Even modest sleep deprivation slows brain wave activity—a change also commonly seen in those who are depressed.[5] Sleep deprivation also causes the brain's neurons to function at a slower speed; that is, they become "depressed."[6] Virtually every aspect of human performance is affected by missing some needed sleep.[7] Getting just six hours each night (some less than the optimal amount) causes significant cognitive declines.[8]

Getting less than optimal amounts of sleep can also cause health problems that further stress the body and make avoiding depression more difficult. The immune system is compromised when someone is not getting enough sleep.[9] Averaging less than six hours per night (or more than nine hours per night) impairs glucose tolerance and increases one's chance of developing diabetes.[10]

A host of other health problems has been shown to result when someone does not get an adequate amount of sleep—bacterial infections,[11] slow wound healing,[12] hypertension[13] and heart disease[14] among others. It is hard to imagine that inadequate sleep can do such harm to the body physically and yet not also damage mental health. No, it does matter. Getting an adequate amount of sleep moves you toward the joyful end of the continuum model.

(2) Are you abusing alcohol or drugs?

Would abusing these substances move you toward depression or joy? Obviously, alcohol and drugs weaken our ability to cope with the problems of life. In fact, people who engage in heavy drinking as adolescents are likely to have unrecognized but permanently reduced learning ability.[15] When the mind is less capable, we are more susceptible to the trials of life. This may help explain why those with prior alcohol problems are more than four times as likely to be currently depressed,[16] a relationship which has been reported over and over.[17]

I have always chosen to let others work with alcoholics. I would like to be of help, but I have found that drug abusers make many promises (to control their drinking, to stop their hitting, to act responsibly, etc.), but their promises are almost worthless. Thus, my personal experience in this area is limited. However many years ago I was asked to investigate and present the psychological research at a seminar on alcohol. What I learned and found most significant was the following fact. Alcohol's effects on the mind are more dramatic in studies that used the most objective measures. For example, rape has long been associated with alcohol abuse. However, surveying several studies involving hundreds of rape cases, Judith Roizen found police reports indicated alcohol use by the rapist in only 13%–37% of cases. But when alcohol content was measured in the urine of apprehended rapists, 50% were found to have been drinking.[18]

But even if we had no research on alcohol's effects, I would encourage minimal use or abstinence for anyone struggling with depression. The Continuum Model requires that we do that which moves us toward joy and avoid that which moves us towards depression. Since alcohol is a depressant, it moves the user in the wrong direction.

Various prescription drugs also move the user toward depression. The FDA–approved package insert for Accutane, an acne–control medicine, warns "Accutane may cause depression."[19] The package inserts for dozens of other drugs have the same warning,[20] so be sure you read the fine print for any drug that you have been prescribed.

(3) Are you watching much television?

You may be surprised to learn that I do not want my clients watching much television. My reasons are consistent with the Continuum Model. We decrease our metabolic rate whenever we lie down and rest. As hard as it may be to believe, television viewing somehow decreases the body's metabolic rate even more dramatically.[21] Watching television also slows down the body more than does reading.[22] I want to see the depressed person moving away from anything that depresses physically or mentally. The "opposite" of watching television in terms of metabolic rate changes is getting physical exercise. Perhaps this is another reason exercise is so beneficial to those seeking to overcome depression.

There are secondary reasons why I am concerned about television viewing. Those who watch more TV are more apt to become obese,[23] develop diabetes[24] and develop heart disease[25] as well as a host of other health problems. Those are not just physical health issues. Obesity has such negative connotations in our society that emotional well–being is put at risk[26]—especially for females.[27] It is reasonable to assume that the embarrassment, shame and guilt often associated with obesity can bring about isolation or rejection and, hence, depression. Diabetes or heart disease may not carry the same negatives that are felt by the obese; nevertheless, having health problems tends to move us toward depression rather than joy.[28]

There is yet another benefit of avoiding television. Television viewing is often a solitary experience that can reduce the amount of time we would otherwise spend in the company of others. Sadly, those who spend much time watching TV have fewer friends.[29]

Time is "hydraulic" which means that the more time we devote to television, the more other activities will be robbed of time. A widely publicized study by the Stanford Institute for the Quantitative Study of Society reported that as Americans began spending more and more time surfing the web, time with people (and even time given to sleep and television) went down.[30] That television displaces socializing time has been known for decades.[31] We did not necessarily need web–surfing studies to confirm that internet use has some consequences which are very similar to TV viewing, but we have them.[32]

BOX #16-1

Entertaining One's Self

Not all television viewing or time in front of a computer monitor is equal. Many of us spend many hours in front of a monitor each day as a part of our work. That is not something which concerns me. My concern is when the viewing is extensive and for our own pleasure (whether it be television shows, video games or web–surfing). That type of viewing is self–centered and leads to less focus on others, moving us away from joy and toward depression. When we spend our free time in isolation, we weaken our mental health—even if the activity is done for our own pleasure. We are not meant to live isolated lives.[1]

Those who watch more television are also more likely to adopt values or experience consequences that make joyfulness more elusive. Cognitive development is negatively affected;[33] academic achievement is diminished;[34] socioeconomic status is harmed;[35] behavioral problems are increased;[36] more sexually permissive behaviors are pursued;[37] dissatisfaction with one's own appearance grows[38] and unhealthy health practices are encouraged.[39] Once someone is depressed, getting out of the house and socializing can become very unappealing. This is where a friend needs to take charge and get the depressed person away from the TV and into a warm, lively social setting.

Those should be reasons enough to avoid too much television if you tend to get down often, but I will add a final fact. This is particularly aimed at adolescents who are at risk. Those adolescents who watch more television are more likely to become underage alcohol users than those who watch less TV.[40] Keep in mind some of the depression problems already noted that can be caused by alcohol.

(4) Are you violating your values?

If you were to yell at your mother, hit your spouse or steal from your employer, you would likely feel an abundance of guilt–induced stress. Good! We need to feel that guilt if we act in a way that is unethical or immoral. I shared earlier that I tell my students that to best help those who are struggling with depression, they need to possess a value system that is compatible with good mental health. Let me share an example of what I see as a value system which could do great harm and, in effect, denies that sexual morality matters. The example comes from a book written by David Viscott, one of America's best known psychiatrists. In his book about marriage entitled *How To Live With Another Person*, he argues that committing adultery is natural.

> Most sexual encounters that do develop outside a relationship are casual, the product of chance, loneliness, separation or curiosity and may have little to do with the other person. . . . That seems to be reality, the way things are, the way they have always been and probably the way they will continue to be. Who is to say whether it is right or not?[41]

Viscott then goes on to share his viewpoint that to insist on sexual fidelity is unrealistic, not because most husbands or wives won't avoid adultery, but because they can't avoid adultery.

> To insist on sexual fidelity is to make a demand most people cannot meet, even if they would agree to enter into a

relationship that placed such a demand on them. The opportunities for sexual interaction are everywhere and people are only human. To demand that your partner promise to be true in a way he may not be able to fulfill may make an insecure partner feel better for the time being but it will not have any effect on the partner's activities and may create a needless sense of betrayal later on.[42]

Who does Viscott say is insecure? The one who expects his or her spouse to be faithful. And expecting a spouse to be faithful creates a "needless sense of betrayal" when adultery occurs? Viscott's values will not discourage adultery. They, in effect, grant permission. That counsel denies reality. The reality is that adultery causes emotional turmoil, divorce, depression and even suicide. One in–depth study of marriages involving adultery found that it led to divorce in 34% of the cases (many more would divorce in time), and in 43.5% of the cases the marriage remained together but the marriages were described as negative or "dysphoric" (unwell or unhappy, from the Greek for "hard to bear").

A marital therapy text I used many years ago had two tables which impressed me then and impress me now as to how hard divorce is on both physical and emotional well being. The statistics are now old, but newer studies[43] continue to reveal the same truths—separation and divorce cause great distress, physical illness, depression and death.

MENTAL HEALTH ADMISSIONS BY MARITAL STATUS[44]

	Psychiatric Outpatient Clinics*		State/County Mental Hospitals*	
	Male	Female	Male	Female
Married	276	423	133	125
Divorced	1,365	1,621	2,168	759

*Rate per 100,000 people per year

RATES OF DEATH BY MARITAL STATUS[45]

	Suicide*		Auto Accidents**		Coronary Disease***		Cancer (Digestive Organs)***	
	Male	Female	Male	Female	Male	Female	Male	Female
Married	18.0	5.5	100	100	159	63	34	22
Divorced/ Separated	69.4	18.4	362	328	330	87	66	29

* Age–adjusted rate per 100,000 people per year
** Standardized rate of 100 for married persons
*** Rate per 100,000 people per year

Over and over in my own experience, I have known of psychiatrists who have sought to downplay the significance of an extramarital affair or who have actually encouraged it. (Remember that Freud taught suppressing sexual urges could result in mental disorders.) The *American Journal of Psychiatry* presented a case study of an anesthesiologist who, following his wife's affair, considered switching his specialty to psychiatry "and began reading extensively in the field."[46] He soon came to see his wife's affair "as something that happens in life that could not be avoided."[47] That is nonsense. Affairs can and should be avoided. If that is not true, we should consider the traditional marriage vows sheer hypocrisy and stop exchanging them.

Whenever I counsel individuals involved in an extramarital affair, I find they want to justify it for all kinds of reasons, but when I clearly state, "What you have done is wrong," they always agree. That illustrates why I maintain that intellectual discussions and analysis ("What unmet childhood need were you trying to meet by having this affair?") actually do harm, but affirming good values can change lives. To acknowledge that adultery is a sin (a word David Viscott and most therapists refuse to use), to ask for forgiveness, to commit to being a better spouse (and to accept specific changes in behavior) can begin to build hope and trust in the offended spouse and can bring emotional healing to the one who committed adultery. (The spouse who committed adultery is generally more depressed than those who come to therapy who have not committed adultery.[48])

But today biological psychiatry so dominates the field that it is believed that prescribing a drug can even bring healing following an extramarital affair. Consider again the case study from the *American Journal of Psychiatry*. The authors correctly identified the wife's adultery as capable of causing the anesthesiologist's depression, but then think about the "treatment" which they describe.

> Dr. A developed a severe depression in reaction to his wife's infidelity. He saw a psychiatrist and was given medication, but after 2 years of treatment with antidepressants, mood stabilizers, neuroleptics and ECT, his response was far from robust.[49]

The doctor had to stop working. (Who could work when filled with the multiple mind drugs he was given and the ECT he underwent?) Two more years of "treatment" followed.

> Over the course of the next 2 years, most sessions dealt with the patient's continuing depressive symptoms, his desire to return to work, his anxiety about doing so, and changes in his medication.[50]

After four years of "treatment," 51–year–old Dr. A asked his daughter not to disturb him and then went to his bedroom and set up a bag and tubing which dripped lethal drugs into his body. He was already dead when his wife returned home from work and found him. In this case it was the physician's wife who committed adultery, but my own counseling experiences and the sparse statistics we have indicate that it is generally the physician who has the extramarital affair, and they do so at rates that are above the average for many other occupations.[51]

Do sexual adventures bring additional joy? No, they lead to stress and depression and may be an important but unrecognized factor in the high rate of suicide among physicians.[52] Isn't it ironic? Pursuing pleasure may bring only a very temporary pleasure followed by, in some cases, a lifetime of pain. Maimonides (1135–1204), the famous Jewish rabbi, philosopher and physician, discussed the importance of right living in his "Diseases of the Soul."

> The ancients maintained that the soul, like the body, is subject to good health and illness. The soul's healthful state is due to its condition, and that of its faculties, by which it constantly does what is right, and performs what is proper, while the illness of the soul is occasioned by its condition, and that of its faculties, which results in its constantly doing wrong, and performing actions that are improper.[53]

Of course, Maimonides was speaking of any violation of good values, not just adultery. Any friend, family member or professional who is willing to confront sin and unhealthy values is proving to be a worthy counselor.

I remember one wife and mother who believed she had a right to get angry, yell, throw things and hit. Her husband asked to meet, and then he told me that they had been to counselors previously and nothing had worked to curb her angry tantrums. "I'm going to ask for your help, and I hope you can help; but if it doesn't work, I'm going to divorce her. I just can't live like this any longer." When I met with her, she knew her husband's position and did not want to be divorced from him, but she also felt desperate. "I don't want to get so angry. I hate myself for it, but I cannot help it. I was born with a temper. I've tried to overcome it all my life. I've been to therapy, but I just cannot overcome it."

I don't believe God made any of us without the ability to avoid sin, and I told her so. We can choose, and it was time she made a commitment not to yell, throw anything or hit her husband. (It is interesting, since she claimed she really could not control it, that she hit only her husband, never any of her children.) I did not even get close to convincing her. When I told her she had to keep a daily record of her mood and behavior (she had to comply or lose her $500 deposit), she said it wouldn't help. I then explained, "If you yell, throw or hit, it will cost you $10 per incident." Her response was, "You don't understand. I do not want to lose my temper. I just can't help it. Losing money won't be of any help at all."

"Well, it may not, but let's make the penalty $20 per incident and see what happens."

"It doesn't matter how much you make it, it won't matter."

"You may be right, but let's make the penalty $50 per incident and see what happens." I'm not sure she was too happy with me when she left, but when she came back a week later, I had a wife and mother who had taken a giant step toward being joyful. She lost $50, but only $50.

"I've thought all my life that I couldn't control my temper. But over and over this week I thought about how much it would cost me to explode, and I did control it." She was genuinely happy over this growth, and so was her husband. I expected her to lose another $50 two or three more times before we finished meeting together, but she never lost another dime. Her marriage was saved and thoughts of suicide (she had previously attempted suicide more than once) were gone.

It is important that anyone counseling another person be firm and clear concerning what values are right and good. Unfortunately our moral compass can be suppressed and almost destroyed if we repeatedly choose to do what is wrong. This is because of a psychological principle known as cognitive dissonance.[54] When our behaviors and our values are in conflict, we will, over time, change our values. But that does not mean that the immoral behavior does not still cause distress which can lead to depression and a ruined life. Being a values advocate is one of the most important roles any therapist can play. Unfortunately, many of my colleagues argue that therapists should be careful not to impose their values on clients. If you express a desire to be unfaithful to your husband or wife, your therapist may choose to be "open–minded" and accepting of your lifestyle choice, but that therapist is failing to help you find joy.

We have an inherent sense of right and wrong, and when we do what is wrong, we hurt ourselves. People who are unkind are not filled with joy. Neither are those who are dishonest or immoral. Doing what is right, especially when it is difficult to do, makes us feel better. That is part of what moves us toward joyfulness and away from depression.

(5) Do you have to make excuses because of your lack of self–discipline?

More than 25% of Americans admit that procrastination is "a significant problem" in their lives.[55] I meet a lot of those Americans every semester. John is my most recent and is a very memorable example. John was in my office to take a test which I had given his psychology class earlier that day. He had called me later that morning and asked if he could make up the exam. "Why were you not here?" "I overslept," he responded. I told him he could come, but when I got off the phone, I noticed he had already been absent six times.

He took the test, and I asked him to wait while I graded it. The grade was a low "F." I said, "John, I'm wondering if it is in your best interest to stay in this course. Your college grade point average is important. You got an A+ on the first quiz, which tells me you are quite intelligent, but you failed this test and have not turned in any assignments. Every absence from this point on will be lowering your grade. It might be best for you to drop the course and take it again next semester."

"Oh, no, sir. I really don't want to drop it. I've already taken this course four times before."

"What? You've taken this psychology course four times already?"

"Yes, sir."

"Who was your instructor?"

"Well, I took it from Dr. Smith once and from you three times."

"Three times?"

"Yes, sir."

"Did you fail each time?"

"Well, I failed once, and I dropped the other times." (I later checked and found that the last time I had him in class, he had failed the quiz and had not submitted any assignments at the point when he dropped.)

"John, you must not be paying for this yourself."

"Yes, sir, I am."

"Well, what is the problem?"

"I just can't seem to make myself study when I should or even get out of bed in time. Sometimes I would wake up almost in time, but I knew if I came I would walk in right in the middle of class. But, I will be here early from now on. I'll never miss another class." John's intentions were good, but when his class next met, John was not there. I got the drop notice a few days later.

I have talked to hundreds of Johns. These are not bad people. And John's A+ on the first quiz told me he was not just a very polite and pleasant student; he really was very intelligent. But his behaviors confirmed to me that he was also a very undisciplined student. Now let me ask you, how do you suppose John felt about himself when he made an A+ on his quiz earlier that semester? When we work hard and achieve success, there is an immediate emotional benefit. It causes a positive expectation effect which brings hope, excitement, elation and joy.[56] But over and over I have sat with someone who espoke harsh, painful words about themselves after they failed. Because of failures caused by their own lack of self–discipline, they often have what are reasonable concerns about the future. Many of these individuals were students who, like John, were failing classes because they could not turn off the TV or get out of bed. Sometimes it is a husband whose marriage is in trouble because he could not resist a sexual opportunity with someone other than his wife. Or it might be a woman who lost another job and, though in financial trouble, was not welcomed at her parents' home because of her inability to get along with family or friends, .

Those who are undisciplined have a much harder life in many, many ways. To some extent, this, like all personality traits, is inborn. Yet, as humans we all have the privilege of being able to make choices. Those who have been hit hard by the consequences of their poor choices and lack of discipline may be feeling (and it is often expressed) "I'm just a loser," but that feeling can be banished if the right choices are made. The employee who is at work on time, who works hard to complete his assignments and gives his employer his best effort will be more likely to reap respect, praise and promotions. The undisciplined employee is more likely to reap criticism and job losses.

Self–discipline is fundamental to an emotionally healthy life. So, how self–disciplined are you? If you would describe yourself as disciplined, you are likely to have fewer problems that could bring about depression than the average American. After all, America is no longer a very disciplined nation. Today 64.5% of our population is overweight or obese,[57] and the inability to control eating has led to an explosion in stomach bypass surgeries, stomach stapling, stomach banding and other surgical procedures aimed at controlling food intake for those who cannot make themselves eat less.[58] But is it possible to control our behavior? We can, sometimes even in areas where most psychiatrists would argue that self–control cannot have any effect.

An example of that involved a woman who was confined to a mental hospital. She was detained because her constant auditory hallucinations were driving her insane. Today drugs would immediately be prescribed, but this case was many years ago when behavior therapy was very popular. So instead of drugs, the woman was asked to keep a daily record of her hallucinations. Giving her something to do, by itself, helped greatly. But then the researchers had an idea. "Perhaps we can lower the number of times she hallucinates if we praise her whenever she has a day with fewer hallucinations." They then began publicly displaying the number of hallucinations she experienced each day and praising any reductions. Sixteen days after the experiment began, the hallucinations came to an end.[59]

Other studies have also reported that the mentally retarded, the psychotic and others who function way below the average college student can overcome hallucinations, tics, hairpulling behaviors, obsessions and compulsions with the aid of positive reinforcements.[60] In fact, behavioral techniques have been compared with mind drugs and found to be superior.[61]

Behavior modification techniques have been used effectively for treating almost every behavior problem you can imagine: temper tantrums, eating problems, autism, bedwetting, academic problems, social problems, delinquency, smoking, drug addiction and on and on it goes.[62] Why does it work? Because it motivates us to change. We avoid punishment or enjoy reward. But wouldn't it be better if we could control our behavior without the external control imposed by stomach bypass surgery or behavior modification techniques? Being able to do so is called self–control or self–discipline, and its benefits are tremendous.

Self–disciplined students are not any more intelligent than their peers,[63] but they are more likely to make better grades and achieve more academic success[64] in public school settings,[65] in college[66] and in graduate school.[67] Self–disciplined students are better liked by their fellow students,[68] and they are preferred by their teachers.[69] Not surprisingly, they also feel better about themselves.[70]

One of the reasons the self–disciplined tend to make better grades is that they are less likely to procrastinate.[71] That may explain why they are also less likely to cheat at school.[72] Self–disciplined students, because they make better grades, are more likely to be admitted to the better four–year institutions and graduate schools. Graduates of these institutions get better jobs and make more money.[73]

Of course, these more disciplined adults are also better able to save money.[74] Thus, impulsive buying is not as great a threat to their diets or to their bank accounts.[75] On the other hand, it is the undisciplined who are more likely to suffer the financial harm and emotional distress associated with long–term unemployment.[76] Failure to control one's emotions (and subsequent aggression) in childhood is especially predictive of long–term unemployment in adulthood.[77]

Smokers are less likely to be disciplined people.[78] The degree of self–discipline also predicts drug abuse during adolescence[79] and the amount of alcohol consumption and abuse during adulthood.[80] It also correlates with dangerous non–marital sexual liaisons.[81] Those who have less self–discipline are more likely to be involved in juvenile delinquency[82] and, later, wife abuse[83] and other criminal activity,[84] including violent crimes. Amazingly, one study that focused on gender and self–control found that when researchers controlled for the amount of self–discipline, the huge male–female gap in crime rates almost disappeared![85]

Interpersonal relationships are superior among those who exercise self–control. The benefits include better relationships with family members and less conflict with that same group.[86] This is probably because self–disciplined people are more conscientious, agreeable, in control of their tempers and emotionally stable.[87]

These benefits are also found among children. Children with less self–control have more conflicts[88] and are more likely to respond with an angry outburst when they do have a conflict.[89] In fact, one study looked at the degree of self–discipline children had at age 4 as measured by delaying gratification and found it predicted the degree to which those young children got along with other teens when they became teens themselves.[90]

It should not be surprising, in view of all the other relationships, that those with more self–discipline also have numerous psychological benefits. The disciplined of our world are less likely to have anxiety, eating disorders, paranoid thinking, a susceptibility to psychotic experiences, obsessions and compulsions, and are less likely to get depressed.[91] They are also less likely to allow various stresses to move them into emotional distress.[92]

Put it all together, and we find that a lack of self–discipline can make it more difficult for us to avoid bad habits, resist temptation, get our work done, make good grades, succeed academically, get better jobs, retain our jobs, make more money, control our weight, get adequate sleep, avoid credit card debt, keep our promises, be on time, get out of bed in the morning, maintain a friend's secret, control our mouths, master our tempers, get along with our family, not hit our spouses and not get depressed. But I have never had someone tell me that her physician asked her to complete a brief two–minute survey on self–discipline[93] or any other stress–inducing source before writing a prescription for an antidepressant. That is irresponsible. It is time we get real about some of the real causes of depression. (See Appendix 4 for a "brief two–minute" measure that covers self–discipline and other factors which can cause depression.)

An Introduction to Question 6

Before we consider the sixth question I want you to be aware of the research concerning physical attractiveness and its effects. That research provides an important foundation of knowledge which is needed as we consider the next question.

Fact: Physically attractive people are treated better and are more popular than those who are not as physically attractive.

From the day we are born, our appearance affects how we are treated by others. Babies who are attractive receive more attention from hospital nursery attendants before they even go home.[94] Adults judge that attractive babies will be smarter, more likable and good.[95] It goes the other way as well—babies prefer attractive faces more than unattractive faces, as evidenced by the fact that they will stare longer at the attractive face.[96]

Children prefer attractive children,[97] and so do adults.[98] When a child gets into trouble on the school playground or in the classroom, it pays to look good. Attractive children receive less severe scoldings and receive less of the blame for problems.[99] Although attractiveness consistently predicts the severity of punishment, adults who are upset are especially prone to mete out severe punishment to children who are unattractive.[100]

How attractive a young woman is can predict with a moderate degree of accuracy how often she will be asked out for a date.[101] And though male attractiveness is less predictive of treatment than female attractiveness, females do prefer to date attractive males.[102] Attractive people are also more socially connected. [103]

Students who are attractive are likely to receive better grades on essays than equivalent essays submitted by unattractive students.[104] Teachers are also more likely to expect academic success in other courses if the student looks relatively handsome or beautiful.[105] Mock jury experiments find that attractive people are more likely to be found "not guilty" or to be given lighter sentences.[106] This is especially true for attractive female defendants, the gender for which appearance is more important.[107]

Appearance makes a difference when it's time to get a job. Simply wearing glasses to an interview can keep men and women from getting hired for a sales position—a position for which attractiveness is apparently deemed important.[108] Not only are attractive people more likely to be hired,[109] they are generally judged to be more qualified for employment[110] and are recommended for employment with a higher suggested salary.[111] Those same people then get better jobs and get promoted more often. That is why they have higher salaries than less attractive employees.[112]

If you go to the doctor, you may get more attention if you look good. At least we know that medical students prefer to treat physically attractive patients.[113] But patients also prefer to be treated by attractive health care providers. They even consider attractive therapists as more competent and genuine, and they are more willing to disclose personal information to them.[114]

Attractive males and females are judged to be more interesting, socially skilled, well–adjusted and successful than the less attractive.[115] They are even assumed to have happier marriages, more fulfilling lives and better character than those who are less handsome or less beautiful.[116] Not surprisingly, those who enjoy better looks are assumed to have better mental health and less depression.[117] In fact, they do.[118] (It helps to be treated better than less attractive individuals all your life.) The relationships found between attractiveness and how we are treated are not just an American phenomenon. Similar studies report similar outcomes in other nations as well.[119]

When I told my wife that I was going to share the research on physical attractiveness, she acted surprised. "But won't that make most of your readers feel worse?" Yes, that is a very real possibility. In fact, a lot of studies make it plain that exposure to attractive people can make women (and to a lesser extent, men) not just more depressed, but distressed and angry. We know, for example, watching television commercials which show women with perfect figures increases viewers' anger, anxiety, body dissatisfaction and depression.[120] The effects are not hugely dramatic, but they are real. TV commercials without the beautiful bodies do not have this effect.

Another study similar to that mentioned above showed commercials with attractive women to half of the women in the study and commercials with unattractive women to the other study participants. Again, it was found that when women were exposed to female models previously rated as highly attractive, they experienced emotional changes.[121] Anger, anxiety, depression and appearance dissatisfaction all increased. But now listen to the rest of the story. The women who watched commercials which used overweight and unattractive women actually began to feel happier and better about their own appearance and body shape.[122]

(6) Do you focus on yourself?

The research I have shared on physical attractiveness may well have made you squirm a little. Some of you may have even felt a little angry or depressed about not being more attractive (or not being treated as well as highly attractive people). So why did I relate that research? I will explain after I share the following story.

A number of years ago I was going over the psychological test results of what would appear to be the ideal young couple (about 26 years old). Both were intelligent, attractive, pleasant and successful, and they enjoyed a good marriage. They had taken time off from their careers to attend graduate school together at that time, and I was doing the testing and counseling with those involved in the graduate school's holistic approach to education. As I went over the test's results, I gently suggested to the wife that it appeared she might be struggling with low self–esteem. Those words brought an instant surge of tears and pain. She was not just crying; she was weeping uncontrollably. The amount of pain and sadness experienced by those who do not feel especially well–liked or loved can be intense, and it is amazingly common.

Now, I want you to appreciate how "above average" this young wife was—intelligent, attractive, pleasant, with a good husband and with a good future. She seemed so sweet and likable, but inside that happy exterior she was miserable. In the 25 years since I counseled that couple, I have learned a painful truth. Many if not most people are suffering—even kind, loving and good people. Many people do not feel like they fit in as well as others fit in. Many people often feel neglected and left out and excluded. Those truths apply to people who are at all different levels of physical attractiveness as well as every educational, intellectual or financial level. I do not know what causes more people more daily pain. It also causes anger.

I hear on a regular basis from wives in tears over not being adequately loved, and yet as they describe their own misery, they also express anger and even hostility toward a husband who is not very loving or a mother– in–law who, they are convinced, has never really accepted them. They may say that their co–workers exclude them or express anger at not being invited over by other acquaintances. Depression and anger often go together because feeling excluded (or unloved) hurts and is taken as a personal attack.

A man whose brothers were both successful lawyers said, "I wouldn't be looked down on by my family if I made as much money as my brothers." Do you hear the hurt? But can you also hear the resentment? All around us are people who long to be viewed by others as financially successful, attractive, intelligent or something else that they may or may not have achieved. Why? The answer is that we all want to be loved, and we sense that better looks or more money or more success will make others like us or love us more and give us more attention.

That "intelligent, attractive, pleasant" wife I described earlier was above average on virtually every measure but was miserable inside. Again, I ask, "Why?" The answer is that she was focused on herself. That is what is natural, but doing what is natural can make us miserable. Focusing on ourselves means we are going to compare ourselves to others. That is why viewing TV commercials which show very beautiful women increases anger and depression in women whereas viewing overweight and unattractive women makes them feel better. Rather than pretend that this relationship does not exist (not sharing the research), I believe it should be shared and confronted head on.

This is especially important for young people. Since overcoming the intense focus on self takes many years for most of us, it is young people who are most apt to feel lonely and left out. A study of this very issue among 10–18 year olds found that *over half* felt lonely and left out *often*.[123] (See Box #16–2, "I Feel So Left Out of Things.") That tells me that our schools are filled with children who are suffering emotionally. Are kids aware of how many others feel neglected and excluded? No, and neither are adults. I tell every class I teach these facts because I am very aware that part of the pain comes from feeling like everyone else fits in, everyone else has plenty of friends and "no one has any idea of what I have to go through every day."

This is such an important point and such a difficult issue to confront that I believe it needs further illustration before we discuss the solution. I will illustrate it with a discussion of anorexia nervosa, the eating disorder in

BOX #16–2
"I Feel So Left Out of Things"

Even children in kindergarten can be excluded.[1] That rejection hurts, and it can cause long–term maladjustment and rebellion.[2] The dangers associated with being rejected increase in about the 5th grade as children begin to spend appreciably less time with their parents.[3] As children and teens become focused on their peers, the emotional attachment to parents begins to diminish and not receiving the approval of peers begins to pose an even greater threat.[4] The result is that some 65% of high school students have reported feeling "psychologically isolated."[5]

The principle is simple: the greater the desire for peer approval, the more likely one will find examples of rejection. This is not to say peer rejection is not real and even common. It is. But the point is that feeling "so left out of things" becomes increasingly common as peer approval becomes the focus.[6] It is common among 10–year–olds,[7] and it is common among college students[8]—especially those with a greater focus on self.[9] As children become adults and parents themselves, their focus must shift more to others. That is a healthy change which will lead to fewer feelings of social rejection and loneliness.

which people sometimes literally starve themselves to death. Who would you guess is most likely to develop anorexia nervosa—males or females? It is females by a very wide margin.[124] Why would that be? Do they have a genetic predisposition to starve themselves? Is the female sex more prone to a chemical imbalance in the brain that causes them to enjoy not eating? Such speculation is foolishness though there is no shortage of studies seeking to identify the genetic underpinnings and the chemical imbalances which may be responsible.[125]

No, the rather obvious explanation is that we live in a culture which places tremendous importance on physical attractiveness, especially for girls and women. That is why anorexia nervosa is more prevalent today than it was 60 years ago when teenage girls were not continuously exposed to magazines and television shows which glorify the perfect body and a beautiful face.[126] Now, guess again. Is it 60–, 70– and 80–year–old women who are most susceptible or is it girls of 12, 16 and 20? As you know, the answer is the younger group of mostly teens. But why? I will answer that question with three questions. Who thinks the most about looking good? Who is most apt to dwell on the fact that their noses are too big, their eyes are too close together and their hair is too thin and straight? Who is most apt to spend a lot of time looking at magazines that have lots of articles on how to look "hot" or "sexy"? It is the very group which is most likely to become anorexic.

One study related to eating disorders and the media's role in the increase in that problem provided subscriptions to *Seventeen* magazine for approximately half of a sample of vulnerable, adolescent girls. The girls believed they were receiving the magazine because they won a raffle in which all research participants were entered in appreciation for their willingness to participate in "other" research. The girls spent little extra time each month reading *Seventeen*, but the little extra time they spent with the magazine resulted in some actual attitude changes among them concerning the ideal body.[127] Other researchers have also found mere-exposure to pictures of thin models led to decreases in satisfaction with one's own weight.[128]

Related studies find that women viewing attractive women begin to feel less attractive,[129] and men viewing attractive women (in pornographic photographs) begin perceiving their own mates as less attractive.[130] There is a danger in even looking at those magazines. Every time these teenage girls stare at a beautiful young lady or read an article on looking good or attracting guys, their values are slowly but surely being changed—and the more likely they will become anorexic.[131] My advice is to give up the magazines entirely and adopt and actively voice contrary values: "It is unhealthy to place too much value on beauty. The media has fooled me in the past, but from now on I am going to help influence others not to overly value beauty and fashion by not focusing on those issues." This will not work if it is simply done cognitively. I believe it is true, and I want my clients to believe it is true. I want them to believe that this is the greater moral value.

> **BOX #16–3**
>
> ## An Alternative Approach—Get Beautiful
>
> I know some readers will object to my counsel. They would argue that we must go along with the culture, and the better approach would be pursuing more beauty (nice clothes, perfect make–up, etc.). The logical extension of this view includes lip augmentation, breast augmentation, a transcutaneous facelift, laser resurfacing, nose reduction and other types of cosmetic surgery, orthodontic work and liposuction. (For men this may include muscle–building steroids, hair transplants or an expensive car.) In other words, don't focus less on beauty; focus on it even more.
>
> In fact, more and more Americans are having plastic surgery.[1] Is this the road to joy? There are reports of women reporting better mental health following surgery,[2] but I suspect these women are more likely to say they feel better but are in reality feeling worse. Now they have sought to improve their looks and, if that does not make a significant difference, they could feel rather hopeless.
>
> That may be why we find that Swedish women who had cosmetic surgery were found to have suicide rates 2.9 times what would be expected.[3] The rate reported by a study of Danish women was 3.1 times the expected number.[4] Of course, it is also true that women having cosmetic surgery are more likely to have mental disorders (47.7% in one study)[5] and are more egotistical.[6]
>
> Another line of research which supports my contention that focusing on one's self is unhealthy: women who gaze (not just look) at the mirror invariably feel worse after the mirror gazing than they did before.[7]

One more question related to this issue: Would you guess that anorexic girls are more or less likely to have mothers who carefully diet and who have an above average focus on their own appearance? As you would correctly assume, the answer is "more likely."[132] That fact tells me that the values of those we are around affect us. We need to surround ourselves with people who have sound values so we are not overcome by the values that harm good mental health.

For some, depression will always be a struggle because they cannot bring themselves to accept and live out a most important value whose by–product, ironically, is feeling loved. That important value is: focus on loving and encouraging others and stop focusing on yourself. For many, no counsel is more difficult to accept, but I am fully convinced that dwelling on the lack of friends or the need for more attention from a spouse or dwelling on why a relationship with one's mother–in–law is not ideal will not help and will only cause misery. As we focus on how popular we are or how accepted we are, feelings of disappointment grow. The difficult but better approach is to make a commitment to (1) act in a loving way towards others and then (2) not focus on one's own needs but focus on the needs of others. I never tell anyone that either goal is easy to reach. But I insist that these are the right things to do.

Dale Carnegie's *How To Win Friends and Influence People*, first published in 1936, is the all–time best seller among self–help books. Over 15 million copies have been printed, and it still sells well.[133] Dale Carnegie courses, based upon the book's principles, are still taught all over the nation and around the world. Carnegie shared "Six Ways to Make People Like You" in the form of six rules. Consider how each rule essentially says, "Focus not on yourself, but on others. Make them feel you are glad to see them and that you are interested in them."

Rule 1: Become genuinely interested in other people.
Rule 2: Smile.
Rule 3: Remember that a man's name is to him the sweetest sound in any language.
Rule 4: Be a good listener. Encourage others to talk about themselves.
Rule 5: Talk in terms of the other man's interest.
Rule 6: Make the other person feel important—and do it sincerely.[134]

Carnegie's principles for influencing others and his principles for having a good marriage also encourage the reader essentially to love and encourage others and take the focus off self. What Jesus called the two greatest commandments were also based on this principle: "'Love the Lord your God with all your heart and with all your soul and with all your mind.' This is the first and greatest commandment. And the second is like it: 'Love your neighbor as yourself.'"[135]   The New Testament also teaches Christians, "In humility consider others better than yourselves." That passage then continues, "Each of you should look not only to your own interests, but also to the interests of others."[136]

However, there is a problem with Dale Carnegie's rules and God's commandments. I am convinced they are of little value if only a cognitive acknowledgment is made "to act in a new way so people will like me more." They require a heart commitment to love others and not focus on self because it is the right thing to do. Again, one's values are the key, not cognitive acknowledgment. That means every thought must be taken captive. When we start feeling unloved and neglected, we must immediately commit to getting rid of that thought and focus instead on helping others who may need attention and love.

I think you can see why some people will never take this road. It requires a daily commitment. It is not easy. But it is the road to joy. No pill can provide the feeling of joy that comes from a real commitment to such a life.

Now, let's be sure you see the application to depression. It is no more healthy to focus on being relatively unpopular than it would be to focus on not being as beautiful as the cover girl. Neither do I believe popularity and beauty should be valued highly. What we should value is character and loving others. Once again, this change will never happen cognitively. It requires a transformation of *values*. This view is contrary to the messages we hear daily. Not only do we hear that we need to be sexy; we are told we need nice clothes, a new car, exciting travel and financial security. It is a value system and a philosophy which cannot bring joy.

There is a better way, but unfortunately we can be terribly blind to our own self–centered focus. We may often drop hints that we know more than someone else, brag about an accomplishment, make someone listen to us talk instead of listening to them. We may be hurt when someone does not

Should You Desire Popularity or Personal Character?

A value that needs to be taught to children and adults is that popularity is not important; character is. Character (being loving and kind even to those who are unpopular, honest even when it hurts, unselfish, dependable, disciplined, moral, thoughtful—qualities that in some settings can bring the disdain of others) is within your control, but popularity is not. If you are not a smooth speaker, athletic or very attractive, you are not apt to be very popular. If you stutter or are uncoordinated or are unskilled, you may be ridiculed.

So just as physical attractiveness is not something we control and thus should not be highly valued, we cannot control how popular we will be and, thus, popularity should not be highly valued. Knowing and being convicted of what is truly important can provide some degree of emotional protection for all of us.

greet us warmly when we arrive at an event, but we may fail to encourage others by greeting them warmly. We may feel incensed when we have invited others over and no one can come, or someone does come for dinner and a game but does not ever offer a return invitation. Read back over the list and see why we are hurt, become incensed or even feel excluded. We are focusing on ourselves. Love is blind, and nowhere is love more blind than when it is focused on self. The following case illustrates that truth and the harm which follows.

A Case Study

In 1951 *New York Times* reporter Lucy Freeman wrote a very honest account of the daily turmoil and misery she felt and the six years of psychoanalysis she purchased in hopes of overcoming her unhappiness. It is not a pleasant book to read and has no happy ending, but remarkably it became a national bestseller.

> My desperation made no sense. Ostensibly I possessed all
> a girl needed for happiness. I worked on what I believed

the world's finest newspaper, rubbed shoulders reporter–fashion with great and near–great. By society's standards I was successful—but I felt miserable. I had never known more people—nor been lonelier.[137]

What Lucy Freeman never understood was the importance of not focusing on herself—a fact revealed in dozens of examples throughout her book. She was unwilling to build up and encourage others though she still desperately desired their attention, approval and love. For example, her father chewed gum, a habit she disliked, but rather than feeling pleasure that he was enjoying something he liked or even being gracious enough to ignore his habit, she tried to "get even" by smoking cigarettes in his presence despite his sinus problems. "We finally compromised. He promised he would not chew gum in my presence, a noise that made me want to rip out my hair, if I would not smoke cigarettes in his."[138]

Conflict with her mother was also common. "Mother and I fought some vicious verbal battles. . . . Sometimes Mother would whistle or hum to drown out my words, and I would scream in anguish. (No wonder when I was depressed and the person next to me on a bus started to whistle, I winced and felt like choking him.)"[139] As a young woman Freeman spoke with a quiet voice that could not always be heard. "People would often ask me to repeat when they did not hear. That increased my fury so I could hardly get words out." When meeting a cousin's new husband who could not hear what she said, she shot back, "Why don't you listen, you jerk?"[140]

Lucy Freeman was so self–centered that when she looked back as an adult on a minor, unfortunate mistake, she personalized it and it became a source of personal torture. Her account is also a good illustration of why self–analysis can be dangerous. When Lucy was a child, her mother would often go by her school and pick her up for lunch. Unable to do so one day, she called the school and asked them to get a message to her daughter to eat at school. The message was not delivered until Freeman had been standing out in the icy cold weather for over an hour. The school apologized with a huge lunch.

> But that could not remove the hurt in my heart. I was con-
> vinced Mother had finally forsaken me. She liked my
> brother and sister much better. She never would have left
> either of them standing alone in the street. . . . "Why is it
> always me?" I wondered, then and now . . . . My mother
> hated me. And I hated her.[141]

I have often visited with students who were depressed over a relationship and "catastrophized" minor events in the same way. The key to overcoming this misery is not to avoid making mountains out of molehills. It is to understand the root cause—an intense focus on having *my* needs met rather than focusing on others. Ironically, Freeman wrote that "this book represents all my needs that writing fills—attention, approval, love"[142] just two pages before expressing her philosophy of life: "Each one thinks of himself first whether or not he admits it. It is human to live a life of self–interest."[143] Lucy Freeman sought to do just that and suffered anxiety, depression, conflict and divorce as a result. Despite her many years of psychoanalysis and an entire book in which she analyzes herself, she never saw the real causes of her unhappiness.

Wanting to be appreciated, cared about and loved is natural. But the greater the desire, the less likely we are to feel satisfied with what we receive. That is why learning to focus on appreciating, caring about and loving others rather than getting our own needs met makes sense. Ironically, it is also the best way to be appreciated, cared about and loved.

(7) Do you have clear meaning and purpose in life?

When I began my PhD program, I was determined to study the role of purpose in life in mental health or family functioning. I had already completed a 60–hour masters degree in marriage and family therapy and a

36–hour interdepartmental masters with a psychology emphasis, and yet I knew I had never heard much, if anything, about purpose in life. My professors were outstanding men and women, but a discussion of purpose in life was simply not a part of the curriculum.

I investigated and learned that there were books which addressed that subject. The first of the many books I read was Victor Frankl's *Man's Search for Meaning*.[144] Frankl was a Jewish psychiatrist who was sent to the Nazi concentration camps. Every day he fought to survive by trying to look healthy and capable of work. He used a broken piece of glass to shave often, thinking it would make him look more fit.

He also kept his mind sharp by beginning an observational study, and what Frankl observed among his fellow prisoners became the basis for his future approach to helping others. He noticed a remarkable transformation occurred among his fellow prisoners as the days passed. Many of those who came to the camp afraid and angry but polite became more and more selfish, hostile and uncaring. And yet others who were also afraid and angry upon arrival became more and more unselfish and kind. They would sacrifice the little food they received to feed a dying person. They cared for the sick. They comforted the hopeless.

These were not isolated cases. All the prisoners tended to move in one direction or the other. Within the concentration camp all the familiar goals of life were beyond reach. Physical health, wealth, family, fame, occupational success—even the right to be treated with dignity—were beyond reach. The choices that free people can generally make (when to get up, what to eat, what to do with one's time, where to go, when to go to bed) were all removed. All that remained, the prisoners' only choice, was how to live. Frankl watched as prisoner after prisoner moved toward one of the two extremes. In time, some behaved like animals. Others behaved like saints.

But what made the difference? That was Frankl's question, and his final conclusion was found in a person's reason for living. For some, life was all about themselves, and when all their rights were stripped away, the anger, hostility, emptiness and despair grew daily. For others, life was about far

---

BOX #16–5

Purpose In Life Research

Higher purpose in life is associated with

1. Less depression[1]
2. Fewer suicide thoughts or attempts[2]
3. Less anxiety/general neuroses[3]
4. Fewer mental problems[4]
5. Less schizophrenia[5]
6. Better adjustment to serious illness or tragedy[6]
7. Better ability to overcome obstacles[7]
8. Better recovery after surgery[8]
9. Less death anxiety[9]
10. Less delinquency among adolescents[10]
11. Less crime among adults[11]
12. Less alcohol abuse[12]
13. Less drug abuse[13]
14. Fewer teen pregnancies[14]
15. Overall better mental health[15]
16. A greater sense of well–being[16]
17. Less boredom and greater happiness[17]
18. Less value placed on happiness, pleasure, excitement, freedom and comfort[18]
19. More pro–social behavior[19]
20. Being more religious[20]

---

more than self. Life was about helping and serving and making a difference.
Frankl's conclusion was that nothing was more fundamental. This "will to
meaning" was the primary force of life.

Frankl was concerned that during his lifetime Europe and America were
becoming more self–centered, which, ironically, would lead to a sense of

inner emptiness, a condition he termed "existential vacuum."[145] As America entered the "me decade," Abraham Maslow, another famous interpreter of the human condition, witnessed the same phenomenon and declared "value-lessness" the ultimate disease of his era.[146]

They were right. Compare suicide rates for young people in 1960 (the "me decade" had not yet begun) with 1970 (its beginnings were already having a dramatic impact), with 1980 (its growth and effects were still increasing), with 1990 (the harm was peaking with more and more voices saying we went in the wrong direction). We see similar increases in divorce. Look at the numbers for depression, child abuse, rape or homicide. For every kind of personality or social issue, we saw a dramatic turn for the worse as we entered a period where self and personal rights became a greater focus and unselfishness and service became less important. And yet meaning and purpose in life is a subject that is rarely mentioned in psychology textbooks. I have taught from many psychology texts and have kept them all. But as I went through all those texts, I found that only one mentioned the subject, and even the few paragraphs it devoted to meaning in life were taken out after the second edition.[147]

Psychiatry has the same problem. "It is arguably the main reason people seek psychiatric treatment, yet it is a concept largely ignored in psychiatry," observed two Australian psychiatrists.[148] Dr. Hans Selye, the great endocrinologist who became the father of stress research, called a lack of meaning in life the greatest stressor of all.[149]

So it is that a lack of meaning in life is the single greatest threat to mental health, yet "it is a concept largely ignored in psychiatry." This is one of those great mysteries which I have never understood. I suspect that it is because of its tie to religious faith that the hugely important role of purpose in life has been ignored. However, I also have hope that purpose in life will not continue to be overlooked. Not too surprisingly, the reason for the potential change (which I am now seeing in the research literature) will likely be a Christian pastor.

When Rick Warren published *The Purpose Driven Life*[150] in 2002, no one expected that within two years it would become the greatest selling hardback in the history of America. Over 20 million copies had been sold by 2005, and it is still on the best–selling book lists.[151] Perhaps its success was, in some measure, a reflection of how far we as a nation had moved from living for more noble and meaningful reasons to living for self. The question on the book's cover asks, "What on earth am I here for?" The book's first sentence answers, "It's not about you." That shift from not focusing on self and our pleasures and wants stands in stark contrast to the age of narcissism (self–love) which began in the mid–1960s. That era's expressions ("Do your own thing"), concerns (self–esteem), behaviors (the sexual revolution and the drug culture), therapies (self–awareness and self–help groups), songs ("Why Don't We Do It in the Road"), movies ("Deep Throat") and books (*Looking Out for Number 1*) often reflected a cultural shift—an acceptance of focusing on self.

Between 1970 and 1987 large annual surveys of college freshmen found the desire for financial wealth increased each and every year but one.[152] The rapid rise came to an end in 1987, but the number of college freshmen who indicate that it is "very important" to be quite well off financially remains at a level which is far above the levels that preceded the value changes which were part of and continued past the "cultural revolution" of the 1960s. Perhaps it is in our nature to assume that wealth brings happiness. But the research into this subject reveals it is a false hope.[153] Neither does the pursuit of alcohol and drugs[154] or premarital or extramarital sex bring happiness—or good mental health.[155] But purpose in life can. Its ability to strengthen us mentally is tremendous. Dr. Selye argued that those with clear meaning and purpose could overcome virtually any obstacle. If your spouse were to die, could you carry on? If you had a leg amputated, would it throw you into depression or cause you to consider suicide? Over a century ago Emile Durkheim, founder of sociology and the father of suicide research, identified a lack of meaning as being the first cause among the four types or causes of suicide.[156]

Those who know why they are here, who believe they are here for a definite reason, can overcome all kinds of stressors that might lead to mental instability in another person. But those who do not have a clear, significant purpose for living are at risk for all kinds of mental problems. Gaining new purpose in life can also heal a mind that has already experienced serious declines. Consider the case of JoAnn.

A Case Study

I know JoAnn but not as a client. She is the mother of our friend Tammy. JoAnn had worked for many years in a responsible job that demanded a lot of capability. Upon retirement, she and her husband Paul were encouraged by their daughter to sell their home and move further south so they could be near family. JoAnn had always been a very negative person, and she and Paul had frequent conflict, but she had never had any mental problems. That all changed when they sold their home and headed south.

JoAnn began complaining about their new home from the day they arrived. It was nicer than the home they had sold, but JoAnn was determined not to be happy. It was all she would talk about. She hated her new house. "We were foolish to sell our house. We should never have done it. This house is terrible." After three weeks of constant complaining and distress, JoAnn's mind became completely clouded. She began walking around the house without any clothes. Her daughter was distraught, but her mother was now unable to talk with her rationally. Then one morning Paul called his daughter. "Tammy, you have to do something fast. Your mother is walking down the street, and she doesn't have any clothes on." That experience (and the fact that the psychiatrist who was consulted learned that she had also been carrying a knife around the house) led to her commitment. She was put on Haldol, and within one day her daughter saw a drooling, incoherent woman with whom she could not even hope to communicate. Her mother was completely "zombied." She did not even know who Tammy was.

In hopes of restoring her sanity, Paul moved them back north, but her condition remained desperate. Eleven years of various mind drugs followed during which time JoAnn went from a size 8 to a size 22 and was incapable of caring for herself. But then one day about two years ago a miracle happened. Paul was getting forgetful and was diagnosed as being in the early stages of Alzheimer's disease. JoAnn was barely functioning at that time. Paul had been taking care of her, preparing her meals and driving her where she needed to go. But when JoAnn heard the diagnosis, she immediately announced, "Then I have to get off these drugs. I can't take care of myself, and I sure won't be able to take care of Paul."

That amount of self–awareness amazed me, but it also tells me that even months of antipsychotics followed by years of antidepressants do not necessarily keep a patient from being able to make some good choices. Her doctor was opposed to JoAnn's decision, but she did get off her drugs, and suddenly JoAnn became a new person. She was going to have to care for Paul. She began cooking again. She then decided she would need to drive again since Paul would soon lose his license. She started studying and soon passed the driving test. She even began shedding extra pounds. Suddenly, as the caregiver instead of the one needing care, her mind was as clear as it had ever been. JoAnn even announced one day, "Paul, we need to get out of this house and start going to church again."

I have not seen Paul and JoAnn since they moved back north, but Tammy tells me the transformation is hard even to imagine. Almost overnight her mother regained the personality she had lost for 11 years. In fact, she is a more compassionate and devoted person than she has ever been as she now has the privilege to care for a loving husband who cared for her for so many years. "I want to make the end of his life pleasant. That's the least I can do for him after all the years he cared for me." Paul has had other health problems since, and at a recent doctor's visit JoAnn began to cry when they received his diagnosis of lymphoma. The doctor suggested that he would like to write a prescription for JoAnn for an antidepressant. JoAnn's response was "No way!"

BOX #16–6

Purpose in Life

Gordon W. Allport was one of America's most famous psychologists. Known for his pioneering work in personality, he could have been analyzing how JoAnn's thinking became so confused and how it cleared again when he wrote, "The possession of long–range goals, regarded as central to one's personal existence, distinguishes the human being from the animal, the adult from the child, and in many cases the healthy personality from the sick."[1]

Knowing we are needed can have a powerful, positive effect on the mind. So can choosing to do the right thing. In 1902 William James, the father of American psychology, wrote, "How to gain, how to keep, how to recover happiness is in fact for most men at all times the secret motive of all they do and of all they are able to endure."[157] James may be right, but ironically, making personal happiness the ultimate goal of life seems to be the surest way not to find it. No, an important piece of the puzzle that makes up good mental health is to realize that life is not about us and then to live in a way that proves we really believe it.

(8) Do you have idiopathic depression?

"Idiopathic" means "a disease with no known cause." It is a word I have known for many years because my daughter has idiopathic scoliosis, a condition that required her to wear a hard plastic body–wrapping back brace 23 hours a day for nearly 4 years. America's drug manufacturers spend millions of dollars every year to convince us that depression is also often or typically idiopathic. Why would they want to continually emphasize that depression is not a personal weakness but a mental disease just like diabetes?[158] Why do they repeatedly tell us that "although the exact causes of depression are unknown, it may be due to a chemical imbalance in the brain."[159] Why do they want us to believe that "some types of depression run in families, suggesting that a biological vulnerability can be inherited."[160] Why do they emphasize that "a person may experience symptoms of depression suddenly, for no apparent reason."[161]

The simple reason: they are committed to convincing our nation that biological psychiatry is right, that a chemical imbalance in the brain is the cause of most depression and that antidepressant drugs are the answer. In part because of the success of these public "education" campaigns, I have seen "unexplained" depression also. But I have *never* seen a case of unexplained depression that remained unexplained.

I have gone over seven causes of depression in this chapter, most of which are never discussed with patients before antidepressant prescriptions are written. I did not cover research that shows that being critical rather than generous results in more depression. Neither did I share research on drug interactions, self–disclosure, environmental influences and other issues that are related to this problem and which I cover in lecturing on depression. My purpose in this section is not to be comprehensive. My purpose is to show that there is an abundance of research indicating that depression can stem from many issues that are ignored or downplayed by drug–industry–funded ads and literature. The fact that physicians rarely go over the many factors which we know can move us away from joyfulness and toward depression is a clear indication of the success of the industry's marketing strategy.

The chapter epigraph (the words above the chapter's title) is from The Carpenter's 1971 hit, "Rainy Days and Mondays." I chose it because the words are worth considering. "Nothing is really wrong" we are told, but in just the two stanzas I have shared we also learn that she is "feelin' like I don't belong," feeling like a "lonely clown," and she has "nothing to do" but dwell on her problems ("frown"). It is not uncommon for those who are depressed, when asked why they feel depressed, to respond, "I don't know why." But with enough discussion, the causes will be expressed. (Sometimes offering possibilities may be necessary: "Rejection is far, far more common than most people realize. It hurts, and it often causes depression. Many of those I counsel have experienced rejection from a friend or coworker or a family member. Let me ask you on a scale of 1–10 . . . ") Rejection is a good example of a problem someone may not want to share, but depression related to feelings of rejection, being left out and not really loved are very, very common.

Though many people have average popularity and suffer largely because they are too focused on not being popular enough, some have a value system that differs markedly from their peers or have poor social skills and are thus ignored or shunned. The research indicates that generally peers, teachers and others can quickly pick up on who is popular or accepted and who is rejected.[162] People who are actively rejected know it. No pill will fix that problem.

I am frustrated and angered by the industry's dishonest research studies, essential disregard for the financial costs these ineffective drugs impose on poor families, and the actual physical harm they inflict on millions of users who consume these drugs year in and year out. However by continuing to promote the biochemical theory, the industry harms Americans in another way.

Overcoming depression requires lots of work or changes that the depressed person does not want to make. I will provide an example shortly, but first note how industry messages provide an excuse for depression, lessen personal responsibility and keep doctors from seeking out the real causes of the depression. Take note of these comments from the National Alliance for Research on Schizophrenia and Depression, one of many drug–industry–financed "not for profit" organizations.

> People with cancer aren't expected to heal themselves. People with diabetes can't will themselves out of needing insulin. And yet you probably think, like millions of people do, that you or someone you know should be able to overcome another debilitating disease, depression, through sheer will and fortitude. . . . Recent medical research has

taught us that depression is often biological, caused by a chemical imbalance in the brain. We've even found that depression has a genetic link.[163]

The absolute falsehoods that this ad perpetuates were discussed in Chapter 2. I won't go over those issues again. Instead, note how this ad's message could cause a patient to assume his or her depression is inevitable and cause the physician to ignore the actual causes. Two psychiatrists once wrote in their book on depression that "pent–up anger is the root cause of the vast majority of depressions."[164] If they were right, "the vast majority" of pent up anger is being treated with pills.

Consider a different approach which I will illustrate with a woman who had a major conflict with her next door neighbor. Though they had been friends, the relationship was absolutely over. Or so my client thought. Conflict needs to be resolved, no matter who started the problem. In fact, it generally is not helpful to discuss how the conflict began. That can open old wounds, stir up anger over injustices suffered and move the person you want to help toward depression, not joyfulness. Instead I asked her to make some bread for her own family . . . and for her neighbor.

My client did not even want to consider taking bread to her neighbor. "She would slam the door in my face." I doubted it, but that thought helped control her guilt over not even having eye contact with her old friend. (Yes, they saw each other often when taking out the trash, working in the yard or going to work, but, as we tend to do, they pretended not to see each other. They kept their eyes looking down or scurried back into the house when they noticed the other outside. Simple eye to eye contact can be difficult following a major conflict!) Once again, you can see why I sometimes require a financial deposit when counseling. She did not want to do it, but I told her it was one of her assignments.

When the next week came, my client was anxious to tell me all about it. She had gone next door with shaking knees, miserable, hating the assignment. But when the door opened and the two sets of eyes met, no door was slammed. (I have never had a client come back saying someone slammed the door on them.)

"Hi, Sandra. I was baking some bread and I made several loaves. I thought you might enjoy some while it is still hot."

When you know you have done the right thing, does it move you toward depression or joy? The Continuum Model works because it reflects how our emotions work. In contrast, no number of pills could have made my client feel that good about herself or could have repaired that broken friendship.

A Last Thought

I have already emphasized that I cannot be comprehensive in discussing depression. However, I think you should be. Put yourself to the test. Evaluate yourself. Are you getting enough sleep? Are you a television junkie? Are you being a responsible employee, parent and friend? Are you meeting your obligations? Are you feeling guilty because you are flirting (in very "innocent" ways, of course) with others besides your spouse? Are you generally loving to your spouse but also guilty of little, unkind criticisms when frustrated? Are you guilty of slandering your friends or your family members behind their backs? Are you violating what you know is the right choice in some other area of your life? Are you spending time with others? Are you seeking to help and encourage others? Do you feel angry when you are not getting their attention or invitations in return? Are your values healthy values or are beauty, popularity, prestige and "success" the desires of your heart? Does your lifestyle indicate that you value pleasure and recreation more than service, goodness and love? Do you need to analyze your purpose in life?

Only you know the answers to all the questions. You do not need me or any other professional to ask those questions if you will honestly evaluate yourself. Now you have some choices. You can take an antidepressant to control your anger, unkindness, selfishness or whatever the problems are.

But that will never solve the problems. There is a better road to take. Few are ever willing to commit to taking and staying on that less travelled road, but that is the road that leads to joy. I hope you will choose that path.

"There is one area of biomedicine in which the government allows—even defends—a minimal standard that would be unacceptable anywhere else in research. It is the set of evidentiary requirements maintained by the Food and Drug Administration (FDA) for the approval of new drugs."[1]

—*Jerry Avorn, M.D.*
Professor of Medicine
Harvard Medical School, 2005

Epilogue

About two years ago my wife and I went to a new restaurant for dinner. We will never go back. The center smoking section was about three feet higher than the non–smoking section where we sat but was immediately adjacent to it. We were directly below the smokers, some of their feet being little more than inches from our heads. Perhaps because we were not on the same level, the smokers did not seem to even notice us. They consistently turned their heads our direction and exhaled their smoke. We would have breathed in less smoke if we had been seated next to them in the restaurant's smoking section. For those of you who have had similar experiences, let me comfort you with this fact. Many literature reviews of the research have found that passive smoking (breathing smokers' exhaled smoke) poses no risks to non–smokers. Surprised? Then read on.

Literature reviews are frequently published by scientific journals to bring the reader up to date concerning what the most recent research studies have found on various topics being reviewed. In theory, those who publish the review articles are simply summarizing what other researchers have found. Their own bias should not result in any bias in the literature review. That is the theory. In real life, however, we are all more subtly influenced than we may realize—especially when our job or our income is on the line. This was the finding of Deborah Barnes and Lisa Bero who published an analysis of review articles on passive smoking in the *Journal of the American Medical Association*.

Knowing they might also be less objective than they would like to be, they gathered every review article in English on the health effects of passive smoking written between 1980 and 1995 and then asked two independent reviewers (who were kept in the dark concerning the purpose of the study) to categorize each review's conclusions for 12 criteria. A total of 106 review articles were located, 37% of which concluded that passive smoking is not bad for one's health! If the two independent assessors' rating scores for any article differed by more than .20 points, they discussed their evaluations and sought a consensus. This was rarely necessary as 95% of the time their independent assessments were in agreement. For over three–quarters of the articles the authors did not reveal their source of funding for the research. Thus, Barnes and Bero investigated that issue.

When the results were finally analyzed, the study revealed that 94% of the review articles which concluded passive smoking is not bad for one's health were written by those who had tobacco industry ties. Only 13% of those without tobacco industry ties came to such a conclusion. But even more telling, when only articles of high quality (based on the independent raters' assessments) were examined, tobacco industry ties became the one and only factor associated with a review concluding that passive smoking is not dangerous.[2] A number of other studies have also found that sponsorship can greatly influence a study's conclusions.[3]

Two points concerning this research demand comment. First, money greatly influences research results, a fact I hope you clearly understand by now. Second, (and this is most encouraging) an excellent research design will ultimately overcome outright dishonesty, an innocently but poorly designed research study or blind bias. Truth does prevail in the end. Truth will ultimately convince America that antidepressants and antipsychotics harm rather than help those who are depressed, anxious or suffering severe mental problems.

Randomized, controlled trials which demand use of placebo controls and double–blind designs will continue to show these drugs to be only slightly superior to sugar pills[4] (and then only because mind drugs have more side effects). Yet antidepressants and antipsychotics pose real dangers to physical and mental health. In theory, the growing awareness of the need and importance of quality RCT research combined with the expiration of the patents for all the antidepressants and antipsychotics in current use should mean that the use of these drugs will be greatly diminished before long. (Remember that drug patents are awarded for only 20 years from the time the drug patent is submitted.[5]) After all, once a drug's patent expires and generics become available, the drug companies should no longer be willing to spend the vast sums promoting the chemical imbalance view as they did in the past. With no active promotion, will the truth quickly rise to the surface and mind drugs no longer be requested by Americans?

To conclude so is naive. History tells us that drug companies will not give up the chemical imbalance propaganda. They have too much to lose. As soon as the selective serotonin–reuptake inhibitors go off patent, the pharmaceuticals will adjust the chemical formula (and their advertising and marketing campaigns), and we will learn that serotonin is not the key to healing depression, but it will be GABA or epinephrine or some neurotransmitter we don't even know about today. (Or they may add one of these chemicals to serotonin to provide us with a new type of antidepressant.)

I cannot tell you exactly what will happen in the future, but I can say with confidence that the drug companies will claim to have developed a new and improved antidepressant (changed sufficiently to be awarded a new patent), and this battle will be fought again. My greatest hope for the American people ultimately winning the battle and no longer being fooled lies in five areas.

(1) College and universities will finally recognize that education must be committed to teaching research design as one of the most important and fundamental aspects of being truly educated. If graduates do not have sufficient knowledge of research design to analyze and critique the research upon which their education is based, they will always be in danger of being duped. It is a great flaw in our educational system that these are not skills universally taught. This demands correction, and, when it is corrected, poor research will have far less influence.

(2) An independent board with expertise in scientific research and no ties to the drug companies will design studies used for gaining the approval of new drugs. This is such a simple matter that it would seem our government should have implemented it decades ago. Allowing the pharmaceutical companies to design their own drug studies makes no more sense than allowing a terrorist organization to design a plan for our national security. The cost to our nation for establishing a "drug studies standards board" would be minimal. Properly promoted, it could be seen as a great national service and be eagerly sought by the nation's leading authorities even if no remuneration were given board members. Drug companies could still pay for the studies, and results of each study (not just those with "good" outcomes) could be submitted and made public. Data could then be easily reviewed and appropriate praise or criticism made.

(3) The FDA standards for allowing a drug to enter the marketplace will be raised. Currently, drugs do not have to prove they actually work. They just have to be relatively safe and have better results than a placebo. Any drug that causes headaches or dry mouth or diarrhea could be approved for depression because any drug which caused any of these side effects would prove more effective than sugar pill placebos. The standards today for antidepressants and antipsychotics are a joke. Drugs should be compared to active placebos (placebos which cause side effects) and should be appreciably better than the placebo even if they cause no side effects. (Isn't it immoral to charge expensive prices for drugs that are not actually capable of healing anything?) If drugs cause serious side effects, then their ability to heal needs to be substantial. Of course, if this standard had been in place before Prozac (the first SSRI antidepressant) was approved, it and all the other antidepressants which followed would never have been permitted. Long–term use side effects (as discussed in Chapters 10, 11 & 13) should be considered. Allowing drugs to be approved based on 4–, 6– or 8–week studies needs to come to an end.

(4) Insurance companies will establish an "approved drug list" which demands that drugs meet the standards that the FDA should be requiring. This is already happening to some extent. Eli Lilly's Cymbalta antidepressant was disqualified from appearing on Kaiser Permanente's preferred drugs list for Northern and Southern California because it has not been found superior to the off–patent Prozac.[6] (Lilly claims it is a superior antidepressant, but Kaiser now has a group of pharmacists who are critically reading the drug studies. In the case of Cymbalta, they found its claim of superiority was based on administering higher doses to study subjects than what is recommended on the label, one of the tricks discussed in the "Tricks of the Trade" chapter.[7]) A similar board might also be established by an association of state Medicaid programs, since they also pay for prescription drugs.[8] Money talks, and I hope that one or the other of the major funding sources will use their influence to benefit the public and save dollars, which could lower overall medical costs for everyone.

Change might come from other sources, of course. State attorney general lawsuits might bring about more objective science (but it would likely occur on a case by case basis and is not likely to bring the fundamental reforms that are needed). Congress may pass laws that will quickly bring needed reforms. Cochrane Library's collection of evidence–based databases might become so authoritative that physicians will not be inclined to prescribe any drug that has not received favorable attention from Cochrane Collaboration reviewers.

(5) Physicians and the public will become knowledgeable about drug studies and the drug approval process. It is possible that a growing awareness by physicians and the public of the issues addressed in this book will result in healthy changes. If they become convinced that textbooks are not free of errors, that "big pharma's" massive advertising and other marketing efforts shape opinion and hide truth, that there are many drug trial tricks which can influence drug trial results, that the FDA drug approval process is flawed and that there are better options than mind drugs for good mental health, then progress is possible.

I have written this book in hopes of bringing change in this quarter. And though researching this subject has been a relentless pursuit for years, I am not accepting any profit this book might earn. This matter is so important that a non–profit effort seemed to be the right choice. I am hoping the public will be more inclined to purchase and read this book if they know their dollars will profit a worthy organization (Habitat for Humanity). Yet, I am also realistic. The reality is that this book will not likely have much effect on whether or not America will continue to be fooled. The money keeping our nation in the dark will continue to flow from the drug companies. Textbook publishers will continue to fear that sharing a message which is out of step with conventional wisdom could hurt textbook sales. Drug companies will continue to be the number one source of information on mind drugs for medical school students (our future doctors). No, big change is not coming any time soon.

However, this book can make a difference in the lives of your family and friends if you simply encourage them to read it. Many who might accept an antidepressant prescription from their physician might not do so if they knew more. Family members of those whose thinking becomes confused could keep them from antipsychotics and the resulting tragic life if they knew the truth. I will especially appreciate your passing the book on to your physicians since they are still the ones who write the drug prescriptions. We each have a responsibility to do whatever good we can. I hope you will join me in this effort to keep America from continuing to be fooled.

Getting Off Antidepressants

I personally know of many individuals who simply stopped taking their antidepressant after learning of the dangers these drugs present or because they did not like their side effects. I have also known of a few cases where antipsychotics were abruptly halted. Because of my own knowledge of persons who simply decided to get off their mind drug all at once, I was skeptical of the warnings concerning some severe reactions from stopping abruptly. Minor discontinuation symptoms are known to be common.[1] "SSRI discontinuation syndrome" and "antipsychotic discontinuation syndrome" (or similar labels) have even become recognized medical conditions in the research literature.[2] But very severe reactions are another issue.

As I researched the question, I discovered that, indeed, a small percentage of users have extreme withdrawal reactions, including a five–fold increased risk of suicide.[3] Joseph Glenmullen, MD, a Harvard Medical School professor and psychiatrist, has even written a book on safely getting off antidepressants. *The Antidepressant Solution* has one chapter entitled, "The 5–Step Antidepressant Tapering Program: How to Avoid Uncomfortable or Dangerous Withdrawal Reactions."[4] However when you have never seen a case personally, it does make you have some doubts.

Those doubts ended for me when Angie, the grown daughter of some of our best friends, was given an antidepressant by a physician whom she consulted because she was having a breathing difficulty. It is not surprising that, not being able to find any reason for the occasional breathing problem, he decided her problem might be stress induced. (Stress can cause breathing difficulties, but so can a dust–laden environment, a heart arrhythmia or an allergic reaction to pollen, mold or dog/cat hair. Less common is troubled breathing caused by dozens of other medical conditions—severe anemia, bronchiolitis, Lyme disease, pericarditis and so forth.)

I have known Angie for most of her life. If she were an average person in terms of mental health, then her experience would not be so convincing for me. But not only has she no history of depression or mental problems, she always has a positive attitude and is one of the most personable and pleasant young women I have ever known.

Angie took her antidepressant as her physician instructed her to but after four months decided she should not stay on them any longer. That is when the strangest experience of her life began. She was at home with her young son when she began to crash emotionally. Suddenly she found herself on the floor weeping, and she didn't know why. Life was going well, but she was miserable. She could not explain it. She didn't understand it herself. As she related the experience to me, she said, "I didn't care if I were to die. In fact, that's what I was thinking, 'I just don't care.'" For three days Angie went through this torment, crying relentlessly but not knowing why.

Two years later Angie went to a surgeon for a needed operation. The surgeon informed her that he routinely gave all of his patients an antidepressant following surgery "just to be sure my patients don't develop depression following surgery." Angie did not argue, but she told me, "There was no way I was going to take an antidepressant. I'll never do that again."

This is not the typical reaction, but today we have well-designed research studies which make it clear that severe reactions to these drugs do occur. You need to be aware of this and inform your family and healthcare professional before you begin tapering off your antidepressant.

One last note: After the breathing problem and antidepressant experience, Angie discovered she had gallstones—severe enough to require the removal of her gallbladder at an uncommonly young age. And, yes, gallstones can also cause shortness of breath.

The *British Medical Journal* Controversy

The *British Medical Journal* is considered one of the world's most important and respected medical journals. On New Year's Day 2005, the *BMJ* published an article by Jeanne Lenzer which indicated that Eli Lilly, the maker of Prozac, had failed to disclose documents during a lawsuit that found Prozac could increase the risk of aggressive behavior and suicide.[1]

Overnight tens of millions heard the story as the report was passed along by the news media. The implications for Lilly were horrendous. Lawsuits are often won or lost based on public attitudes and perceptions. Suddenly Lilly was at lawsuit risk for the thousands of Prozac patients who had committed suicide. Lilly's stock dropped over $800 million on the news.[2] Lilly decided it had to take the offensive and on January 13 did so in a big way, spending $800,000 on ads in major publications.[3]

The *BMJ* began an internal investigation, and in their January 29, 2005, issue they printed a correction and apology stating that their investigation "has revealed that all of the documents supplied to the *BMJ* that were either Eli Lilly documents or were in the hands of Eli Lilly had in fact been disclosed during the suit."[4] The correction and apology were also covered by major news outlets. Unfortunately, many of those news reports implied that the suicide and violence link with Prozac was not real. The Associated Press reported that "the *British Medical Journal* has retracted a report that said Eli Lilly and Co. documents suggesting a link between Prozac and a heightened risk of suicide attempts and violence had gone missing for years."[5]

MSNBC did an even worse job. They ran the Reuters' wire report under the heading, "Claim of Prozac Suicide Link Retracted." The Reuters story began, "The *British Medical Journal* has retracted its controversial claims about drug maker Eli Lilly and Co., its drug Prozac and a potential link to suicide."[6] The *BMJ* never declared the "Prozac suicide link retracted"; they retracted their statement that documents "went missing." Eli Lilly knew it, but their statement to Reuters sought to convince the public that there was no link.

In the end the public's perception of Eli Lilly's integrity was aided by the events, and Lilly was able to be generous to itself and the *BMJ* in the press release which followed its apology. "It is Lilly's policy to be honest in our dealings with the public, the media, regulatory bodies and our customers. We accept the apology and retraction with the understanding that both our organizations are committed to providing doctors and patients with accurate information about medications."[7]

Has Lilly been honest? Peter Breggin has again provided a public service by placing on the web a discussion of the facts. Go to http://www.breggin.com and select the box entitled "Dr. Breggin Analyzes the Eli Lilly Prozac–Induced Suicide and Violence Documents Now in Possession of the *British Medical Journal* (*BMJ*)." Even a casual reading of Dr. Breggin's review makes it plain that Lilly has consistently sought to keep the whole truth of this matter from ever seeing the light of day.

The Real Reasons for the Decline in Mental Hospital Population

There are many reasons the number of patients in state and county mental hospitals declined after 1955. (My college lecture on this subject includes a total of 18.) Three of the major factors are considered here.

An Artificially Inflated Mental Hospital Population

Mental hospitals' population decline after 1955 occurred primarily because the institutional population in 1955 was artificially inflated and because it was not until then that the public became aware that these institutions were a national disgrace and needed dramatic reform. Understanding the decline in the number of mental hospital patients following 1955 must start with the question, "Why did the number of patients increase at rates that far exceeded the growth in the nation's population?"

The population of the United States increased by 656% from 1850 to 1950, but the mental hospital population increased 10,835% during these same years.[1] A small proportion of this surge was likely due to actual increases in mental instability.[2] However most of the increase was due to a host of other factors, including a trend throughout most of the last two centuries to commit family members who had lost their minds. The 1840 census reported that 16,457 citizens were insane though only 2,561 of these were in asylums or hospitals, a mere 14.7%.[3] And included in this small number were those who were not insane but "mentally deficient."[4] Though asylums or mental hospitals have existed for centuries, they grew in number as they became a more acceptable means of dealing with an unstable family member and as states began paying the bills.

Another trend also emerged as mental hospitals became supported by the states. More and more people were placed into mental hospitals who were societal problems but not necessarily mentally unstable. An 1890 law, the

State Care Act of 1890, eliminated almshouses across the nation. Consequently the only place a large number of older people could go was to state hospitals.[5] It was also the only place left for alcoholics, vagrants, the mentally retarded and those with pellagra or epilepsy. The number of first admissions to state hospitals for senility rose from 18% in 1920 to 31% in 1940.[6]

A 1950 study of all state mental hospitals also concluded that the hospitals' populations included large but unknown numbers of "persons with mental deficiency, with convulsive disorders, with chronic alcoholism and other drug addiction, or with persistent sex deviation."[7] In 1958 the president of the American Psychiatric Association noted that "the current movement in our field" was to remove those not seriously disturbed from the mental hospitals and place them in various community settings.[8] If those in state and county mental hospitals in 1955 who were not mentally unstable were all released at once, the drop in the number of patients would have been hugely greater than the drop that actually occurred between 1955 and 1960.

A National Disgrace Leads to Releases From Mental Hospitals

When the postwar public became aware of the conditions found in mental hospitals, families became less inclined to commit family members with mental disorders. When Pearl Harbor was attacked by the Japanese on December 7, 1941, it brought an ambivalent America into the war many had hoped to avoid. The war resulted in the deaths of more people (a total of 16 million not counting civilian deaths), the destruction of more buildings and property, the accumulation of the greatest debts and the overall greatest changes of any war in human history. It was hard to focus on what was happening in mental institutions during this period. However when the war came to an end, problems at home began to receive greater scrutiny.[9]

Few Americans who had not reached adulthood by 1936 can appreciate what a cultural phenomenon *Life* magazine was for many years. An *Encyclopaedia Britannica* article on the history of publishing calls *Life* "the most influential" picture magazine ever published in America.[10] When it was released in November 1936, the publisher hoped it would achieve a circulation of about 250,000.[11] But the response was dramatic. The first issue

394

sold out. The fourth issue sold over half a million copies. Some newsstands began allowing customers to pay in advance to reserve upcoming issues. A million copies were being sold each week, only four months after publication began.[12]

Within two years *Life* reported it had "more readers every week than any other magazine in history."[13] And its influence was unique. George Gallup reported that "the biggest publicity break a movie can get is a two–page layout of stills in *Life*."[14] Henry R. Luce biographer James Baughman reported that "within days of a *Life* advertisement for the Chrysler Highlander automobile, dealers reported being out of the model. Consumers clutching copies of *Life* had literally rushed into showrooms."[15]

Life's circulation continued to rise, reaching 6 million homes by 1960.[16] But of particular significance for our topic is the fact that *Life*'s readers, and therefore its influence, were disproportionately among professional people. A 1955 study found that professional people, which would include physicians and psychiatrists, were much more likely to be subscribers to *Life* than was the average American.[17]

When the war came to an end, *Life* published an article entitled "Bedlam 1946." It was a devastating 13–page exposé which included 15 photographs, some of which were given titles such as "Neglect," "Restraint," "Useless Work," "Nakedness," "Overcrowding," "Forced Labor," "Idleness" and "Despair." The author, Albert Maisel, declared,

> Through public neglect and legislative penny–pinching, state after state has allowed its institutions for the care and cure of the mentally sick to degenerate into little more than concentration camps. . . . Court and grand–jury records document scores of deaths of patients following beating by attendants. Hundreds of instances of abuse, falling just short of manslaughter, are similarly documented. And reliable evidence from hospital after hospital, indicates that these are but a tiny fraction of the beatings that occur, day after day, only to be covered by a conspiracy of mutually protective silence. . . . Yet, beatings and murders are hardly

the most significant of the indignities we have heaped upon most of the 400,000 guiltless patient–prisoners of over 180 state mental institutions.

We feed thousands a starvation diet . . . . We jam–pack men, women and sometimes even children into hundred–year–old firetraps in wards so crowded that the floors cannot be seen between the rickety cots, while thousands more sleep on ticks, on blankets, or on the bare floors. We give them little and shoddy clothing at best. Hundreds—of my own knowledge and sight—spend 24 hours a day in stark and filthy nakedness. Those who are well enough to work slave away in many institutions for 12 hours a day, often without a day's rest for years on end. . .

Hundreds are confined in "lodges"—bare, bedless rooms reeking with filth and feces—by day lit only through half–inch holes in steel–plated windows, by night merely black tombs in which the cries of the insane echo unheard from the peeling plaster of the walls. . . . Restraints, seclusion, and constant drugging of patients become essential in wards where one attendant must herd as many as 400 mentally deranged charges. . . . Thousands who might be restored to society linger in man–made hells for a release that comes more quickly only because death comes faster to the abused, the beaten, the drugged, the starved and the neglected. In some mental hospitals, for example, tuberculosis is 13 times as common as in the population at large.[18]

The *Life* exposé spurred sales of what became a national bestseller. The 1946 novel, *The Snake Pit*, was an autobiographical tale of Mary Jane Ward's experiences with mental illness and mental hospitals. As her young newlywed character Virginia begins suffering from confusion, depression and memory loss, including some uncertainty concerning her own identity, she is placed in a psychiatric hospital by her loving husband in hopes of helping her recover. She does, but only after being slowly shocked back to reality. In the hospital she did not have enough food, toilet paper or covers for the cold of night. On the other hand, there was no shortage of odors, isolation, wrappings in wet sheets and electroshock. The book's title can be understood from a passage deep within the story.

> Long ago they lowered insane persons into snake pits; they thought that an experience that might drive a sane person out of his wits might send an insane person back into sanity.[19]

Two years later, *The Snake Pit* was made into an award–winning movie starring Olivia de Havilland, one of Hollywood's most popular actresses. All over America audiences were horrified as most saw the insides of a mental hospital for the first time. That same year, 1948, Albert Deutsch, a social historian who had for many years been writing about mental hospitals, published another book on mental hospitals, and it received considerable attention.[20] *The Shame of the States* described conditions in several state mental hospitals in words similar to those found in *Life*'s "Bedlam 1946" article. (In fact, it was Deutsch who had taken many of the photographs found in that article.) The chapter titles reveal the reason for the book's title: "Byberry—Philadelphia's Bedlam"; "Cleveland—A Hell for the Sick"; "New York's Isle of Despair."

When the 41st annual meeting of the states' governors met in June of 1949, they directed the Council of State Governments to begin a comprehensive study of "mental hygiene and the care and treatment of the mentally ill" and to have it completed by June of 1950. The introduction of the completed, 12–month study announced that this was an issue about which the public was demanding change. They had read the magazines. They had read the books. They had seen the movie.

> Never before has there been so much public interest in mental health and in the facilities provided for the care and treatment of the increasing numbers who are being admitted to our mental hospitals. The problems of mental illness have not been overcome, but in every state there is a growing demand for more effective mental health and hospital programs.[21]

In 1950 the need for community–based outpatient clinics was under-stood, but most states simply did not have the funds needed to establish these facilities throughout their states, and state hospital populations contin-ued to grow each year. By May of 1958, the number of patients in state mental hospitals had been dropping for over two years, but that fact would take three years to become apparent from the published reports produced by the Census Bureau. Many assumed that despite the horror stories, books and movies, the situation was only growing worse.

The result was a startling admission by the president of the American Psychiatric Association at the organization's annual meeting, "I do not see how any reasonably objective view of our mental hospitals today can fail to conclude that they are bankrupt beyond remedy. I believe therefore that our large mental hospitals should be liquidated as rapidly as can be done in an orderly and progressive fashion."[22] The superintendents of most state hos-pitals were psychiatrists, and when the president of the psychiatrists' profes-sional organization declared in such forceful language that "large mental hospitals should be liquidated," the last stronghold of opposition was sur-rendered.[23]

Patients Were Moved to Nursing Homes

Consider again the number of patients in state mental hospitals in 1951 compared with 1960 (p. 285). The total number was actually larger in 1960 despite the advent of antipsychotic drugs. The major declines actually fol-lowed 1965, the year the federal government began two new programs we still know as Medicare and as Medicaid.[24] If the government had decided that those in mental hospitals would be eligible for benefits but those in nursing homes would be ineligible, there would have been an immediate shift in patient populations out of nursing homes and into mental hospitals all across the nation. However the new programs decided it would be just the opposite of that: coverage for nursing home residents but no coverage for those in state mental hospitals. The number of state mental hospital patients declined more between 1965 and 1966 than at any time previous-ly.[25] The next year saw an even greater decline.[26] The following year's decline was greater still.[27] Obviously, any state could save large sums by transferring state mental hospital patients to nursing homes, and that is exactly what they did.

Many other factors added to the decline which continued throughout the 1970s, 1980s and 1990s. Today psychiatric hospitals, general hospitals with psychiatric wards and community mental health centers have largely replaced the role played by large state mental hospitals. Research demonstrating that mental hospitalization led to worse patient outcomes than any of several other forms of outpatient care[28] only confirmed what many professionals had come to believe—traditional mental hospitals were not the answer. That conclusion means that even when individuals are sent by a court to a state mental hospital, they are evaluated frequently in hopes they will not remain at the institution long.

Clearly the decline in the nation's mental hospital population involves several factors not mentioned in most general psychology textbooks (if any). The pivotal role credited to Thorazine is blatantly false.

Personal Assessment Inventory–M

The very significant benefit that can be derived from this inventory can only be obtained if you are completely open and honest. All responses will be kept completely confidential.

1. How would you rate the amount of stress you are under at this time?
   Very great   Much   Some   Very little   None

2. How often do you get 6 to 8 hours of sleep at night?
   Never   Rarely   Occasionally   Often   Usually/Always

3. How often do you abuse alcohol?
   Daily   Often   Occasionally   Rarely   Never

4. How much television or video entertainment do you watch on an average day?
   3 hrs. +   2–3 hrs.   1–2 hrs.   Less than 1 hr.   Little or none

5. How often do you flirt or make suggestive comments with someone other than your spouse?
   Daily   Often   Occasionally   Rarely   Never

6. How often do you feel guilty as a result of being unloving to your spouse (impatient, harsh, critical, etc.)?
   Daily   Often   Occasionally   Rarely   Never

7. How much stress do you feel related to your financial situation?
   Very great   Much   Some   Very little   None

8. How much stress do you have over an unresolved issue or a violation of your values which is causing you to feel guilt (use of obscenities, telling a lie, stealing, a sexual event, viewing pornography, etc.)?
   Very great   Much   Some   Very little   None

9. Have you or your spouse had an extramarital affair? (Circle "Yes" even if you have no absolute proof of your spouse having an affair but you believe it has likely occurred.)
   Yes   No

10. How much self–discipline do you have?
    Very great   Much   Some   Very little   None

11. How often are you late for appointments?
Daily   Often   Occasionally   Rarely   Never

12. How often do you lose your temper?
Daily   Often   Occasionally   Rarely   Never

13. How often are you in a bad mood?
Daily   Often   Occasionally   Rarely   Never

14. How satisfied are you with how much affection your spouse shows you?
Miserable   Unhappy   Dissatisfied   Content   Pleased

15. How do you feel about your personal appearance?
Miserable   Unhappy   Dissatisfied   Content   Pleased

16. How often do you feel "left out" by others?
Daily   Often   Occasionally   Rarely   Never

17. How often do you feel lonely?
Daily   Often   Occasionally   Rarely   Never

18. How much conflict do you have in your marriage?
Very great   Much   Some   Very little   None

19. How much conflict do you have between yourself and other family members?
Very great   Much   Some   Very little   None

20. How much conflict is there between yourself and other acquaintances?
Very great   Much   Some   Very little   None

21. How often are you in a negative mood?
Daily   Often   Occasionally   Rarely   Never

22. How would you describe your self-esteem?
Very poor   Poor   Uncertain   Good   Very good

23. How would you describe your degree of selfishness?
Very great   Much   Some   Very little   None

24. How would you describe yourself in terms of being critical or generous?
Very critical   Critical   Mixed   Generous   Very generous

25. To what extent do you agree with the following statement: I believe my life has been of no great benefit to others?
Strongly agree   Agree   Uncertain   Disagree   Strongly disagree

26. To what extent do you agree with the following statement: I feel my existence is almost meaningless?
Strongly agree   Agree   Uncertain   Disagree   Strongly disagree

27. To what extent do you agree with the following statement: I believe my life is ultimately about my finding happiness?
Strongly agree   Agree   Uncertain   Disagree   Strongly disagree

28. To what extent do you agree with the following statement: I have made almost no progress toward achieving the goals I have for my life.
Strongly agree   Agree   Uncertain   Disagree   Strongly disagree

Note: A printable copy of this inventory for marrieds as well as a form for singles are available at the *America Fooled* website (www.americafooled .com). The forms may be freely used by physicians and others who are in a helping role. No "total score" or comparative scores are used with the Personal Assessment Inventory. This is a common sense inventory whose usefulness would be diminished and purposes distorted if responses were all quantified. The better approach is to use the inventory to determine if depression and anxiety are likely related to specific concerns that should be addressed and which might otherwise be overlooked. For example, if someone is buried in debt and has creditors calling constantly, the resultant stress and worry could cause that person to become depressed even if his or her "total score" was very normal. Likewise, if someone responded to item #15, "How often do you feel 'left out' by others?" by circling "daily," then you have uncovered an issue that all by itself could lead to stress, unhappiness, depression or even more severe mental problems.

LIST OF BOXES

BOX ENDNOTES

Preface

Box #P–2: "It's So Easy To Be Fooled" Answers
1. The show ran from September 30, 1960, to September 2, 1966 (Adams, T. R. [1994]. *The Flintstones: A Modern Stone Age Phenomenon.* Kansas City, MO: Andrews & McMeel.
    2. Countless studies find that age is the strongest predictor of cancer risk. See, for example, general articles (Misra, D.; Seo, P. H. & Cohen, H. J. [2004]. Aging and cancer. *Clinical Advances in Hematology & Oncology, 2,* 457–465; Lynch, J. & Smith, G. D. [2005]. A life course approach to chronic disease epidemiology. *Annual Review of Public Health, 26,* 1–35) or articles by specific type of cancer (Kim, S. P.; Feinglass, J., et al. [2004]. Merging claims databases with a tumor registry to evaluate variations in cancer mortality: Results from a pilot study of 698 colorectal cancer patients treated at one hospital in the 1990s. *Cancer Investigation, 22,* 225–233; Kalady, M. F.; Peterson, B., et al. [2004]. Pancreatic duct strictures: Identifying risk of malignancy. *Annals of Surgical Oncology, 11,* 581–588).
    3. The date is given on the web at http://www.foodreference.com/html/html/yearonly timeline1951–2000.html.
    4. Fergusson, D.; Swain–Campbell, N. & Horwood, J. (2004). How does childhood economic disadvantage lead to crime? *Journal of Child Psychology & Psychiatry & Allied Disciplines, 45,* 956–966.

Box #P–3: Schizophrenia Defined
1. The word literally means "split mind," the choice of Swiss physician Eugen Bleuler (1857–1939) who was seeking to emphasize that the mental abilities are split away from the person and to avoid Emil Kraepelin's term *dementia praecox.* He had probably been using the term for a few years, but it was properly introduced and discussed in his 1911 book *Dementia Praecox or The Group of Schizophrenias,* trans. J. Zinkin (1950). New York: International Universities Press.
    2. American Psychiatric Association (2000). *Diagnostic and Statistical Manual of Mental Disorders,* 4th ed., text revision. Washington, D.C.: American Psychiatric Association, p. 298.

Chapter 2 — Are Mental Problems Mental Diseases?

Box #2–1: Is It Possible to Measure Serotonin and Dopamine Levels or Not?
1. Smith, D. (April 12, 2005). Personal correspondence.

Box #2–2: A Flaw in Chemistry?
1. "What You Don't Know About Mental Illness Could Fill a Booklet," American Mental Health Fund.

2.   Ibid.
3.   "Depression: A Flaw in Chemistry, Not Character," National Alliance for Research on Schizophrenia and Depression.

Box #2–3: Comparing Apples and Apples?
1.   Much of the research on identical/fraternal twins was done very early (1930s and 1940s) but was of surprisingly good quality. Identical twins raised in separate environments were found to be slightly less alike in height and weight than those raised together but were still more similar than fraternal twins. They also looked more alike, a finding that we would expect (Newman, H.; Freeman, F. & Holzinger, K. [1937]. *Twins: A Study of Heredity and Environment*. Chicago: University of Chicago Press).
2.   The identical twins were extremely similar in height with a correlation coefficient of .93 (using a 0 to 1 scale with 1 being a perfect correlation). Fraternal twins (same sex) had a correlation coefficient of only .64 (ibid.).
3.   Ibid.
4.   Newman, Freeman & Holtzinger found intelligence scores of identical twins had a correlation coefficient of .88 (not much different than the correlation between two testings of the same individuals). The correlation coefficient for fraternal (same sex) twins was .63 (ibid.).
5.   Ibid.
6.   Ibid. This was also reported by Wilson (Wilson, P. T. [1934]. A study of twins with special reference to heredity as a factor determining differences in environment. *Human Biology, 6*, 324–354.
7.   Shields, J. (1954). Personality differences and neurotic traits in normal twin school-children. *Eugenics Review, 45*, 213–246 in Joseph, J. (2003). *The Gene Illusion: Genetic Research in Psychiatry and Psychology Under the Microscope*. Ross–on–Wye, Herefordshire, UK: PCCS Books. A study by Einar Kringlen reported that identical twins' level of closeness was "extremely strong" in 65% of all cases—a level found in only 19% of fraternal twins (Kringlen, E. [1967]. Heredity and environment in the functional psychoses: An epidemiological–clinical study. Oslo: Universitetsforlaget in ibid).
8.   Ibid.
9.   Ibid.
10. Ibid.

Box #2–4: In Search of the Holy Grail
1.   Norton, N. & Owen, M. J. (2004). Can we find the genes that predispose to schizo-phrenia? Ch. 3 (pp. 17–22) in McDonald, C.; Schulze, K., et al., eds. *Schizophrenia: Challenging the Orthodox*. London: Taylor & Francis, p. 17.
2.   Ibid.
3.   Ibid.

Box #2–5: Hyping Genetics
1.   Petursson, H.; Stefansson, H., et al. (2004). Genes for schizophrenia can be detect-ed—data from Iceland implicates *neuregulin* 1. Ch. 4 (pp. 23–29) in McDonald, C.; Schulze, K., et al., eds. *Schizophrenia: Challenging the Orthodox*. London: Taylor & Francis.
2.   Ibid., p. 27.

Chapter 3 — How Psychiatrists and Doctors Are Fooled

Box #3–1: Textbooks Have Errors?

1. Rathus, S. A. (1984). *Psychology*, 2nd ed. New York: CBS College Publishing, p. 456. The four errors on that page are as follows:

  a. Three times as many men commit suicide as women. Correction: He is not too far off the mark for 1984, but he should have given 3.59 (or rounded it to 4, not 3) (U.S. Bureau of the Census [1988]. *Statistical Abstract of the U.S.*, 108th ed. Washington, D.C., Table 118).

  b. Men prefer to use guns or hang themselves when committing suicide, but women prefer sleeping pills. Correction: The number one method of committing suicide for both males and females is the use of firearms (U.S. Bureau of the Census [1982–83]. *Statistical Abstract of the U.S.*, 103rd ed. Washington, D.C., Table 121). Note: The use of gas, if subtracted from the pills category, results in more suicides than firearms. Also see 1987 data from the National Center for Health Statistics in Buda, M. & Tsuang, M. T. (1990). The epidemiology of suicide: Implications for clinical practice (Ch. 2) in Blumenthal, S. & Kupfer, D., eds. *Suicide Over the Life Cycle*. Washington, D.C.: American Psychiatric Press, p. 22. The total firearm suicide rate in 1987 for females was 2,597 compared with 1,695 suicides by means of "drugs, meds, biologicals, solid or liquid substances."

  c. Young blacks and native Americans are more than twice as likely as whites to commit suicide. Correction: The young black suicide rate was not higher but much lower than the young white suicide rate throughout the 1970s and 1980s. This is the most surprising error, as the rates were not even close during that era. (They are more similar today.) For 1980, for example, the rate per 100,000 for 15- to 19-year-old white males was 15.0, but only 5.6 for black males. For females in that age category the rates were 3.3 and 1.6 for whites and blacks respectively (U.S. Bureau of Census [1990]. *Statistical Abstract of the U.S.*, 110th ed. Washington, D.C., Table 125).

  d. Suicide is especially common among physicians, lawyers and psychologists. Correction: The suicide rate for male physicians is essentially equivalent to the rate of suicide for males age 25 and older if one specialty (psychiatry) is removed from the physician category (Holmes, V. F. & Rich, C. L. [1990]. Suicide among physicians. Ch. 22 in Blumenthal, S. J. & Kupfer, D. J., eds. *Suicide Over the Life Cycle*. Washington, D.C.: American Psychiatric Press, pp. 599–618.

2. See http://www.pierce.ctc.edu/mcoffey/M121TBE.html for a listing of the errors. The text is Stewart, J.; Redlin, L. & Watson, S. (2001). *Precalculus, Mathematics for Calculus*, 4th ed. New York: Brooks Cole.

3. What is most surprising about these historical and scientific errors is that the State of Texas, in order to insure fewer errors than all those pointed out in the past in embarrassing media stories, required publishers to certify that their textbooks were error free before they could be adopted (Texas Education Code, Section 31.151). The state (which sets the standard for many other states) then gave grants to Texas Tech and Texas A&M universities to review the textbooks for errors. All these and *several hundred* additional errors were later uncovered after the requirement was put in place. (Most were found by Educational Research Analysts and John Hubisz, a physics professor working under a Packard Foundation grant.)

Box #3–2: Biological Thinking Can Get Silly
 1. Myers, D. (2002). *Exploring Psychology*, 5th ed. New York: Worth Publishers, p. 477.
 2. Ibid.
 3. Ibid.
 4. Ibid.

Box #3–3: Comparison of Old & New Approaches to Families of Schizophrenic Patients
 1. Leff, J. (1989). Family factors in schizophrenia. *Psychiatric Annals, 19*, 542–547, p. 544. (*Psychiatric Annals* is a publication of SLACK, Inc.)

Box #3–4: The Benefits of Playing the Game
 1. Krimsky, S. & Rothenberg, L. S. (2001). Conflicts of interest policies in science and medical journals: Editorial practices and author disclosures. *Science & Engineering Ethics, 7*, 205–218.
 2. Barnes, D. E. & Bero, L. A. (1998). Why review articles on the health effects of passive smoking reach different conclusions. *JAMA, 279*, 1566–1570.
 3. Taylor, D.; Mir, S., et al. (2002). Co–prescribing of atypical and typical antipsychotics: Prescribing sequence and documented outcome. *Psychiatric Bulletin, 26*, 170–172.
 4. Reuters News Service (July 18, 1998). Researchers say drug companies, politics cheat mental health research. These quotes and more of the article are found on the Connecticut Volunteers in Psychotherapy website available at http://www.ctvip.org/web2c.html.
 5. The study is available on the web at http://www.cspinet.org/new/200407123.html.

Box #3–6: Confirmation Bias—Why Doctors Increase Dosages and Try Other Antidepressants
 1. Examples of studies which have found this phenomenon include Anderson, C. A.; Lepper, M. R. & Ross, L. (1980). Perserverance of social theories: The role of explanation in the persistence of discredited information. *Journal of Personality & Social Psychology, 39*, 1037–1049; Lord., C. G.; Lepper, M. R. & Preston, E. (1984). Considering the opposite: A corrective strategy for social judgment. *Journal of Personality & Social Psychology, 37*, 2098–2109.
 2. Kirsch, et al. reported that in 12 trials investigating the dose–response relationship, mean improvement scores on the Hamilton Depression Rating Scale were 9.57 points for the lowest dosages and 9.97 for the highest dosages—a non–significant difference (Kirsch, I.; Moore, T. J., et al. [2002]. The emperor's new drugs: A meta–analysis of antidepressant medication data submitted to the U.S. Food and Drug Administration. *Prevention & Treatment, 5*, Article 23. Available on the web at http://www.journals.apa.org/prevention/volume5/pre0050023a.html. Some studies report better depression relief with lower dosing and some with higher dosing, but no clear pattern emerges. This would seem to indicate variables other than the medication are responsible for reported changes.
 3. Freemantle, N.; Anderson, I. M. & Young, P. (2000). Predictive value of pharmacological activity for the relative efficacy of antidepressant drugs: Meta–regression analysis. *British Journal of Psychiatry, 177*, 292–302.

Chapter 4 — Advertising Works

Box #4–1: Don't Be Fooled—Don't Buy the Purple Pill Nexium

1.   World Trade Organization (WTO) members have trade guidelines that require 20–year patent laws for pharmaceuticals. Most countries were in compliance by 2000, and all members were required to comply by 2005.

2.   The $219 million figure is from TNS/CMR as reported by Christine Bittar (Oct. 11, 2004). Act two from the purple pill. *Brandweek, 45*, Special Section, M54.

3.   This story has been carefully investigated and told by several investigative reporters and several books by those with expertise in drug development. Jerry Avorn, a Harvard professor and chief of the Division of Pharmacoepidemiology and Pharmacoeconomics at Brigham and Women's Hospital in Boston, explains the "sameness" of Prilosec and Nexium using the left–hand, right–hand illustration in his 2004 book *Powerful Medicines: The Benefits, Risks, and Costs of Prescription Drugs*. New York: Alfred A. Knopf. Endnote 4 below references a well–researched and enlightening article though they note AstraZeneca's claim that Nexium is superior to Prilosec without an adequate critique. The *Physicians' Desk Reference* discusses the Prilosec/Nexium comparison trials. There are four studies which examined erosive esophagitis healing rates and resolution of heartburn. Three of the four studies allowed 20mg of Prilosec to be compared with 40mg of Nexium. Only one study did simple equivalent comparisons. That study (study 1) at week 4 found Prilosec did better than Nexium by less than 1% (69.5% vs. 68.7%, respectively) at healing erosive esophagitis and did worse by less than 1% (64.1% vs. 64.3%) at resolving heartburn at day 14 (*Physicians' Desk Reference*, 59th ed. [2005]. Montvale, NJ: Thomson PDR, p. 622). The differences are statistically insignificant, and even the dishonest 40mg of Nexium versus the 20mg of Prilosec comparisons had amazingly small differences. Increasing the dosage has little benefit and likely increases risk. For an interesting overview of AstraZeneca's motivation to secure a patent for Prilosec as an OTC medicine, see Abboud, L. (June 23, 2003). AstraZeneca to settle fraud charges—Prilosec gets FDA approval for over–the–counter sales; Risk for successor Nexium? *Wall Street Journal*, A.2.

4.   Berenson, A. (Mar. 2, 2005). Where has all the Prilosec gone? *NY Times*, C.1. An unusual decision by the FDA is allowing AstraZeneca to sell the Prilosec as a nonprescription drug without generic competition until 2006 (though Prilosec as a more expensive prescription drug does have generic competition). Thus, if there are shortages of the less expensive OTC Prilosec, AstraZeneca will make more from the alternatives.

Box #4–2: Would Your Physician Prescribe Nexium?

1.   Prices are based on 30 20mg capsules of Nexium and 30 20mg capsules of Prilosec OTC from my local pharmacy (Mar. 22, 2005). The Prilosec OTC capsules come in a 28–capsule package, so I adjusted the $18.99 price upwards.

2.   Harris, G. (Aug. 20, 2003). Two fronts in heartburn market battle. *NY Times*, C.1.

3.   From February 2002 through January 2003 the number of Nexium prescriptions rose from 15.1 million to 21.3 million (NDC health information reported by Bittar, C. [Oct. 11, 2004]. Act two from the purple pill. *Brandweek, 45*, Special section, M54).

4.   Prilosec is also used with animals. Prilosec's official chemical name and a clear description of its mode of action are found in an Australian application for veterinary uses. This is available at http://www.aprma.gov.au/gazette/gazette0202p19.pdf.

Box #4–3: A *British Medical Journal* Editorial: Direct–to–Consumer Advertising
   1. Mansfield, P. R.; Mintzes, B., et al. (2005). Direct to consumer advertising. *British Medical Journal, 330*, 5–6.

Box #4–4: Isolated Explosive Disorder
   1. Isolated Explosive Disorder was included in the *DSM*'s 3rd edition but not its 4th edition which reveals how these "medical diagnoses" are very subjective matters. The 4th edition (*DSM–IV*) retained the "Intermittent Explosive Disorder" label (American Psychiatric Association [1994]. *Diagnostic and Statistical Manual of Mental Disorders*, 4th ed. Washington, D.C.: APA., pp. 609ff).
   2. See endnote 1 above for an example. The first two *DSM*s were strongly psychodynamic (Freudian). The 3rd edition abandoned this bias in favor of a chemical imbalance (biological psychiatry) view. It was also more behaviorally oriented. The 4th edition is similar to the 3rd, though it has even more diagnoses (approximately 300 more than the 1st edition) and has a "checklist" approach to diagnosing mental disorders. The current edition has a 2002 text revision. It is known as the *DSM–IV–TR* (*Diagnostic and Statistical Manual*, 4th ed., Text Revision).
   3. American Psychiatric Association (1994). *Diagnostic and Statistical Manual of Mental Disorders*, 4th ed. Washington, D.C.: APA, pp. 91ff.
   4. See endnote 6.
   5. See endnote 6.
   6. The Health Insurance Portability and Accessibility Act (HIPAA) requires insurance companies to accept the *World Health Organization's International Statistical Classification of Diseases and Related Health Problems, 9th ed. Clinical Modification* (*ICD–9–CM*) whose diagnostic labels are almost but not wholly identical to the *DSM* labels. For example, both used an identical code (315.4) and label for Developmental Coordination Disorder (*DSM–IV*, pp. 53ff) for many years. However when the *ICD–10* was published, they chose to change the name to Clumsy Child Syndrome (under F82, "Specific developmental disorder of motor function" in the *ICD–10*). New disorders that make it into the *DSM* have often made it into the *ICD* and vice versa. Academic Underachievement Disorder and Undersocialized Disorder are both *ICD* classifications. (Available on the web at the World Health Organization's *ICD* site at http://www3.int/icd/vol1htm2003/fr–icd.htm.) The *ICD* is now in its 10th edition.
   7. Ibid., pp. 615ff.
   8. Ibid., pp. 243ff.
   9. Ibid., pp. 662ff.

Chapter 7 — Tricks of the Trade

Box #7–3: *British Medical Journal* Policy on Advertisements
   1. Smith, R. (2003). Medical journals and pharmaceutical companies: Uneasy bedfellows. *British Medical Journal, 326*, 1202–1205, p. 1203.

Chapter 8 — Do Antidepressants Work?

Box #8–1: More on the *JAMA* Article—Mystery Solved
   1. Wagner, K. D.; Ambrosini, P., et al. (2003). Efficacy of Sertraline in the treatment of children and adolescents with major depressive disorder. *JAMA, 290*, 1033–1041.
   2. Ibid., p. 1041.

Box #8–2: How Safe Are New Drugs? It Takes Years to Know
1. Lasser, K. E.; Allen, P. D., et al. (2002). Timing of new black box warnings and withdrawals for prescription medications. *JAMA, 287*, 2215–2220.
2. Ibid., p. 2218.

Box #8–3: The Emperor's New Drugs: A Biological Psychiatrist Objects
1. Michael E. Thase was one of the many authors who wrote the study that resulted in the "Is academic medicine for sale?" editorial by Marcia Angell, then editor of the *New England Journal of Medicine*. It involved the antidepressant nefazodone (Serzone) made by Bristol Meyers Squibb (see Keller, M. B.; McCullough, J. P., et al. [2000]. A comparison of nefazodone, the cognitive behavioral–analysis of psychotherapy, and their combination for treatment of chronic depression. *New England Journal of Medicine, 342*, 1462–1470 and Dr. Angell's editorial, Angell, M. [2000]. Is academic medicine for sale? *New England Journal of Medicine, 342*, 1516–1518.) If you will enter into Medline's PubMed search engine both "Thase" and the name of Wyeth's antidepressant Effexor (use "vanlafaxine," Effexor's generic name), it will yield many of Thase's studies with Wyeth ties. The summary (abstract) of a 1996 article on antidepressants includes this sentence, "An overview of antidepressant options is presented, with a particular focus on venlafaxine." Many of the studies in which he has been involved have been with Wyeth employees (see, e.g., Entsuah, A. R.; Huang, H. & Thase, M. E. [2001]. Response and remission rates in different subpopulations with major depressive disorder administered venlafaxine, selective serotonin reuptake inhibitors, or placebo. *Journal of Clinical Psychiatry, 62*, 869–877 and Thase, M. E.; Entsuah, R., et al. [2005]. Relative antidepressant efficacy of venlafaxine and SSRIs: Sex–age interactions. *Journal of Women's Health, 14*, 609–616). Dr. Thase has often had papers presented at the European College of Neuropsychopharmacology (see Entsuah, R.; Cantillon, M. & Thase, M. [2001]. Venlafaxine and selective serotonin reuptake inhibitors in depression: Comparison among age and gender variables. *European Neuropsychopharmacology, 11*, 197). See Chapter 5 (Analyzing an Antidepressant Ad) for a discussion of how transportation costs and honoraria, etc., are paid by the pharmaceutical companies. Richard Entsuah, Wyeth employee, is also discussed in that chapter. (See especially the section entitled, "The First 'Proof.'")
2. Thase, M. E. (2002). Antidepressant effects: The suit may be small, but the fabric is real. *Prevention & Treatment, 5*, Article 32, posted July 15, 2002. Available on the web at http://www.journalsapa.org/prevention/volume5/pre0050032c.html. The quote comes out of the article's 13th full paragraph.

Box #8–4: Antidepressant Testimonials
1. Each of these testimonials was found on the web. Although the antidepressant used for the first, second and last testimonials is omitted, each can still be located most likely by placing quotation marks at the front and end of a passage and "googling" the quote in the Google search engine. Spelling and grammatical errors have been corrected for the quoted text.

Box #8–5: A Flawed Study of Placebo Effects
1. Hróbjartsson, A. & Gøtzsche, P. C. (2001). Is the placebo powerless?: An analysis of clinical trials comparing placebo with no treatment. *New England Journal of Medicine, 344*, 1594–1602, p. 1594.
2. Kirsch, I. (2002). Yes, there *is* a placebo effect, but is there a powerful antidepressant drug effect? *Prevention & Treatment, 5*, Article 22, p. 2. Available on the web at http://journals.apa.org/prevention/volume5/pre0050022i.html.

3. See Moerman, D. E. & Jonas, W. B. (2002). Deconstructing the placebo effect and finding meaning and response. *Annals of Internal Medicine, 136*, 471–476; Papakostas, Y. G. & Daras, M. D. (2001). Placebos, placebo effect, and the response to the healing situation: The evolution of a concept. *Epilepsia, 42*, 1614–1625; Wampold, B. E.; Minami, T., et al. (2005). The placebo is powerful: Estimating placebo effects in medicine and psychotherapy from randomized clinical trials. *Journal of Clinical Psychology, 61*, 835–854. Also see the eight criticisms that appeared in the next volume of the *New England Journal of Medicine* (2001, *345*, 1276–1279) and five critiques that appeared in *Advances in Mind–Body Medicine* (2001, *17*, 293–312).

Box #8–6: Can Placebos Produce Endorphins?

1. Schwarz, L. & Kindermann, W. (1992). Changes in beta–endorphin levels in response to aerobic and anaerobic exercise. *Sports Medicine, 13*, 25–36; Goldfarb, A. H. & Jamurtas, A. Z. (1997). Beta–endorphin response to exercise: An update. *Sports Medicine, 24*, 8–16.

2. Sher, L. (1997). The placebo effect on mood and behavior: The role of the endogenous opioid system. *Medical Hypotheses, 48*, 347–349; Amanzio, M. & Benedetti, F. (1999). Neuropharmacological dissection of placebo analgesia: Expectation–activated opioid systems versus conditioning–activated specific sub–systems. *Journal of Neuroscience, 19*, 484–494; Petrovic, P.; Kalso, E., et al. (2002). Placebo and opioid analgesia: Imaging a shared neuronal network. *Science, 295*, 1737–1740.

3. de la Fuente–Fernandez, R.; Ruth, T. J., et al. (2001). Expectation and dopamine release: Mechanism of the placebo effect in Parkinson's disease. *Science, 293*, 1164–1166; de la Fuente–Fernandez, R.; Schulzer, M. & Stoessl, A. J. (2002). The placebo effect in neurological disorders. *Lancet Neurology, 1*, 85–91; de la Fuente–Fernandez, R.; Schulzer, M. & Stoessl, A. J. (2004). Placebo mechanisms and reward circuitry: Clues from Parkinson's disease. *Biological Psychiatry, 56*, 67–71.

4. Pollo, A.; Vighetti, S., et al. (2003). Placebo analgesia and the heart. *Pain, 102*, 125–133, p. 125.

Chapter 9 — The FDA Drug Approval Process

Box #9–1: NIH Policies on Outside Financial Ties for Employees

1. Steinbrook, R. (2004). Financial conflicts of interest and the NIH. *New England Journal of Medicine, 350*, 327–330, p. 328.

Box #9–2: What Gets Published?

1. Melander, H.; Ahlqvist–Rastad, J., et al. (2003). Evidence b(i)ased medicine: Selective reporting from studies sponsored by pharmaceutical industry: Review of studies in new drug applications. *British Medical Journal, 326*, 1171–1173.

2. Lexchin, J.; Bero, L. A., et al. (2003). Pharmaceutical industry sponsorship and research outcome and quality: Systematic review. *British Medical Journal, 326*, 1167–1170.

3. Kjaegard, L. L. & Als–Nielsen, B. (2002). Association between competing interests and authors' conclusions: Epidemiological study of randomised clinical trials published in the *BMJ*. *British Medical Journal, 325*, 249–253.

4. Djulbegovic, B.; Lacevic, M., et al. (2000). The uncertainty principle and industry–sponsored research. *Lancet, 356*, 635–638.

5. Als–Nielsen, B.; Chen, W., et al. (2003). Association of funding and conclusions in randomized drug trials. *JAMA, 290*, 921–928.

6. Bhandari, M.; Busse, J. W., et al. (2004). Association between industry funding and statistically significant pro–industry findings in medical and surgical randomized trials. *Canadian Medical Association Journal, 170*, 477–480.

7. Yaphe, J.; Edman, R., et al. (2001). The association between funding by commercial interests and study outcome in randomized controlled drug trials. *Family Practice, 18*, 565–568.

8. Stern, J. M. & Simes, R. J. (1977). Publication bias: Evidence of delayed publication in a cohort study of clinical research projects. *British Medical Journal, 315*, 640–645.

9. Krzyzanowska, M. K.; Pintilie, M. & Tannock, I. F. (2003). Factors associated with failure to publish large randomized trials presented at an oncology meeting. *JAMA, 290*, 495–501.

10. Ioannidis, J. P. (1998). Effect on the statistical significance of results on the time to completion and publication of randomized efficacy trials. *JAMA, 279*, 281–286.

11. MacLean, C. H.; Morton, S. C., et al. (2003). How useful are unpublished data from the Food and Drug Administration in meta–analysis? *Journal of Clinical Epidemiology, 56*, 44–51.

Box #9–3: The "Diseases" Which Prozac is FDA–Approved to Help Cure
1. In 1997 the FDA ruled that all drugs had to have a "Geriatric Use" section on their labels. In other words the FDA divides the population into children, adults and geriatric adults. Prozac was the first drug to receive approval to list "geriatric depression" on its label. Geriatric depression is not a *DSM–IV TR* listed disorder.

Chapter 10 — Physical Side Effects of Antidepressants

Box #10–1: A Window Into the Future?
1. Latorre, P.; Modrego, P. J., et al. (2001). Parkinsonism and Parkinson's disease associated with long–term administration of sertraline. *Journal of Clinical Pharmacy & Therapeutics, 26*, 111–112.

Chapter 11 — Psychological Side Effects of Antidepressants

Box #11–1: A Tragic Lesson for Lilly's Chairman
1. Leigh Thompson memo (Feb. 7, 1990), exhibit 98 in Forsyth vs Eli Lilly as found in Healy, D. (2004). *Let Them Eat Prozac*. New York: New York University Press, p. 133.
2. For the messages and their sources (the Fentress and the Forsyth trials), see ibid., p. 132 and ref. 12, p. 316.
3. Ibid., p. 85.

Box #11–2: Alcohol Also Blunts (Disinhibits)
1. The actual rate is likely ten or more times the rate for matched non–alcoholics. See the old but valuable study by Lemere (*American Journal of Psychiatry, 109*, 674–676) found in Hendin, H. (1995). *Suicide in America*. New York: W. W. Norton & Co., p. 148.

2. Welte, J.; Abel, E. & Wieczorek, W. (1988). The role of alcohol in suicides in Erie County, New York, 1972–1984. *Public Health Reports, 103*, 648–652 in Lester, D. (1992). *Why People Kill Themselves*, 3rd ed. Springfield, IL: Charles C. Thomas, p. 199.

3. Varadaraj, R. & Mendonca, J. (1987). A survey of blood alcohol levels in self–poisoning cases. *Advances in Alcohol & Substance Abuse, 7*, 63–69 in Welte, J., et. al (ibid.).

4. Birckmayer, J. & Hemenway, D. (1999). Minimum–age drinking laws and youth suicide, 1970–1990. *American Journal of Public Health, 89*, 1365–1368.

5. The alcohol–violence relationship has been reported for rape, murder, spousal abuse and other acts of violence. See Bushman, B. J. (1997). Effects of alcohol on human aggression. *Recent Developments in Alcoholism, 13*, 227–243; Collins, J. J. & Messerschmidt, M. A. (1993). Epidemiology of alcohol–related violence. *Alcohol Health & Research World, 17*, 93–100. However, this is not a simple relationship. One animal study found that it is at low intoxication levels but not high intoxication levels that animals are aggressive (Miczek, K. A.; Weerts, E. M. & Debold, J. F. [1993]. Alcohol, benzodiazepine–GABAA receptor complex and aggression. *Journal of Studies of Alcohol Supplement, 11*, 170–179). And a study of college students speculated that alcohol effects vary based on the stability of the individual drinker (Bailly, M. D. & King, A. R. [2004]. A failure to replicate alcohol–induced laboratory aggression among college men without evidence of personality disturbance. *Psychological Reports, 94*, 1089–1096). The classic study by Lang and his colleagues (Lang, A. R.; Goeckner, D. J., et al. [1975]. Effects of alcohol on aggression in male social drinkers. *Journal of Abnormal Psychology, 84*, 508–518) found *expectations* concerning alcohol's effects were most predictive of behavioral changes.

6. Muehlberger, C. W. (1956). Medicolegal aspects of alcohol intoxication. *Michigan State Bar Journal, 35*, 38–42 in Bushman, B. J. & Cooper, H. M. Effects of alcohol on human aggression: An integrative research review. *Psychological Bulletin, 107*, 341–354.

Chapter 12 — Fooled, Fooled and Fooled Again: The History of Treating Mental Problems

Box #12–1: "He's Gone Battie!"
1. Battie, W. (1758). *A Treatise on Madness*. London: J. Whiston & B. White in Hunter, R. & Macalpine, I. (1963). *Three Hundred Years of Psychiatry, 1535–1860*. London: Oxford University Press, p. 405.
2. Ibid., p. 408.
3. Ibid., p. 405.

Box #12–2: Hippocrates on the Origin of Madness
1. Ducey, C. & Simon, B. *Ancient Greece and Rome*, p. 15 in Howells, J. G., ed. (1975). *World History of Psychiatry*. New York: Brunner/Mazel, pp. 1–38.

Box #12–3: Do Hysterical Women Need a Hysterectomy?
1. *Webster's New World Dictionary of the American Language*, 2nd College Ed., Guralnik, D. B., ed. (1986). New York: Prentice Hall Press, p. 693.
2. Jarvis, E. R. (1850). On the comparative liability of males and females to Insanity and their comparative curability and mortality when insane. *Journal of Insanity, 7*, 155 in Barker–Benfield, G. J. (1976). *The Horrors of the Half–Known Life*. New York: Harper & Row, p. 56.
3. Ibid., p. 83.

4. The book E. H. Clarke's *Sex in Education, or A Fair Chance for the Girls* went through numerous editions, an indication of its unexpected and enduring popularity. Dr. Clarke believed that if the female used her brain much, blood flow to the brain would increase but inadequate blood flow to the uterus would result, leading to atrophy (1873, Boston: James R. Osgood & Company).
5. Barker–Benfield, G. J. (1976). *The Horrors of the Half-Known Life*. New York: Harper & Row, p. 122.
6. Ibid., p. 121.
7. Henry, W. O. (1907). To what extent can the gynecologist prevent and cure insanity in women? *JAMA, 48*, 997–1002.
8. Ibid., p. 1002.

Box #12–4: Lucy—The Other Chimpanzee

1. Valenstein, E. S. (1986). *Great and Desperate Cures*. New York: Basic Books, pp. 96–97.

Box #12–5: The Lobotomy: So Simple a Psychiatrist Can Do It

1. Exact numbers are impossible to determine. Freeman claimed he had either performed or supervised over 3,500 prefrontal lobotomies. Valenstein, whom I have learned to trust for his scholarly research in this area, estimates that there were likely about 40,000 done in the United States alone (Valenstein, E. S. [1973]. *Brain Control: A Critical Examination of Brain Stimulation and Psychosurgery*. New York: John Wiley & Sons, p. 55).
2. Kalinowsky, L. B. & Hoch, P. H. (1952). *Shock Treatments, Psychosurgery and Other Somatic Treatments in Psychiatry*, 2nd ed. New York: Grune & Stratton. See pp. 228–230 for the instructions for a transorbital lobotomy.
3. Ibid., p. 228.
4. Ibid.

Box #12–6: A Thorazine "Trip" Described

1. The psychiatrist was Cornelia Quarti who at that time was employed at a psychiatric hospital in Villejuif, France. Quarti's comments were translated by Judith Swazey (Swazey, J. [1974]. *Chlorpromazine in Psychiatry: A Study of Therapeutic Innovation*. Cambridge: The MIT Press, pp. 117–118).

Box #12–7: Dramatic Effect of Thorazine

1. Coleman, J. C.; Butcher, J. N. & Carson, R. C. (1980). *Abnormal Psychology and Modern Life*, 6th ed. Glenview, IL: Scott, Foresman & Company, p. 622.

Box #12–8: SmithKline & French's "Research"

1. Winkelman, N. W. (1954). Chlorpromazine in the treatment of neuropsychiatric disorders. *JAMA, 155*, 18–21.
2. SmithKline & French's marketing strategy is discussed by Ann Braden Johnson in her book *Out of Bedlam: The Truth About Deinstitutionalization* (1990, New York: Basic Books). See Chapter 3.

Box #12–9: The "Miracle" of Antipsychotics: What Students Learn (Textbook Quotes)

1. Myers, D. (2005). *Exploring Psychology*, 6th ed. New York: Worth Publishers, p. 530.

2. Ibid.
3. Coon, D. (2004). *Introduction to Psychology,* 10th ed. Belmont, CA: Thomson Learning, p. 652.
4. Ibid.

Box #12–10: The Frontal Lobes
1. Ratey, J. J. (2001). *A User's Guide to the Brain.* New York: Pantheon Books, p. 309.
2. Czerner, T. B. (2001). *What Makes You Tick?: The Brain in Plain English.* New York: John Wiley & Sons, p. 69.
3. Restak, R. M. (2001). *The Secret Life of the Brain.* Washington, D.C.: John Henry Press & Dana Press, p. 34.
4. Restak, R. M. (1994). *The Modular Brain.* New York: Charles Scribner's Sons, p. 106.
5. Winston, R. (2003). *The Human Mind.* London: Bantam Press, p. 105.

Chapter 13 — Side Effects of Antipsychotics

Box #13–1: Using Animals for Drug Research
1.   A survey of registered British facilities found nearly 80% of animal experiments used rats and mice and 5% used other rodents (guinea pigs almost always being the "other rodents"). Experiments also used birds (8% of all cases), fish (5%) and rabbits (3%). Dogs, cats and primates were used in well under 1% of all experiments using animals. In 1992 animals used in the United Kingdom numbered 2.94 million. The number would have increased significantly since then, and that number would be but a fraction of all experiments conducted in the United States (Wolfensohn, S. & Lloyd, M. [1994]. *Handbook of Laboratory Animal Management and Welfare.* Oxford: Oxford University Press, p. 10).
2.   Several books chronicle the advances made in medicine which have used animals as an essential step in the discovery process. One work that focuses especially on the contribution of animals in mental health research is Carroll, M. E. & Overmier, J. B., eds. (2001). *Animal Research and Human Health: Advancing Human Welfare Through Behavioral Science.* Washington, D.C.: American Psychological Association.
3.   The American Psychological Association has published a book on this topic entitled *Laboratory Animals in Research and Teaching: Ethics, Care, and Methods,* edited by C. K. Akins, S. Panicker and C. L. Cunningham (2004, Washington D. C.: APA).

Box #13–2: The *Physicians' Desk Reference* and Tardive Dyskinesia
1.   *Physicians' Desk Reference,* 59th ed. (2005). Montvale, NJ: Thomson PDR, p. 663.

Chapter 14 — What Really Causes Severe Mental Problems (Schizophrenia)

Box #14–1: Psychiatry Today—Ignoring the Research
1.   Norton, N. & Owen, M. J. (2004). Can we find the genes that predispose to schizophrenia? (pp. 17–22) in McDonald, C.; Schulze, K., et al., eds. *Schizophrenia: Challenging the Orthodox.* London: Taylor and Francis, p. 17.

Box #14–2: Some Effects of 2 Hours of Mother–Pup Separation
1. Schanberg, S. (1995). The genetic basis for touch effects in Field, T. M., ed. *Touch in Early Development.* Mahway, NJ: Lawrence Erlbaum Associates, p. 69.

Chapter 15 — The Continuum Model

Box #15–1: Moral Treatment—1954
1. John Butler, MD, superintendent of The Connecticut Retreat for the Insane, conducted his asylum using moral treatment principles. He describes his own experience and that of others in his book *The Curability of Insanity* (1887, New York: G. P. Putnam's Sons).
2. Hunt, M. M. (Sept. 1954). They go home in Kansas. *Reader's Digest, 65*, 47–50, p. 47.
3. Ibid., p. 48.
4. This 80% figure is Karl Menninger's number, and he is quoted in the article as saying that 85% would soon leave well enough to function on their own (ibid., p. 50).
5. Ibid., p. 47.

Box #15–2: A Survivor's Close Call With Disaster
1. Bassman, R. (2001). Overcoming the impossible: My journey through schizophrenia. *Psychology Today, 34*, 34–40, pp. 35–36.

Chapter 16 — An Effective Guide for Avoiding and Overcoming Depression

Box #16–1: Entertaining One's Self
1. Studies from many seemingly unrelated areas of research point to the emotional dangers arising from isolation. See, for example, Arlinger, S. (2003). Negative consequences of uncorrected hearing loss: A review. *International Journal of Audiology, 42* (Suppl. 2), 2S17–2S20; Ouimet, M. A.; Primeau, F. & Cole, M. G. (2001). Psychosocial risk factors in poststroke depression: A systematic review. *Canadian Journal of Psychiatry, 46*, 819–828.

Box #16–2: "I Feel So Left Out of Things"
1. Gazelle, H. & Ladd, G. W. (2003). Anxious solitude and peer exclusion. *Child Development, 74*, 257–278.
2. Dill, E. J.; Vernberg, E. M., et al. (2004). Negative affect in victimized children. *Journal of Abnormal Child Psychology, 32,* 159–173; Crick, N. R. (1996). The role of overt aggression, relational aggression and prosocial behavior in the prediction of children's future social adjustment. *Child Development, 67*, 2317–2327; Davies, P. T. & Forman, E. M. (2002). Children's patterns of preserving emotional security in the interparental subsystem. *Child Development, 73*, 1880–1893.
3. Larsen, R. & Richards, M. H. (1991). Daily companionship in late childhood and early adolescence. *Child Development, 62*, 284–300.
4. Steinberg, L. & Silverberg, S. B. (1986). The vicissitudes of autonomy in early adolescence. *Child Development, 57*, 841–851.
5. Collier, R. M. & Lawrence, H. P. (1951). The adolescent feeling of psychological isolation. *Education Theory, 1*, 106–115 cited by Brennan, T. (1982). Loneliness at adolescence in Peplau, L. A. & Perlman, D., eds. *Loneliness: A Sourcebook of Current Theory.* New York: John Wiley & Sons, p. 272.

6.   Brennan & Auslander stated 54% of the youths they studied reported such (Brennan, T. & Auslander, N. [1979]. *Adolescent Loneliness: An Exploratory Study of Social and Psychological Pre–Dispositions and Theory* [Vol. 1]. Prepared for the National Institute of Mental Health, Juvenile Problems Division, Grant No. R01–MH289 12–01, Behavioral Research Institute cited by Brennan, T. [1982]. Loneliness at adolescence in Peplau, L. A. & Perlman, D., eds. *Loneliness: A Sourcebook of Current Theory.* New York: John Wiley & Sons, pp. 269–290).

7.   Ibid.

8.   Phillips, M. & Pedersen, D. J. (1972) cited by Brennan, T. (1982). Loneliness at adolescence in Peplau, L. A. & Perlman, D., eds. *Loneliness: A Sourcebook of Current Theory.* New York: John Wiley & Sons, pp. 269–290; LeRoux, A. & Connors, J. (2001). A cross–cultural study into loneliness amongst university students. *South African Journal of Psychology, 31,* 46–52. This study reports that culture does make a significant difference in the degree of loneliness experienced but notes several studies which have found high levels of loneliness among college students.

9.   Twenge, J. M. & Campbell, W. K. (2003). Isn't it fun to get the respect that we're going to deserve? Narcissism, social rejection, and aggression. *Personality & Social Psychology Bulletin, 29,* 261–272.

Box #16–3: An Alternative Approach—Get Beautiful

1.   In 2003 Americans spent $9.4 billion on cosmetic surgeries. A total of 8.3 million surgical and nonsurgical cosmetic procedures were performed in 2003, nearly half (45%) for people between 35 and 50 years of age (Rheault, M. [Sept. 2004]. Cosmetic changes. *Kiplinger's Personal Finance, 58,* 22).

2.   Klassen, A.; Fitzpatrick, R., et al. (1999). Contrasting evidence of the effectiveness of cosmetic surgery from two health related quality of life measures. *Journal of Epidemiology & Community Health, 53,* 440–441.

3.   Kuck–Koot, V. C. M.; Peeters, P. H. M., et al. (2003). The total and cause specific mortality among Swedish women with cosmetic breast implants: Prospective study. *British Medical Journal, 326,* 527–528.

4.   Jacobsen, P. H.; Hölmich, L. R., et al. (2004). Mortality and suicide among Danish women with cosmetic breast implants. *Archives of Internal Medicine, 164,* 2450–2455.

5.   Ishigooka, J.; Iwao, M., et al. (1998). Demographic features of patients seeking cosmetic surgery. *Psychiatry & Clinical Neurosciences, 52,* 283–287.

6.   Dunofsky, M. (1997). Psychological characteristics of women who undergo single and multiple cosmetic surgeries. *Annals of Plastic Surgery, 39,* 223–228.

7.   Veale, D. (2001). Mirror, mirror on the wall, who is the ugliest of them all?: The psychopathology of mirror gazing in body dysmorphic disorder. *Behaviour Research & Therapy, 39,* 1381–1393.

Box #16–5: Purpose in Life Research

1.   Mascaro, N. & Rosen, D. H. (2005). Existential meaning's role in the enhancement of hope and prevention of depressive symptoms. *Journal of Personality, 73,* 985–1014; van Selm, M. & Dittmann–Kohli, F. (1998). Meaninglessness in the second half of life: The development of a construct. *International Journal of Aging & Human Development, 47,* 81–104; Debats, D. L.; Drost, J. & Hansen, P. (1995). Experiences of meaning in life: A combined qualitative and quantitative approach. *British Journal of Psychology, 86,*

359–375; Kinnier, R. T.; Metha, A. T., et al. (1994). Depression, meaninglessness, and substance abuse in "normal" and hospitalized adolescents. *Journal of Alcohol & Drug Education, 39*, 101–111; Lester, D. & Badro, S. (1992). Depression, suicidal preoccupation and purpose in life in a subclinical population. *Personality & Individual Differences, 13*, 75–76.

2. Lester, D. & Badro, S., ibid.; Heisel, M. J. & Flett, G. L. (2004). Purpose in life, satisfaction with life, and suicide ideation in a clinical sample. *Journal of Psychopathology & Behavioral Assessment, 26*, 127–135; Moore, S. L. (1997). A phenomenological study of meanng in life in suicidal older adults. *Archives of Psychiatric Nursing, 11*, 29–36.

3. Mostul, B. L. (1981). The relationship of ambiguity tolerance to trait anxiety, self-esteem, purpose in life and religious orientation (Doctoral dissertation, California School of Professional Psychology). *Dissertation Abstracts International, 41*, 2738; Pearson, P. R. & Sheffield, B. F. (1974). Purpose–in–life and the Eysenck Personality Inventory. *Journal of Clinical Psychology, 30*, 562–564; Ruffin, J. E. (1984). The anxiety of meaninglessness. *Journal of Counseling & Development, 63*, 40–42; Yarnel, T. D. (1971). Purpose–in–Life Test: Further correlates. *Journal of Individual Psychology, 27*, 76–79.

4. Antonovsky, A. (1987). *Unraveling the Mystery of Health: How People Manage Stress and Stay Well*. San Francisco: Jossey–Bass; Debats, D. L. (1996). Meaning in life: Clinical relevance and predictive power. *British Journal of Clinical Psychology, 35*, 503–516; Fava, G. A.; Rafanelli, C., et al. (2001). Psychological well–being and residual symptoms in remitted patients with panic disorder and agoraphobia. *Journal of Affective Disorders, 65*, 185–190.

5. Hablas, R.; Hutzell, R. R. & Bolin, E. (1980). Life purpose and subjective well–being in schizophrenic patients. *International Forum for Logotherapy, 3*, 44–45; Yarnel, T. D. (1971). Purpose–in–Life Test: Further correlates. *Journal of Individual Psychology, 27*, 76–79; Chaudhary, P. N. & Sharma, U. (1976). Existential frustration and mental illness: A comparative study of purpose in life in psychiatric patients and normals. *Indian Journal of Clinical Psychology, 3*, 171–174.

6. Taylor, E. J. (1993). Factors associated with meaning in life among people with recurrent cancer. *Oncology Nursing Forum, 20*, 1399–1405; Thompson, N. J.; Coker J., et al. (2003). Purpose in life as a mediator of adjustment after spinal cord injury. *Rehabilitation Psychology, 48*, 100–108; Ulmer, A.; Range, L. M. & Smith, P. C. (1991). Purpose in life: A moderator from bereavement. *Omega Journal of Death & Dying, 2*, 279–289.

7. Nilsen, A. R. (2005). The tenacious women of LaVerne: A case study of factors that enable resilient doctoral students from nontraditional backgrounds to overcome adversity and meet their goals (California). *Dissertation Abstracts International: Section A. Humanities & Social Sciences, 65*, 2519.

8. Smith, B. W. (2004). The role of purpose in life in recovery from knee surgery. *International Journal of Behavioral Medicine, 11*, 197–202; Smith, B. W. & Zautra, A. J. (2000). Purpose in life and coping with knee–replacement surgery. *Occupational Therapy Journal of Research, 20*, 96S–99S.

9. Viswanathan, R. (1996). Death anxiety, locus of control, and purpose in life of physicians: Their relationship to patient death notification. *Psychosomatics: Journal of Consultation Liaison Psychiatry, 37*, 339–345; Rappaport, H.; Fossler, R. J., et al. (1993). Future time, death anxiety, and life purpose among older adults. *Death Studies, 17*, 369–379; Ardelt, M. (2003). Effects of religion and purpose in life on elders' subjective well–being and attitudes toward death. *Journal of Religious Gerontology, 14*, 55–77.

10. Familetti, M. M. (1975). A comparison of the meaning and purpose in life of delinquent and non–delinquent high school boys (Doctoral dissertation, U.S. International University). *Dissertation Abstracts International, 36,* 1825; Worthen, R.; Johnson, B., et al. (1973). Adolescent adjustment related to the Purpose in Life Test. *Journal of Community Psychology, 1,* 209–211.

11. Reker, G. T. (1977). The purpose–in–life test in an inmate population: An empirical investigation. *Journal of Clinical Psychology, 33,* 688–693.

12. Waisberg, J. L. & Porter, J. E. (1994). Purpose in life and outcome of treatment for alcohol dependence. *British Journal of Clinical Psychology, 33,* 49–63.

13. Kinnier, R. T.; Metha, A. T., et al. (1994). Depression, meaninglessness, and substance abuse in "normal" and hospitalized adolescents. *Journal of Alcohol & Drug Education, 39,* 101–111; Padelford, B. L. (1974). Relationship between drug involvement and purpose in life. *Journal of Clinical Psychology, 30,* 303–305.

14. Hudspeth, D.; Canada, R. M., et al. (1998). Purpose in life and teenage pregnancy. *Family Therapy, 25,* 51–59.

15. Debats, D. L. (1996). Meaning in life: Clinical relevance and predictive power. *British Journal of Clinical Psychology, 35,* 503–516; Kish, G. B. & Moody, D. R. (1989). Psychopathology and life purpose. *The Forum for Logotherapy, 3,* 44–45; Reker, G. T.; Peacock, E. J. & Wong, P. T. P. (1987). Meaning and purpose in life and well–being: A life-span perspective. *Journal of Gerontology, 42,* 44–49; Weber, J. P. (1996). Meaning in life and psychological well–being among high school freshmen and seniors. *Dissertation Abstracts International: Section B. The Sciences & Engineering, 57,* 2912.

16. Moomal, Z. (1999). The relationship between meaning in life and mental well–being. *South African Journal of Psychology, 29,* 36–41; Zika, S. & Chamberlain, K. (1992). On the relation between meaning in life and psychological well–being. *British Journal of Psychology, 83,* 133–145.

17. Bhogle, S. & Prakash, I. J. (1993). Indicators of subjective well–being in a nonclinical adult sample. *Psychological Studies, 38,* 135–141; French, S. & Joseph, S. (1999). Religiosity and its association with happiness, purpose in life, and self–actualisation. *Mental Health, Religion & Culture, 2,* 117–120; Robak, R. W. & Griffin, P. W. (2000). Purpose in life: What is its relationship to happiness, depression and grieving? *North American Journal of Psychology, 2,* 113–119; MacDonald, D. A. & Holland, D. (2002). Spirituality and boredom proneness. *Personality & Individual Differences, 32,* 1113–1119.

18. Crandall, J. E. & Rasmussen, R. D. (1975). Purpose in life as related to specific values. *Journal of Clinical Psychology, 31,* 483–485; Paloutzian, R. F. (1981). Purpose in life and value changes following conversion. *Journal of Personality & Social Psychology, 41,* 1153–1160.

19. Shek, D. T. L. (1994). Meaning of life in adolescent antisocial and prosocial behavior in a Chinese context. *Psychologia: An International Journal of Psychology in the Orient, 37,* 211–218.

20. French, S. & Joseph, S. (1999). Religiosity and its association with happiness, purpose in life, and self–actualisation. *Mental Health, Religion & Culture, 2,* 117–120; Wuthnow, R. (1978). *Experimentation in American Religion: The New Mysticisms and Their Implications for the Churches.* Berkeley: University of California Press.

Box #16–6: Purpose in Life

1. Allport, G. W. (1955). *Becoming.* New Haven: Yale University Press, pp. 50–51.

ENDNOTES

Book Jacket

1. Brooks, B. W.; Chambliss, C. K.; et al. (2005). Determination of select antidepressants in fish from an effluent–dominated stream. *Environmental Toxicology & Chemistry, 24*, 464–469; Fernand, R. & Murray, J. (2005). Drugged waters: Studies detect wide variety of pharmaceuticals in surface and groundwaters and a recent survey conducted in Scotland reveals that 44% of the general public toss unused prescriptions down the drain. *Water and Waste Water International, 20*, 17–18; Eilperin, J. (June 23, 2005). Pharmaceuticals in waterways raise concern; Effect on wildlife, humans questioned. *Washington Post*, A.3.

2. Pfizer website available at http://www.pfizer.com/are/investors_releases/2005pr/mn_2005_0419.cfm.

3. *L.A. Times* (July 21, 2005). Pfizer's, Wyeth's profits climb; solid sales of key drugs boost results in the second quarter; Roche also reports an increase, C.3.

4. Martinez, M.; Abboud, L. & Davies, P. (July 22, 2005). Drug makers' results reflect woes; Merck's profit drops 59%; Lilly, Shering–Plough post losses on litigation charges. *Wall Street Journal*, B.3.

5. Abboud, L. (July 27, 2005). The next phase in psychiatry; largest ever studies on drugs for depression, schizophrenia could transform treatment. *Wall Street Journal*, D.1.

Preface

1. Schopenhauer, A. (1896). On the wisdom of life: Aphorisms. *Essays of Arthur Schopenhauer: Book VII: The Art of Controversy*, trans. Saunders, T. B. Project Gutenberg ebook #10731.

2. The Tom Cruise interview was aired on the "Today" show June 24, 2005.

3. The full conversation is available on the web at http://www.drudgereport.com/flash3tc.htm.

4. American Psychiatric Association Press Release (June 27, 2005). APA responds to Tom Cruise's Today Show interview. Available on the web at http://www.psych.org/news_room/press_release/05–39APAResponds_TomCruiseTodayShowInterview.pdf.

5. Hesman, T. (July 1, 2005). Cruise's aversion to antidepressants at odds with scientific evidence. *St. Louis Post–Dispatch* (via Knight–Ridder/Tribune News Service). Source: InfoTrac OneFile Article CJ133708420.

6. Ibid.

7. Ibid.

8. These statistics are reported in Myers, D. G. (2005). *Exploring Psychology*, 6th ed. New York: Worth Publishers, p. 489. Myers does not reference these statistics. (It is likely that the 1989 report by Wickramaratne, Weissman, et al. referenced below in this endnote is the source. It uses the National Institute of Mental Health Epidemiologic Catchment Area data. However, several other similar reports also use this data set as well.) This and many other similar studies are open to three primary criticisms: namely, these studies involve self–reports; they use retrospective designs; and depressed subjects are more likely to have died, impacting older cohorts the most severely. These issues have been discussed by others. (See the *JAMA* and the *Journal of Clinical Epidemiology* articles below for reasonable arguments supporting the notion that depression has been increasing with each successive 20th century cohort group.) However, it should be noted that some degree of recall of

depression is unreliable (Thompson, R.; Bogner, H. R.; et al. [2004]. Personal characteristics associated with consistency of recall of depressed or anhedonic mood in 13-year follow-up of the Baltimore Epidemiological Catchment Area survey. *Acta Psychiatrica Scandinavica, 109*, 345–354). For studies which find depression increased and emerged at earlier ages with each successive cohort see Klerman, G. L. & Weissman, M. M. (1989). Increasing rates of depression. *JAMA, 261*, 2229–2235; Robins, L. N.; Helzer, J. E., et al. (1984). Lifetime prevalence of specific psychiatric disorders in three sites. *Archives of General Psychiatry, 41*, 949–958; Wickramaratne, P. J.; Weissman, M. M., et al. (1989). Age, period and cohort effects on the risk of major depression: Results from five United States communities. *Journal of Clinical Epidemiology, 42*, 333–343; Klerman, G. L.; Lavori, P. W., et al. (1985). Birth–cohort trends in rates of major depressive disorder among relatives of patients with affective disorder. *Archives of General Psychiatry, 42*, 689–693.

9.   Weissman, M. M.; Bland, R. C., et al. (1996). Cross–national epidemiology of major depression and bipolar disorder. *JAMA, 276*, 293–299. Also see Keene, J. J.; Galasko, G. T. & Land, M. F. (2003). Antidepressant use in psychiatry and medicine: Importance for dental practice. *Journal of the American Dental Association, 134*, 71–79 which found 2 to 3 times as many women as men taking antidepressants. *Psychopharmacology Update* (2005, *16*, 7) reported that an estimated 10% of women and 4% of men 18 and older were taking antidepressants in the 1999–2000 period.

10.   For depression by country, see Weissman, et al. (ibid.). For the U.S., see Demyttenaere, K.; Bruffaerts, R., et al. (2004). Prevalence, severity and unmet need for treatment of mental disorders in the World Health Organization Mental Health Surveys. *JAMA, 291*, 2581–2590. For antidepressant use in Taiwan, see Su, T. P.; Chen, T. J., et al. (2002). Utilization of psychotropic drugs in Taiwan: An overview of outpatient sector in 2000. *Zhonghua Yi Xue Za Zhi* (Taipei), *65*, 378–391. For Korean treatment of depression which, like the rest of the region, is said to be in its infancy, see Hickie, L. (2004). Treatment guidelines for depression in the Asia Pacific region: A review of current developments. *Australas Psychiatry, 12* (Suppl.), S33–S37. Also see Lee, M. S. (2004). A preliminary study of undergraduate education on depression in medical schools in the Asia Pacific region. *Australas Psychiatry, 12* (Suppl.), S28–S32. For Canada, see Patten, S. B. (2004). The impact of antidepressant treatment on population health: Synthesis of data from two national data sources in Canada. *Population Health Metrics, 2*, 9. This electronic resource is available for free on the internet. Go to PubMed for a link. For antidepressant (psychotropic) drug use in Europe, see Alonso, J.; Angermeyer, M. C., et al. (2004). Psychotropic drug utilization in Europe: Results from the European Study of the Epidemiology of Mental Disorders (ESEMeD) project, Table 4. *Acta Psychiatrica Scandinavica Supplementum, 109* (Suppl. 420), 55–64, p. 59.

11.   A 1952 paper in French which described the action of isoniazid on depression is considered the first description of an antidepressant. See Healy, D. (2002). *The Creation of Psychopharmacology*. Cambridge, MA: Harvard University Press, p. 88. For a detailed history by the leading scholar on the development of antidepressant drugs, see Healy, D. (1997). *The Antidepressant Era*. Cambridge, MA: Harvard University Press.

12.   The suicide rate per 100,000 for 5–14 year olds in 1950 was .2. In 2000 the rate was .7. For 15–24 year olds it rose from 4.5 to 10.2 during that period (U.S. Census Bureau, Death rates from suicide, by sex and race: 1950 to 2000, Table 110. *Statistical Abstract of the U.S.: 2004–2005*. Washington, D. C.: U.S. Printing Office, p. 86). For statistics on the dramatic increases in antidepressant use among youth, see Zito, J. M.; Safer, D. J., et al. (2002). Rising prevalence of antidepressants among U.S. youths. *Pediatrics, 109*, 721–727.

13.   Cutler, D. M.; Glaeser, E. L. & Norberg, K. E. (2000). Explaining the rise in youth

suicide. NBER Working Paper #7713. Cambridge, MA: National Bureau of Economic Research, p. 7. Available on the web at http://www.nber.org/papers/w7713.

14. Garnet, L. R. (May 7, 2000). Debate about effects of Prozac continues as drug patent nears expiration. *The Boston Globe*, n.p. Source: InfoTrac OneFile Article CJ12207 4456.

15. Dear Abby (April 29, 1995). *The Victoria Advocate*, D.6.

16. Ibid.

17. Jablensky, A; Sartorius, N., et al. (1992). Schizophrenia: Manifestations, incidence, and course in different cultures: A World Health Organization ten–country study. *Psychological Medicine, 20* (Monograph Suppl.), 1–97. For a 2004 report which also surveyed mental health internationally see Demyttenaere, K.; Bruffaerts, R., et al. (2004). Prevalence, severity and unmet need for treatment of mental disorders in the World Health Organization Mental Health Surveys. *JAMA, 291*, 2581–2590. The World Health Organization (WHO) has been conducting international studies of mental health for over three decades. The pattern of those in third–world countries having better outcomes and shorter duration of schizophrenia has now been found repeatedly. The 1992 report discovered 38% of schizophrenics in developing countries were symptom free at follow–up compared with 22% in developed nations. A more recent study of schizophrenia in Finland found a schizophrenia recovery rate of only 1 out of 59 patients (1.7%). It may be our drug approach which seriously impedes recovery. See Lauronen, E.; Koskinen, J., et al. (2005). Recovery from schizophrenic psychoses within the northern Finland 1966 birth cohort. *Journal of Clinical Psychiatry, 66*, 375–378. Also note the better outcomes longitudinally for schizophrenia in Madras, India. See Thara, R. (2004). Twenty–year course of schizophrenia: The Madras Longitudinal Study. *Canadian Journal of Psychiatry, 49*, 564–569. Also see Hopper, K.; Wanderling J. (2000). Revisiting the developed versus developing country distinction in course and outcome of schizophrenia: Results from the ISoS, the WHO collaborative followup project: International Study of Schizophrenia. *Schizophrenia Bulletin, 26*, 835–846.

18. Jablensky, et al., ibid. As noted in an article authored by Eli Lilly employees, "Continuous therapy [is] commonly recommended by published treatment guidelines" (Loosbrock, D. L.; Zhao, Z., et al. [2003]. Antipsychotic medication use patterns and associated costs of care for individuals with schizophrenia. *Journal of Mental Health Policy & Economics, 6*, 67–75). An abundance of research makes it clear that some of the undesirable "positive" symptoms of schizophrenia are controlled with medication. But if this is due to a brain–damaging effect (it is) and if actual cure rates are reduced (they are), the dubious morality of treating schizophrenics with antipsychotics becomes apparent.

19. It is considered unethical today to do double–blind, placebo controlled studies of long–term results comparing antipsychotics versus placebos. However, such studies, now older, have found that placebos (which do not shrink the brain like antipsychotics) do, in fact, lead to higher recovery rates. An example is found in Rappaport, et al.'s well–designed study (Rappaport, M; Hopkins, H. K., et al. [1978]. Are there schizophrenics for whom drugs may be unnecessary or contraindicated? *International Pharmacopsychiatry, 13*, 100–111). Robert Whitaker's book *Mad in America* (2002, Cambridge, MA: Perseus) does an excellent job of discussing the misleading analysis found in many antipsychotic studies which seeks to make relapse while on antipsychotics infrequent (see pp. 199–203). He notes that "by one estimate, more than 80 percent of the 257,446 schizophrenia patients discharged from hospitals in 1986 had to be rehospitalized within two years, a rehospitalization rate much higher than for 'never–exposed' patients, or—as can be seen by the data above—for those gradually withdrawn from [antipsychotics]" (pp. 202–203).

20. These issues are all discussed and documented in Chapter 13, Side Effects of

Antipsychotics.
21. See endnote 135 in Chapter 12 (Fooled, Fooled and Fooled Again) for several references.

Chapter 1 — Introduction

1. Graham, D. (2004). Blowing the whistle on the FDA: An interview with Dr. David Graham. *Multinational Monitor, 25*, 22.
2. The National Institutes of Health ended the estrogen–only part of the Women's Health Initiative in March 2004 because of higher stroke rates, though they found no higher breast cancer and heart disease rates. However, dosages were lower than what was commonly used, and the picture is still clouded. The Million Women Study (a study of approximately 1 in 4 British women, ages 50–64), however, found increased risk of breast cancer for both estrogen and estrogen–progesterone, and a slightly greater risk for estrogen obtained from pregnant mare urine than synthesized estrogen. Duration of use proved to be an important variable (Million Women Study Collaborators [2003]. Breast cancer and hormone–replacement therapy in the Million Women Study. *Lancet, 362*, 419–427).
3. I suspect most women who took Premarin were unaware of the origin of the estrogen in their daily pill. In fact, the urine of pregnant mares contains incredibly high levels of estrogen (hundreds of times the normal level). To manufacture Premarin, mares' urine is captured and the estrogen is extracted—a process that is undoubtedly far more complicated than that statement reveals. Also simplified in this account is the complexity of what we call estrogen. Barbara Seaman has written a very interesting and personal book entitled *The Greatest Experiment Ever Performed on Women.* A single sentence from her book makes it clear that "estrogen" is not a single hormone but a general term for an entire group of hormones. "Premarin is a mixture of over ten different estrogens—including estrone (which we make in our bodies) and equilin and equilenin (horse estrogen, which of course we don't make in our own bodies" (Seaman, B. [2003]. *The Greatest Experiment Ever Performed on Women: Exploding the Estrogen Myth.* New York: Hyperion, p. 239). Estrogen can also be synthesized or be extracted from plants. The estrogen derived from pregnant mares' urine is associated with greater cancer risks than is estrogen derived from these other sources. This is likely due to the nature of horse estrogen which is not easily metabolized by humans, "and as a result that form of estrogen stays in the body, producing a more potent and long–lasting effect on our estrogen receptors" (ibid., p. 240).
4. Seaman states, "The British doctor who published his estrogen formula in 1938 spent many years thereafter warning the world that these drugs, although containing great promise, put women at serious peril for endometrial and breast cancer" (ibid., p. 5). While there was clearly sufficient evidence to cause concern by the 1960s, the danger was still being discounted. See, for example, the 1963 debate involving a National Cancer Institute researcher who noted animal studies which found breast cancer rates increased in animals exposed to hormones. The *NY Times* reported his concern that even birth control pills should not be taken long term "in the absence of proof that they are not potential stimulators of cancer in humans." (It should be noted that early birth control pills did have much higher amounts of estrogen than those used today.) The other side of the debate was taken by a professor of surgery from the Temple University Hospital and Medical School who noted that many obstetricians and gynecologists were cautious about prescribing hormones to women who had had breast cancer. He was reported to have declared that "in his experience even a previous operation for breast cancer was no necessary bar to the use of hormone drugs" (Schmeck, H. M. [Oct. 23, 1963]. Expert cautions on hormone use. *NY Times*, p. 26).
5. The *New York Times* began a story in 1959 with the following sentence: "Female

hormones, given in doses too small to produce undesirable side effects, may prolong the lives of heart–attack victims, it was reported here today" (Schmeck, H. M. [June 6, 1959]. Report finds female hormone extends cardiac victims' lives. *NY Times*, p. 22).

6. I have simplified the story. In fact, Premarin became the nation's #1 patented drug by 1966 and remained near the top of the "most popular drugs" list until 1975 when the *New England Journal of Medicine* reported that a dramatic (4 to 14 times) increase in endometrial cancer was found in women on Premarin seven years or longer.

7. Progestin was added to between 10 and 14 of each month's supply of estrogen pills.

8. Shairer, J.; Lubin, J., et al. (2000). Menopausal estrogen and estrogen–progestin replacement therapy and breast cancer risk. *JAMA, 283*, 484–491. This study reported that those on estrogen only had between a 1% and 3% increase in breast cancer risk for each year of use. Those who were on an estrogen–progestin combination (what was considered the safe pill) faced increases in breast cancer ranging from 8%–12% for each year of use.

9. My mother was part of a research study. As I scoured the literature I found that the University of California, Irvine had a research focus on breast cancer. Much of the research utilized patients in Orange County, CA, where the third and fourth years of UCI's medical school and professors are located. That was where my mother was treated. Obviously, it will strike readers as unethical for a physician who is aware that my mother would be more likely to survive if she had a lumpectomy rather than a mastectomy not to share that information. But this is one of the dilemmas of conducting research. When the findings come from a large, well–designed study, the study is often stopped in order to give each patient the best possible treatment. But researchers are sometimes wrong about what constitutes the best possible treatment. Thus, doing what may seem unethical is a regular part of medical research. In the long run it does save lives. But, obviously, I was not going to allow my mother to be one of the guinea pigs.

10. Estrogen supplementation became known as estrogen replacement therapy (ERT). However, once estrogen was no longer the only hormone taken, the ERT label was replaced with HRT. The term "hormone therapy" may replace HRT. (See the argument for this term in Barrett–Connor, E.; Grady, D. & Stefanick, M. L. [2005]. The rise and fall of menopausal hormone therapy. *Annual Review of Public Health, 26*, 115–140.)

11. Hulley, S.; Grady, D., et al. (1998). Randomized trial of estrogen plus progestin for secondary prevention of coronary disease in postmenopausal women. *JAMA, 280*, 605–613.

12. Roussouw, J. E.; Anderson, G. L., et al. (2002). Risks and benefits of estrogen plus progestin in healthy post–menopausal women. *JAMA, 288*, 321–333. These risks were not minor. The risk of coronary heart disease, the number one killer of women, was 29% higher when the study was prematurely stopped (after 3.3 years because breast cancer rates rose above a predetermined "stop" level). There was also a 41% increased risk of stroke and 113% increase of having a pulmonary embolism. The RCT results are remarkable in that so many earlier (non–RCT) studies found estrogen to reduce the incidence of these events.

13. Colditz, G. A. (2005). Estrogen, estrogen plus progestin therapy, and risk of breast cancer. *Clinical Cancer Research, 11*, 909s–917s. Though estrogen plus progestin clearly increases breast cancer risk, not all studies suggest estrogen alone is a risk. There is yet to be full agreement in the literature. Obesity, age, other sample variables and the type of estrogen used could explain this. For a review which reports increased risk for estrogen plus progestin (an increased risk of 2.3% for each year of use after 5 years) but no estrogen only increased risk, see Barrett–Connor, E.; Grady, D. & Stefanick, M. L. (2005). The rise and fall of menopausal hormone therapy. *Annual Review of Public Health, 26*, 115–140.

14. Archer, D. F. (2004). Neoplasma of the female reproductive tract: Effects of hor-

mone therapy. *Endocrine, 24,* 259–263. Use of estrogen alone in women who have a uterus has consistently found an increased incidence of endometrial cancer. However, adding a progestin will eliminate this risk and may even prove somewhat protective (for this one cancer). HRT influences on ovarian cancer are inconsistent (and thought to be minimal), though one review found a 50% increase among ever users of HRT and greater risk with increased duration. For this, see Riman, T.; Nilsson, S. & Persson, I. R. (2004). Review of epidemiological evidence for reproductive and hormonal factors to the risk of epithelial ovarian malignancies. *Acta Obstetricia Et Gynecologica Scandinavica, 83,* 783–795.

15. Shumaker, S. A.; Legault, C., et al. (2003). Estrogen plus progestin and the incidence of dementia and mild cognitive impairment in post–menopausal women. *JAMA, 289,* 2651–2662. Also Rapp, S. R.; Espeland, M. A., et al. (2003). Effect of estrogen plus progestin on global cognitive function in postmenopausal women: The Women's Health Initiative Memory Study: A randomized controlled trial. *JAMA, 289,* 2663–2672. We still do not have and will probably never have human studies that determine risks by dosing levels. The Women's Health Initiative (WHI) ended the estrogen–only arm of their study in March 2004 before the study's completion date had been reached. The concern which stopped the study short was over an increased rate of stroke. However they reported no increase in breast cancer or heart disease (unlike the estrogen–progesterone arm of the WHI). There was evidence of a dose–response effect for Prempro and likely the same is true for Premarin, but the question is also impossible to answer definitively without putting lives at risk. The review by Barrett–Connor, et al. reported both estrogen and estrogen plus progestin decreased osteoporosis, but only estrogen plus progestin reduced colon cancer (Barrett–Connor, E.; Grady, D. & Stefanick, M. L. [2005]. The rise and fall of menopausal hormone therapy. *Annual Review of Public Health, 26,* 115–140).

16. Lorenz, K. (1937). The companion in the bird's world. *Auk, 54,* 245–273.

17. The results of Lorenz's experiments are known by most psychology majors since they are reported in virtually every introductory psychology textbook. The Klopfer study which utilized a superior design is almost unknown. The point is that textbooks tend to report the same studies, and those that are discussed are those that become well known. For Klopfer's study, see Klopfer, P. H. (1971). Mother love: What turns it on? *American Scientist, 59,* 404–407. The exact results were as follows: Among 15 mother goats allowed to have 5 minutes of maternal contact with their offspring following birth, 14 of 15 accepted their kids when returned after 1–3 hours. Among the 15 mother goats who did not have 5 minutes of contact with their offspring following birth, only one accepted the kid upon its return.

18. I am not saying the errors will come to an end—only that the frequency will be greatly reduced. Even RCTs can be poorly designed. They can be performed on an inadequate number of people or not conducted for an adequate length of time. They may have erroneous endpoints (lower blood pressure or lower cholesterol) instead of the more logical endpoints (fewer heart attacks or deaths). If the "random" assignment is not done properly or if researchers are not blinded (they know who has been assigned to each group), the end results can be hugely impacted. If two competing drugs are compared but no placebo is included, researchers may conclude one of the drugs is very effective when a placebo may have been as effective or even more effective than either drug. Unfortunately, RCTs are not always possible to conduct. They tend to be very expensive and sometimes are impractical or even unethical to carry out. For an excellent discussion of research design issues see Trisha Greenhalgh's *How to Read a Paper: The Basics of Evidence Based Medicine,* 2nd ed. (2001, London: BMJ Books).

19. The first large RCT study was published in 1998 and was referred to in endnote 11,

Hulley, S., et al. (1998).

20. Cano, A. (1994). Compliance to hormone replacement therapy in menopausal women controlled in a third level academic centre. *Maturitas, 20*, 91–99. Cano found that 9% never had their prescriptions filled. Even life–saving medications may never be filled or may not be taken regularly. Wang and his colleagues found a correlation of only .15 between self–reported compliance by patients and actual compliance as determined by the number of days covered by filled prescriptions (Wang, P. S.; Benner, J. S., et al. [2004]. How well do patients report noncompliance with antihypertensive medications? A comparison of self–report versus filled prescriptions. *Pharmacoepidemiology & Drug Safety, 13*, 11–19). Among those treated with antipsychotic drugs, the literature reveals noncompliance rates ranging from 20% to 89% (Rijcken, C.A. [2004]. Refill rate of antipsychotic drugs: An easy and inexpensive method to monitor patients' compliance by using computerized pharmacy data. *Pharmacoepidemiology & Drug Safety, 13*, 365–370).

21. These characteristics are noted in the following studies: Matthews, K. A.; Kuller, L. H., et al. (1996). Health prior to use of estrogen replacement therapy: Are users healthier than non–users? *American Journal of Epidemiology, 143*, 971–978; Levy, B. G.; Ritchie, J. M., et al. (2003). Physician specialty is significantly associated with hormone replacement therapy use. *Obstetrics & Gynecology, 101*, 114–122; Ettinger, B.; Fugate, W. N., et al. (2000). The North American Menopause Society 1998 menopause survey: Part II. Counseling about hormone replacement therapy: Association with socioeconomic status and access to medical care. *Menopause, 7*, 143–148; Friedman–Koss, D. (2002). The relationship of race/ethnicity and social class to hormone replacement therapy: Results from the Third National Health and Nutrition Examination Survey 1988–1994. *Menopause, 9*, 264–272; Brown, A. F. (1999). Ethnic differences in hormone replacement prescribing patterns. *Journal of General Internal Medicine, 14*, 663–669. Even the Type A personality which was found to be more common among the women taking estrogen and is usually associated with more heart disease was found to be associated with several factors resulting in less heart disease. See Buller, J. C.; Kritz–Silverstein, D., et al. (1998). Type A behavior pattern, heart disease risk factors, and estrogen replacement therapy in postmenopausal women: The Rancho Bernardo Study. *Journal of Women's Health, 7*, 49–56. Finally, I believe it is important to note that even Wyeth's product insert for Prempro noted (albeit in very fine print) that research on estrogen and heart disease utilized women who were more physically active, thinner and less likely to have diabetes. These three factors by themselves would make any honest observer, knowledgeable about research design, recognize that whatever their study found, it would be essentially worthless data. These major factors must be controlled for by random assignment.

22. This study examined the *Physicians' Desk Reference*, five textbooks, and other sources of information available to physicians and noted that it was generally recommended to give estrogen only to women in good health (Hemminki, E. & Sihvo, S. [1993]. A review of postmenopausal hormone therapy recommendations: Potential for selection bias. *Obstetrics & Gynecology, 82*, 1021–1028).

23. *Time* (Oct. 16, 1964). Durable unendurable women, p. 72. The article further states that estrogen could prevent the vaginal dryness that is a problem for some women. Kistner believed that this problem was responsible for many extramarital affairs among middleaged husbands. "If we can prevent or retard these changes of senescence, we can help to keep the women happier and their husbands as well."

24. Lagercrantz, H. & Slotkin, T. A. (1986). The "stress" of being born. *Scientific American, 254*, 100–107.

25. Zhao, Z. Y.; Xie, Y., et al. (2002). Aging and the circadian rhythm of melatonin: A

cross–sectional study of Chinese subjects 30–110 years of age. *Chronobiology International, 19,* 1171–1182. Also Nair, N. P.; Hariharasubramanian, N., et al. (1986). Plasma melatonin: An index of brain aging in humans? *Biological Psychiatry, 212,* 141–150.

26. Dabbs, J. M. (2000). *Heroes, Rogues, and Lovers: Testosterone and Behavior.* New York: McGraw–Hill. See pp. 15–17 especially.

27. Magri, F; Sarra, S., et al. (2004). Qualitative and quantitative changes in melatonin levels in physiological and pathological aging and in centenarians. *Journal of Pineal Research, 36,* 256–261.

28. Luboshitzky, R.; Yanai, D., et al. (1998). Daily and seasonal variations in the concentration of melatonin in the human pineal gland. *Brain Research Bulletin, 47,* 271–276.

29. Dabbs, J. M. (2000). *Heroes, Rogues, and Lovers.* New York: McGraw–Hill. See p. 160. However, there are strong advocates for hormone replacement therapy in the male despite an awareness that few excellent (RCT) studies exist. See, for example, Heaton, J. P. (2002). Point: Urologists should take an active role in the diagnosis and treatment of hypogonadism in the aging male. *Canadian Journal of Urology, 9,* 1677–1680.

30. *Time* (April 1, 1966). Pills to keep women young, pp. 50–51.

31. Ibid., p. 50.

32. Ibid.

33. This is a general statement. For example, the *New England Journal of Medicine* releases the coming week's issue to the media on Fridays so reporters can interview the authors and prepare their reports for the news release day on Wednesday.

34. The statistic is based on *Look*'s claim of "Now more than 7,500,000 circulation," *Look* (Jan. 11, 1966), p. 2.

35. Wilson, R. A. (Jan. 11, 1966). A key to staying young. *Look, 30,* 66–73.

36. Ibid., p. 66.

37. Wilson forced the hand of countless doctors by describing those who refused to give estrogen as either calloused or ignorant. He described his conversation with a woman referred by one of his own patients. "'Have you discussed your symptoms with your family doctor?' I asked her. 'He couldn't care less!' she said bitterly. This woman's experience reflects the traditional attitude of many physicians, who simply refuse to recognize menopause for what it is—a serious, painful, and often crippling disease. . . . Yet one cannot accuse the average practitioner of willful neglect if he fails to treat menopause properly. If he is not yet aware that menopause is a disease caused by a deficiency of ovarian hormones, the doctor could easily be misled by its symptoms" (ibid., p. 66).

38. Ibid., p. 70. His book *Feminine Forever* also adds neuroses and "other personality disorders" to the psychological dangers of having too little estrogen (Wilson, R. [1966]. *Feminine Forever.* New York: M. Evans & Co., p. 133).

39. Wilson, R. A. (Jan. 11, 1966). A key to staying young. *Look, 30,* 66–73, p. 68.

40. Ibid., p. 70.

41. Ibid.

42. Wilson, R. A. (Oct. 27, 1962). The roles of estrogen and progesterone in breast and genital cancer. *JAMA, 182,* 327–331.

43. All these companies have changed names following mergers or acquisitions. The Upjohn Company, for example, became Pharmacia and Upjohn. They then dropped the Upjohn and were known simply as Pharmacia. Pharmacia was then acquired by Pfizer in 2002. The price of that acquisition ($60 billion) should make it clear how much money is being made by drug companies.

44. Dr. Wilson's book *Feminine Forever* (1966, New York: M. Evans & Co.) after 200 pages of estrogen promotion has a note which reads, "The Wilson Research Foundation, of which I am President, will provide additional information on the subject of menopause prevention to any woman seeking it as well as professional information to any doctor who inquires." He then gives the Foundation's mailing address (p. 206).

45. The financial arrangements were made public by the *New Republic* reporters. However, the involvement of family members is less known. Mrs. Wilson as the wife of a gynecologist, an estrogen user and a woman who herself had experienced menopause may have proved an especially effective speaker. Robert Wilson's son Ronald felt she was employed in part because his father suffered from an almost lifelong problem with laryngitis (phone interview, Jan. 18, 2005).

46. I would not argue that Wilson was not a true believer in the value of estrogen. Clearly he was. But I believe he was blinded to the dangers of estrogen by his desire to help (or perhaps his desire to be honored). He did not just discount the danger. He thought and spoke in absolutist language. The first sentence of his 1962 *JAMA* article as cited in *Feminine Forever* begins, "There is no convincing proof that estrogen has ever induced cancer in the human being" (p. 101). The first sentence of the conclusion reads, "Estrogen does not induce cancer" (1966, New York: M. Evans & Co., p. 105).

47. Borel, H. D. (1966). The book that ends menopause. *Science Digest, 59*, 26–28.

48. *Science News* (Nov. 26, 1966). Goddard rebukes drug tester, *90*, 450.

49. Wilson, R. (1966). *Feminine Forever*. New York: M. Evans & Co., p. 113.

50. Robert Wilson's son Ronald very willingly allowed me to interview him on two occasions (Jan. 18 and Jan. 29, 2005), graciously sharing very personal details of this story which I had not known previously, including facts surrounding both his mother's and father's deaths.

51. The sales figures and profits for Premarin found in this section are recorded in Love, S. M. (1997). *Dr. Susan Love's Hormone Book*. New York: Random House, pp. 28–29, 36.

52. Smith, D. C.; Prentice, R., et al. (1975). Association of exogenous estrogen and endometrial carcinoma. *New England Journal of Medicine, 293*, 1164–1167; Ziel, H. K. & Finkle, W. D. (1975). Increased risk of endometrial carcinoma among users of conjugated estrogens. *New England Journal of Medicine, 293*, 1167–170. The first study reported the 4.5 times elevated risk. The second study examined women taking a conjugated estrogen (Premarin) and found an even higher risk—5.6 times more endometrial cancer for women on Premarin between 1 and 4.9 years and 13.9 times more for those with seven or more years of exposure.

53. Thom, M. H.; White, P. J., et al. (1979). Prevention and treatment of endometrial disease in climacteric women receiving estrogen therapy. *Lancet, 2*, 455–457.

54. National Institutes of Health (1984). *Osteoporosis Consensus Development Conference Consensus Statement 1984 (April 2–4)*, 5. Bethesda, MD: U.S. Government Printing Office, 1–6. The consensus statement is on the web at http://consensus.nih.gov/cons/043/ 043_statement.htm#8_Speaker.

55. I would question their "independence" even today. I cannot prove drug company influence, but I was surprised by what I found on their website. In contrast with the National Institutes of Health 1984 consensus statement which now has in large, uppercase type "THIS DOCUMENT IS NO LONGER VIEWED BY NIH AS GUIDANCE FOR CURRENT MEDICAL PRACTICE" (Point: The estrogen replacement, recommended in 1984, is now known to be unsafe), the National Osteoporosis Foundation (NOF) still lists estrogens as

Endnotes, Ch. 2, Are Mental Problems Mental Diseases?

"approved by the U.S. Food and Drug Administration (FDA) for the prevention and/or treatment of osteoporosis." They also list a number of drugs which can be prescribed for osteoporosis—and include brand names. (They do provide something akin to a label insert for each drug and some of the estrogen risks are listed there.) Another fact which makes me wonder about current funding is a headline on their homepage that reads, "Advisory Panel Lists Drugs It Wants New Law To Cover." That headline takes the reader to a *NY Times* article which noted that former NOF president, Dr. C. Conrad Johnston, was pushing to get more osteoporosis medications approved by Medicare (Pear, R. [Jan. 4, 2005]. Advisory panel lists drugs it wants new law to cover. *NY Times*, A.12). The most important question to answer is how much funding still comes from drug companies? I repeatedly asked that question of the NOF's communications office by phone and by email and never received a reply.

56.   Ghostwriting is still practiced and is discussed further in Chapter 6.

57.   A 1992 meta–analysis of observational studies concluded that there was some breast and uterine cancer risk but that the heart disease and hip fracture benefits were so substantial they outweighed concerns about cancer (Grady, D; Rubin, S. M., et al. [1992]. Hormone therapy to prevent disease and prolong life in postmenopausal women. *Annals of Internal Medicine, 117*, 1016–1037).

58.   Hulley, S.; Grady, D., et al. (1998). Randomized trial of estrogen plus progestin for secondary prevention of coronary heart disease in postmenopausal women. *JAMA, 280*, 605–613.

59.   Schairer, C. (2000). Menopausal estrogen and estrogen–progestin replacement therapy and breast cancer risk. *JAMA, 283*, 485–491.

60.   Wyeth press release (Dec. 20, 2001). This press release is still on the web though it came out several years ago. See http://www.wyeth.com/news/Pressed_and_Released/pr12_20_2001_425.asp?archive=2001.

61.   Roussouw, J; Anderson, G., et al. (2002). Risks and benefits of estrogen plus progestin in healthy post–menopausal women, *JAMA, 288*, 321–333.

Chapter 2 — Are Mental Problems Mental Diseases?

1.   Swift, J. (Nov. 9, 1710). *The Examiner*, #15.

2.   On–line Medical Dictionary. Available at http://cancerweb.ncl.ac.uk/cgi–bin/omd?functional+psychosis.

3.   Pedrosa–Sanchez, M. & Sola, R. G. (2003). Modern day psychosurgery: A new approach to neurosurgery in psychiatric disease. *Revista de Neurologia, 36*, 887–897.

4.   Paralysis is the symptom giving the condition its proper medical name—general paresis. The condition was a major cause of mental problems early in the 20th century, being responsible for approximately 10–15% of all patients found in mental hospitals at that time (Barondes, S. H. [1993]. *Molecules and Mental Illness*. New York: Scientific American Library, p. 12). Once the T. pallidum bacterium was isolated, an animal host was sought which would allow the bacterium to survive so experiments could be conducted to determine what chemicals could destroy T. pallidum without injury to its host. Rabbits were found to be effective hosts, and a new drug (arsphenamine) developed by a German microbiologist was found to be an effective T. pallidum eradicating agent. Dr. Paul Ehrlich won much fame for this discovery. The story was even told in the 1940 film "Dr. Ehrlich's Magic Bullet."

5.   Cummings, J.; Benson, D. F. & LoVerme, Jr., S. (1980). Reversible dementia. *JAMA, 243*, 2434–2439.

6.   Kaiser, D. (1996). Commentary: Against biologic psychiatry. *Psychiatric Times, 13*. Available on the web at http://www.psychiatrictimes.com/p961242.html.

7. Breggin, P. R. (2001). *The Anti–Depressant Fact Book*. Cambridge, MA: Perseus, p. 21.

8. Valenstein, E. S. (1998). *Blaming the Brain: The Truth About Drugs and Mental Health*. New York: The Free Press, pp. 4, 96.

9. Glenmullen, J. (2000). *Prozac Backlash*. New York: Simon & Schuster, p. 196.

10. Whitaker, R. (2002). *Mad in America*. Cambridge, MA: Perseus, p. 291.

11. Kemker, S. S. (1995). Residency and psychiatry: Assumptions we learn (Ch. 6) in Ross, C. & Alvin, P., eds. *Pseudoscience in Biological Psychiatry: Blaming the Body*. New York: John Wiley & Sons, p. 242.

12. Horwitz, A. V. (2002). *Creating Mental Illness*. Chicago: University of Chicago Press, p. 156.

13. Dean, C. E. (Nov. 22, 1997). *Minnesota Star Tribune*. Cited at http://home.att.net/~LetFreedomRing/spirituality/prosantibraindisease.html.

14. Mosher, L. R. (Dec. 4, 1998). Letter to Dr. Rodrigo Munoz, American Psychiatric Association president, announcing Mosher's resignation from the APA. Dr. Mosher placed his letter on the web. It is available at http://www.moshersoteria.com/resig.pdf.

15. Borges, E. M. (1995). A social critique of biological psychiatry (Ch. 5) in Ross, C. A. & Pam, A., eds. *Pseudoscience in Biological Psychiatry*. New York: John Wiley & Sons, p. 211.

16. Ross, C. A. (1995). Errors of logic in biological psychiatry (Ch. 2) in ibid., p. 90.

17. Myers, D. (2005). *Exploring Psychology*, 6th ed. New York: Worth Publishers, p. 499.

18. Limosin, F; Rouillon, F., et al. (2003). Prenatal exposure to influenza as a risk factor for adult schizophrenia. *Acta Psychiatrica Scandinavica, 107*, 331–335. However, Battle and colleagues reported a higher incidence of schizophrenia among those born during the winter but did not find the schizophrenia to be related to flu or measle outbreaks (Battle, Y. L.; Martin, B. C., et al. [1999]. Seasonality and infectious disease in schizophrenias: The birth hypothesis revisited. *Journal of Psychiatric Research, 33*, 501–509). The lack of a clear consensus within these numerous studies is not pointed out in the Myers' textbook or other textbooks that cite the influenza–schizophrenia link though contrary findings have long been reported (Kendell, R. E. & Kemp, I. W. [1989]. Maternal influenza in the etiology of schizophrenia. *Archives of General Psychiatry, 46*, 878–882). More recent reviews continue to discuss the inconsistent results of these studies (Ebert, T. & Kotler, M. [2005]. Prenatal exposure to influenza and the risk of subsequent development of schizophrenia. *Israel Medical Association Journal, 7*, 35–38.

19. Torrey, E. F.; Rawlings, R. R., et al. (1996). Birth seasonality in bipolar disorder, schizophrenia, schizoaffective disorder and stillbirths. *Schizophrenia Research, 21*, 141–149.

20. Davies, G.; Welham, J., et al. (2003). A systematic review and meta–analysis of northern hemisphere season of birth studies in schizophrenia. *Schizophrenia Bulletin, 29*, 587–593.

21. Mednick, S. A.; Huttunen, M. O. & Machon, R. A. (1994). Prenatal influenza infections and adult schizophrenia. *Schizophrenia Bulletin, 20*, 263–267.

22. Mental retardation is even increased by prenatal exposure to influenza (Takei, N; Murray, G., et al. [1995]. Prenatal exposure to influenza epidemics and risk of mental retardation. *European Archives of Psychiatry & Clinical Neuroscience, 245*, 255–259).

23. Livingston, R.; Adam, B. & Bracha, H. (1993). Season of birth and neurodevelopmental disorders. *Journal of the American Academy Child/Adolescent Psychiatry, 32*, 612–616.

24.   Susser, E.; Neugenbauer, R., et al. (1996). Schizophrenia after prenatal famine: Further evidence. *Archives of General Psychiatry, 53*, 25–31. It has been known for decades that malnutrition during the prenatal period can result in a slowing in the division of brain cells and 20% fewer brain cells at birth than would occur if nutrition were adequate (Wyden, B. [Dec. 7, 1971]. Growth: 45 crucial months. *Life*, 93ff).

25.   Zornberg, Buka, et al. (2002). At issue: The problem of obstetrical complications and schizophrenia. *Schizophrenia Bulletin, 26*, 249–256.

26.   Ichiki, M.; Kunugi, H., et al. (2000). Intrauterine physical growth in schizophrenia: Evidence confirming excess of premature birth. *Psychological Medicine, 30*, 597–604.

27.   Jones, P. B.; Rantakallio, P., et al. (1998). Schizophrenia as a long–term outcome of pregnancy, delivery, and perinatal complications: A 28–year follow–up, *American Journal of Psychiatry, 55*, 355–364.

28.   Kunugi, H.; Nanko, S., et al. (1996). Perinatal complications and schizophrenia. *Journal of Nerve & Mental Disease, 184*, 542–546; Hultman, C. M.; Ohman, A., et al. (1997). Prenatal and neonatal risk factors for schizophrenia. *British Journal of Psychiatry, 170*, 128–133; Dalman, C.; Thomas, H. V., et al. (2001). Signs of asphyxia at birth and risk of schizophrenia: Population–based case–control study, *British Journal of Psychiatry, 179*, 403–408.

29.   Brown, A. S.; Cohen, P., et al. (2000). Nonaffective psychosis after prenatal exposure in rubella. *American Journal of Psychiatry, 157*, 438–443.

30.   Myers, D. (2005). *Exploring Psychology*, 6th ed. New York: Worth Publishers, p. 491.

31.   Ibid., p. 498.

32.   Kassin, S. (2004). *Psychology*, 4th ed. Upper Saddle River, NJ: Pearson Education, p. 50.

33.   Healy, D. (2004). *Let Them Eat Prozac: The Unhealthy Relationship Between the Pharmaceutical Industry and Depression*. New York: New York University Press, p. 12.

34.   *American Heritage Dictionary of the English Language*, 4th ed. (2000). Boston: Houghton Mifflin Company.

35.   An interesting overview of the discovery of neurotransmitters is provided by neuropsychologist Elliot Valenstein (Valenstein, E. S. [2002]. The discovery of chemical neurotransmitters. *Brain & Cognition, 49*, 73–95).

36.   Webster, R. A.; Brown, D., et al. (2001). *Neurotransmitters, Drugs, and Brain Function*. New York: Oxford University Press.

37.   Acetylcholine, GABA, epinephrine, norepinephrine, histamine, dopamine, serotonin, endorphins, and enkephalins are just a few of the better known neurotransmitters (Van de Graaff, K. M. & Rhees, R. W. [2001]. *Schaum's Easy Outlines: Human Anatomy and Physiology* [ed. Wilhelm, P. B., abridgement]. New York: McGraw Hill, p. 76).

38.   Valenstein, E. S. (1998). *Blaming the Brain*. New York: The Free Press, p. 4.

39.   Ibid., p. 5.

40.   Ibid., see p. 222. This is an excellent source for this and other neurotransmitter facts. See Chapter 8 for an overview. There you will learn that several widely believed neurotransmitter concepts are simply false. Alternately, search the National Library of Medicine's PubMed database for research studies on this topic. For example, the following study found that some of those with schizophrenia had low dopamine levels (Okubo, Y.; Suhara, T., et al. [1997]. Decreased prefrontal dopamine D_1 in schizophrenia revealed by PET. *Nature, 385*, 634–636).

41.   Okubo, Y.; Suhara, T., et al. (1997), ibid.

42. Valenstein, E. S. (1998). *Blaming the Brain.* New York: The Free Press, p. 5. For example, dopamine output in response to stress can be blunted by taking various drugs that are not designed to affect dopamine levels (Dazzi, L; Spiga, F., et al. [2001]. Inhibition of stress– or anxiogenic drug–induced increases in dopamine release in the rat prefrontal cortex by long–term treatment with antidepressant drugs. *Journal of Neurochemistry, 76,* 1212). This study found a 90% rise in dopamine in the prefrontal cortex of rat brains when the rats were exposed to electric shocks. Taking estrogen can cause dopamine levels to rise (Walker, Q. D.; Rooney, M. B., et al. [2000]. Dopamine release and uptake are greater in female than male rat striatum as measured by fast cyclic voltammetry. *Neuroscience, 95,* 1061–1070). Drinking coffee can cause dopamine and serotonin levels to rise (Solinas, M; Ferre, S., et al. [2002]. Caffeine induces dopamine and glutamate release in the shell of the nucleus accumbens. *Journal of Neuroscience, 22,* 6321–6324; Chen, M. D.; Lin, W. H., et al. [1994]. Effect of caffeine on the levels of brain serotonin and catecholamine in the genetically obese mice. *Zhonghua Yi Xue Za Zhi,* Taipei, *53,* 257–261.) The English language abstract is available online at the National Library of Medicine's PubMed site, http://www.ncbi.nlm.nih.gov.

43. Dazzi, L; Spiga, F., et al. (2001). Inhibition of stress– or anxiogenic drug–induced increases in dopamine release in the rat prefrontal cortex by long–term treatment with antidepressant drugs. *Journal of Neurochemistry, 76,* 1212.

44. Bethea, C. L.; Streicher, J. M., et al. (2005). Serotonin–related gene expression in female monkeys with individual sensitivity to stress. *Neuroscience, 132,* 151–166.

45. Pruessner, J. C.; Champagne, F., et al. (2004). Dopamine release in response to a psychological stress in humans and its relationship to early life maternal care: A positron emission tomography study using [11C]raclopride. *Journal of Neuroscience, 24,* 2825–2831.

46. Field, T; Diego, M. A., et al. (2004). Massage therapy effects on depressed pregnant women. *Journal of Psychosomatic Obstetrics & Gynaecology, 25,* 115–122.

47. Volkow, N. D.; Wang, G. J., et al. (2002). Nonhedonic food motivation in humans involves dopamine in the dorsal stratium and methylphenidate amplifies this effect. *Synapse, 44,* 175–180.

48. Ibid.; Small, D. M.; Zatorre, R. J., et al. (2001). Changes in brain activity related to eating chocolate: From pleasure to aversion. *Brain, 124,* 1720–1733.

49. Faherty, C. J.; Raviie, S. K., et al. (2005). Environmental enrichment in adulthood eliminates neuronal death in experimental Parkinsonism. *Brain Research.Molecular Brain Research, 134,* 170–179. The serotonin effect involved rats and found effects are dependent on obtaining regular exercise as reported by Greenwood, B. N.; Foley, T. E., et al. (2005). Wheel running alters serotonin (5–HT) transporter, 5–HT(1A), 5–HT(1B), and alpha (1b)–adrenergic receptor mRNA in the rat raphe nuclei. *Biological Psychiatry, 57,* 559–568.

50. Lechin, F; Pardey–Maldonado, B., et al. (2004). Circulating neurotransmitters during the different wake–sleep stages in normal subjects. *Psychoneuroendocrinology, 29,* 669–685.

51. Yamamoto, T; Ohkuwa, T., et al. (2003). Effects of pre–exercise listening to slow and fast rhythm music on supramaximal cycle performance and selected metabolic variables. *Archives of Physiology & Biochemistry, 111,* 211–214.

52. Moore, H; Rose, H. J. & Grace, A. A. (2001). Chronic cold stress reduces the spontaneous activity of ventral tegmental dopamine neurons. *Neuropsychopharmacology, 24,* 410–419.

53. Wong, D. F.; Wagner, H. N., et al. (1984). Effects of age on dopamine and serotonin receptors measured by positron tomography in the living human brain. *Science, 226,* 1393–1396.

54.   Just the direct–to–consumer advertising portion of drug promotion, a small part of annual drug promotion spending, amounted to $2.46 billion in 2000 (Rosenthal, M. B.; Berndt, E. R., et al. [2002]. Promotion of prescription drugs to consumers. *New England Journal of Medicine, 346,* 498–505).

55.   PET scan studies that are not considering the effects of mind drugs on patient outcome specifically exclude those on psychotropic medication or note that medication has not been taken for a certain length of time. The study cited in the following endnote is an example of this. However, non–human studies make it clear that drugs can dramatically shrink the brain. Dorph–Petersen and colleagues reported macaque monkeys given antipsychotics for 17–27 months in doses matching typical human doses experienced 8–11% reduction in brain weight.   See Dorph–Petersen, K. A.; Pierri, J. N., et al. (March 9, 2005). The influence of chronic exposure to antipsychotic medications on brain size before and after tissue fixation: A comparison of Haloperidol and Olanzapine in macaque monkeys. *Neuropsychopharmacology.* (Epublished ahead of print. Abstract available at Medline.)

56.   Zubieta, J. K.; Heitzeg, M. M., et al. (2005). Regional cerebral blood flow responses to smoking in tobacco smokers after overnight abstinence. *American Journal of Psychiatry, 162,* 567–577.

57.   Myers, D. (2005). *Exploring Psychology,* 6th ed. New York: Worth Publishers, p. 486.

58.   For alcohol: Boileau, I; Assaad, J. M., et al. (2003). Alcohol promotes dopamine release in the human nucleus accumbens. *Synapse, 49,* 226–331. For smoking: Brody, A. L.; Olmstead, R. E., et al. (2004). Smoking–induced ventrial striatum dopamine release. *American Journal of Psychiatry, 161,* 1211–1218. For amphetamines: Drevets, W. C.; Gautier, C., et al. (2001). Amphetamine–induced dopamine release in human ventral striatum correlates with euphoria. *Biological Psychiatry, 49,* 81–96. For pleasure: Small, D. M.; Jones–Gotman, M. & Dagher, A. (2003). Feeding–induced dopamine release in dorsal striatum correlates with meal pleasantness ratings in healthy human volunteers. *Neuroimage, 19,* 1709–1715. For smiling: Wild, B.; Erb, M., et al. (2003). Why are smiles contagious? An fMRI study of the interaction between perception of facial affect and facial movements. *Psychiatry Research, 123,* 17–36. For seeing an unhappy face: Iidaka, T; Okada, T., et al. (2002). Age–related differences in the medial temporal lobe responses to emotional faces as revealed by fMRI. *Hippocampus, 12,* 352–362; Nomura, M; Ohira, H., et al. (2004). Functional association of the amygdala and ventral prefrontal cortex during cognitive evaluation of facial expressions primed by masked angry faces: An event–related fMRI study. *Neuroimage, 21,* 352–363. For fear: Sabatinelli, D; Bradley, M. M., et al. (2005). Parallel amygdala and inferotemporal activation reflect emotional intensity and fear relevance. *Neuroimage, 24,* 1265–1270; Schienle, A; Schafer, A., et al. (2005). Gender differences in the processing of disgust– and fear–inducing pictures: An fMRI study. *Neuroimage, 16,* 277–280.

59.   My "stealing pencils" example is based on a study reported in the *American Journal of Psychiatry.* It noted that some patients have a "syndrome that includes indecisiveness, disorganization, perfectionism, procrastination, and avoidance." They then tried to determine if patients with a tendency to gather things (pencils, pens, books, paper, etc.) can be identified by PET scans. And, indeed, they concluded they could be! (Saxena S; Brody, A. L., et al. [2004].   Cerebral glucose metabolism in obsessive–compulsive hoarding. *American Journal of Psychiatry, 161,* 1038–1048.)

60.   I suspect some textbook authors know this is a myth but assume their publishers would not allow them to explain what would admittedly harm textbook sales. The discipline

has so bought into the chemical imbalance myth that to challenge it would bring rejection when textbooks are being selected by professors.

61. Pfizer. Understanding the family connectedness in mental illness, *The Pfizer Journal*. Available on the web at http://www.thepfizerjournal.com.

62. Myers, D. (2005). *Exploring Psychology*, 6th ed. New York: Worth Publishers, p. 489.

63. Ibid., p. 499.

64. Myers, D. (2002). *Exploring Psychology*, 5th ed. New York: Worth Publishers, p. 493.

65. Mirsky, A. F.; Bieliauskas, L. A., et al. (2000). A 39-year followup of the Genain quadruplets. *Schizophrenic Bulletin, 26*, 699–708.

66. Genain is the name given this family by their principle investigator, David Rosenthal of the National Institute of Mental Health.

67. The facts of this case can all be found in the "official" report. See Rosenthal, D., ed. (1963). *The Genain Quadruplets: A Case Study and Theoretical Analysis of Heredity and Environment in Schizophrenia*. New York: Basic Book Publishers.

68. Ibid., p. 85

69. Ibid., p. 84.

70. Coleman, J. C.; Butcher, J. N. & Carson, R. C. (1980). *Abnormal Psychology and Modern Life*, 6th ed. Glenview, IL: Scott, Foresman & Company, p. 400.

71. Breggin, P. R. (1991). *Toxic Psychiatry*. New York: St. Martin's Press, pp. 106–107.

72. Myers, D. (2005). *Exploring Psychology*, 6th ed. New York: Worth Publishers, p. 499.

73. Tryon, R. C. (1940). Genetic differences in maze learning in rats. *Yearbook of the National Society for Studies in Education, 39*, 111–119.

74. Kamin, L. (1974). *The Science and Politics of IQ*. New York: Halsted Press.

75. Gillie, O. (Oct. 24, 1976). Crucial data faked by eminent psychologist. *Sunday Times,* London, pp. 1–2.

76. Lewontin, R. C. (1993). Biology as ideology: The doctrine of DNA. *Harper Perennial*, p. 33.

77. See Myers, D. (2005). *Exploring Psychology*, 6th ed. New York: Worth, p. 499.

78. The early and famous Kallmann study so defined "reared apart," a fact noted by Alvin Pam. See Pam, A. (1995). Biological psychiatry: Science or pseudoscience? *(*Ch. 1) in Ross, C. A. & Pam, A., eds. *Pseudoscience in Biological Psychiatry: Blaming the Brain*. New York: John Wiley & Sons, p. 19.

79. Joseph, J. (2001). Don Jackson's 'A critique of the literature on the genetics of schizophrenia: A reappraisal after 40 years.' *Genetic, Social & General Psychology Monographs, 127*, 27–57, p. 28.

80. Ibid., p. 45.

81. Carlson, N. R. (1984). *Psychology: The Science of Behavior*. Boston: Allyn & Bacon, p. 681.

82. Tienari, P.; Wynne L. C., et al. (2003). Genetic boundaries of the schizophrenia spectrum: Evidence from the Finnish Adoptive Family Study of Schizophrenia, *American Journal of Psychiatry, 160*, 1587–1594.

83. Breggin, P. R. (1991). *Toxic Psychiatry*. New York: St. Martin's Press, p. 97.

84. Ibid., p. 98.

85. Many books and articles address this subject. The best book is Jay Joseph's *The Gene Illusion: Genetic Research in Psychiatry and Psychology Under the Microscope.*

Endnotes, Ch. 2, Are Mental Problems Mental Diseases?

(2003, Ross–on–Wye, Herefordshire, UK: PCCS Books). Ty Colbert's *Blaming Our Genes* (2001, Tustin, CA: Kevco) is an easy to understand volume that summarizes much of Jay Joseph's work. Also see the following articles: Lidz, T. (1976). Commentary on a critical review of recent adoption, twin, and family studies of schizophrenia: Behavioral genetics perspectives. *Schizophrenia Bulletin, 2*, 401–412; Lidz, T. & Blatt, S. (1983). Critique of the Danish–American studies of the biological and adoptive relatives of adoptees who became schizophrenic. *American Journal of Psychiatry, 140*, 426–435; Lidz, T.; Blatt, S. & Cook, B. (1981). Critique of the Danish–American studies of the adopted–away offspring of schizophrenic parents. *American Journal of Psychiatry, 138*, 1063–1068; Kendler, K. S. & Gruenberg, A. M. (1984). An independent analysis of the Danish adoption study of schizophrenia. *Archives of General Psychiatry, 41*, 555–564.

86.   I had read enough in previous years to know that these adoption studies do not prove a genetic link. However, it was Jay Joseph's book that enlightened me to the degree this study was manipulated and can truly be called junk science. Yet, the facts mentioned in this first point are still not discussed in any psychology textbook I have ever examined. See Joseph's *The Gene Illusion* (endnote 85), especially p. 181 for Kety's admission that each rater's definition of schizophrenia "varied by virtue of [their] training and experience" and p. 201 for the "five–minute doorstep interview" fact. Chapters 6 and 7 (pp. 134–239) cover the genetics of schizophrenia, including the studies considered here.

87.   Mednick, S. A. & Hutchings, B. (1977). Some considerations in the interpretation of the Danish adoption studies in relation to asocial behavior (pp. 159–164) in Mednick, S. A. & Christiansen, K., eds., *Biosocial Bases of Criminal Behavior*. New York: Gardner Press.

88.   Soyka, M.; Albus, M., et al. (1993). Prevalence of alcohol and drug abuse in schizophrenic inpatients. *European Archives of Clinical Neuroscience, 242*, 362–372. This study, like many newer studies, reports a higher incidence of alcohol and drug abuse among schizophrenics. For a study indicating that drug abuse commonly precedes the onset of the first psychiatric treatment for schizophrenia, see the following article. (The article is in French, but the abstract, available on the Medline site, is in English and provides more detail than is found in most abstracts.) Dervaux, A; Laqueille, X., et al. (2003). [Cannabis and schizophrenia: Demographic and clinical correlates.] *Encephale, 29*, 11–17.

89.   Low birth weight babies have about a 6–point difference in IQ scores than would otherwise be expected (Aylward, G. P.; Pfeiffer, S. I., et al. [1989]. Outcome studies of low birth weight infants published in the last decade: A meta–analysis. *Journal of Pediatrics, 115*, 515–520). However, if the baby has very low birth weight (less than 1,500 grams), she is much more likely to need special education—nearly half requiring such in one study (Ross, G.; Lipper, E. G. & Auld, P. A. M. [1991]. Educational status and school–related abilities of very low birth weight premature children. *Pediatrics, 8*, 1125–1134). Very low birth weight is also associated with emotional, behavioral, social and language difficulties (Klebanov, P. K.; Brooks–Gunn, J. & McCormick, M. C. [1994]. Classroom behavior of very low birth weight elementary school children. *Pediatrics, 94*, 700–708).

90.   For lower intelligence being associated with schizophrenia see David, A. S.; Malmberg, A., et al. (1997). IQ and risk for schizophrenia: A population–based cohort study. *Psychological Medicine, 27*, 1311–1323. For lower occupational status being associated with schizophrenia see Clark, R. E. (1948). The relationship of schizophrenia to occupational income and occupational prestige. *American Sociological Review, 13*, 325–330. For the relationship between social isolation and schizophrenia see Done, D. J.; Crow, T. J., et al. (1994). Childhood antecedents of schizophrenia and affective illness: Social adjustment at ages 7 and 11. *British Medical Journal, 309*, 699–703.

91.   Tienari, P; Wynne, L. C., et al. (2003). Genetic boundaries of the schizophrenia spectrum: Evidence from the Finnish Adoptive Study of Schizophrenia. *American Journal of Psychiatry, 160,* 1587–1594.

92.   See, for example, Kosslyn, S. M. & Rosenberg, R. S. (2005). *Fundamentals of Psychology: The Brain, The Person, The World.* Boston: Pearson Education which states, "Twin, family, and adoption studies point to the influence of genetic factors in the development of schizophrenia" (p. 437). The authors then cite one book and two journal articles. The book uses the Danish Adoption Study as evidence, as does the first journal article. The second article is the Finnish Adoptive Family Study of Schizophrenia. This is, indeed, a house of cards!

93.   Tienari, P.; Wynne, L. C., et al. (2004). Genotype–environment interaction in schizophrenia spectrum disorder: Long–term follow–up study of Finnish adoptees. *British Journal of Psychiatry, 184,* 216–222, p. 216.

94.   Joseph, J. (2003). *The Gene Illusion: Genetic Research in Psychiatry and Psychology Under the Microscope.* Ross–on–Wye, Herefordshire, UK: PCCS Books, p. 229. A brief comment on just one of Dr. Joseph's criticisms, "they changed . . . ways of counting" is needed. To determine how often schizophrenia appears in identical versus fraternal twins, each study of this issue needs to be considered. These studies have come up with hugely different findings. For example, a study by Luxenberger found 59% of identical twins both developed schizophrenia but none of the fraternal twins developed schizophrenia. Kallman's famous study reported that 69% of identical twins both developed schizophrenia and 11% of fraternal twins did so. But Gottesman and Shields found only 4% of identical twins both became schizophrenics at some point, but over twice as many (9%) of the fraternal twins became schizophrenics. Those opposite findings alone should indicate something is wrong here. But then the real problem begins. The studies are all added up and averaged. That yields an average of about 38% (i.e., 38% of identical twins will both become schizophrenics). But, if you want to be less than honest, you can use a statistical procedure (the proband method), and all of a sudden the rate jumps up to approximately 50%. And that is the rate generally found in the drug company literature and in the psychology textbooks. Joseph provides a very helpful discussion of the "pairwise" vs. the "proband" methods of calculating concordance rates. Concerning the proband method he states, "It is difficult to understand how this method could have gained the level of acceptance that it has . . ." (ibid., p. 143). All of these and other twin studies are discussed by Joseph in this outstanding work. See p. 142 of *The Gene Illusion* for a table summarizing the studies.

Chapter 3 — How Psychiatrists and Doctors Are Fooled

1.   From transcript of interview by Brian Lamb on C–SPAN's "Q&A" program, June 19, 2005. The entire transcript is available on C–SPAN's website at http://www.q–and–a.org/Transcript/?ProgramID=1027&QueryText=bethany+mclean.

2.   McLean, B. & Elkind, P. (2003). *The Smartest Guys in the Room.* New York: Portfolio, p. 233.

3.   Lee, S. (Dec. 26, 2001). The dismal science: Enron's success story. *Wall Street Journal,* A.11.

4.   Malkiel, B. (Jan. 16, 2002). Watchdogs and lapdogs. *Wall Street Journal,* A.16.

5.   McLean, B. & Elkind, P. (2003). *The Smartest Guys in the Room.* New York: Portfolio.

6.   The ad follows p. 1136 of the September 1979 issue (Vol. 36) of *Archives of General Psychiatry* and is promoting Norpramin.

7.   Ross, C. A. (1995). Errors of logic in biological psychiatry (Ch. 2) in Ross, C. A. & Pam, A., eds. *Pseudoscience in Biological Psychiatry: Blaming the Brain*. New York: John Wiley & Sons, p. 107.

8.   Neimark, J. (1994). The Harvard professor and the UFOs. *Psychology Today, 27,* 46–90 passim.

9.   Boggs believed he had to eat chicken to bat well and did so daily for 20 years. He ran his sprints each evening at 7:17 exactly. He would never step on the foul line when coming onto the field but believed it was critical to touch it as he left the field. He always wrote the Hebrew word *chai* (life) with his bat in the dirt after he entered the batting box.

10. Pam, A. (1990). A critique of the scientific status of biological psychiatry. *Acta Psychiatrica Scandinavica, 82* (Suppl. 362), 1–35.

11. Kemker, S. S. (1995). Psychiatric education: Learning by assumption (Ch. 6) in Ross, C. A. & Pam, A., eds. *Pseudoscience in Biological Psychiatry: Blaming the Brain.* New York: John Wiley & Sons, pp. 241–242.

12. Herbert, J. D. (2003). The science and practice of empirically supported treatments. *Behavior Modification, 27,* 412–430.

13. Breggin was discussing University of Washington–Seattle psychiatrist Gary J. Tucker. See Breggin, P. (1991). *Toxic Psychiatry*. New York: St. Martin's Press, p. 12.

14. Guze, S. B. (1989). Biological psychiatry: Is there any other kind? *Psychological Medicine, 19,* 315–323, p. 322.

15. Ibid., p. 315.

16. Ibid.

17. Goodwin, D.; Schulsinger, F., et. al (1973). Alcohol problems in adoptees raised apart from alcoholic parents. *Archives of General Psychiatry, 28,* 238–243.

18. Wood, S. E.; Wood, E. G. & Boyd, D. (2004). *Mastering the World of Psychology*. Boston: Pearson Education, p. 305.

19. Kosslyn, S. M. & Rosenberg, R. S. (2005). *Fundamentals of Psychology: The Brain, The Person, The World*, 2nd ed. Boston: Pearson Education, p. 81.

20. The statement is given the following reference: Goedde, H. W. & Agarwal, D. P. (1987). Aldehyde dehydrogenase polymorphism: Molecular basis and phenotypic relationship to alcohol sensitivity. *Alcohol & Alcoholism* (Suppl. 1), 47–54. The abstract for this article is available without cost on the National Library of Medicine's Medline site. It simply does not report what the textbook indicates it reports.

21. Whittaker, J. O. (1965). *Introduction to Psychology*. Philadelphia: W. B. Saunders, p. 21.

22. Goodwin, D.; Schulsinger, F., et al. (1973). Alcohol problems in adoptees raised apart from alcoholic parents. *Archives of General Psychiatry, 28, 238–243*.

23. Plomin, R.; Corley, R., et al. (1990). Individual differences in television viewing in early childhood: Nature as well as nurture. *Psychological Science, 1,* 371–377.

24. Loehlin, J. C. (1976). *Heredity, Environment and Personality: A Study of 850 Sets of Twins*. Austin, TX: University of Texas Press.

25. Carmelli, D.; Swan, G. E., et al. (1992). Genetic influence on smoking: A study of male twins. *New England Journal of Medicine, 327,* 829–833.

26. Brunner, H. G.; Nelen, M., et al. (1993). Abnormal behavior associated with a point mutation in the structural gene for monoamine oxidase A. *Science, 262,* 578–580. Also see Brennan, P. A.; Mednick, S. A. & Jacobsen, B. (1996). Assessing the role of genetics in crime using adoption cohorts. *Ciba Foundation Symposia, 194,* 115–123. It is important to note that I am not arguing that there are not differences in genetics that then influence behavior. Being born male or female, naturally strong, coordinated and athletic or not, being born

with high intellectual capacity or low intellectual capacity all impact behavior. The problem comes from a view that attributes so much genetic influence to behavior that humans become less human and responsibility is reduced. Heath and Martin, for example, argue that 53% of a person's choice to continue smoking may be genetic. In other words, smoking is less of a personal choice than it is a behavior that some people are predestined to adopt and continue (Heath, A. C. & Martin, N. G. [1993]. Genetic models for the natural history of smoking: Evidence for a genetic influence on smoking persistence. *Addictive Behavior, 18,* 19–34).

27.   Ross, C. A. (1995). Errors of logic in biological psychiatry (Ch. 2) in Ross, C. A. & Pam, A., eds. *Pseudoscience in Biological Psychiatry: Blaming the Body.* New York: John Wiley & Sons.

28.   Ibid., p. 87.

29.   Maidment, R.; Livingston, G., et al. (2004). Changes in attitudes to psychiatry and intention to pursue psychiatry as a career in newly qualified doctors: A follow–up of two cohorts of medical students. *Medical Teacher, 26,* 565–569; Mahoney, R; Katona, C., et al. (2004). Shortage specialties: Changes in career intentions from medical student to newly qualified doctor. *Medical Teacher, 26,* 650–654.

30.   Zarin, D. A.; Pincus, H. A., et al. (1998). Characterizing psychiatry with findings from the 1996 National Survey psychiatric practice. *American Journal of Psychiatry, 155,* 397–404. The phenomenon is occurring in other nations also as medical students reject psychiatry as an option (Goldacre, M. J.; Turner, G., et al. [2005]. Career choices for psychiatry: National surveys of graduates of 1974–2000 from UK medical schools. *British Journal of Psychiatry, 186,* 158–164).

31.   Leger, G. R. (2005). Determinants of physicians' decisions to specialize. *Health Economics, 14,* 721–735.

32.   Ross, C. A. (1995). Errors of logic in biological psychiatry (Ch. 2) in Ross, C. A. & Pam, A., eds. *Pseudoscience in Biological Psychiatry: Blaming the Body.* New York: John Wiley & Sons, p. 86.

33.   The American Psychological Association's website (http://www.apa.org) has an abundance of articles and arguments in favor of prescribing privileges (enter "prescribing privileges" into their search engine).

34.   See the article by the former American Psychiatric Association president entitled "APA armed and ready to fight psychologist–prescribing bills" (Riba, M. [2004]. *Psychiatric News, 39,* 3).

35.   Lavoie, K. L. & Fleet, R. P. (2002). Should psychologists be granted prescription privileges? A review of the prescription debate for psychiatrists. *Canadian Journal of Psychiatry, 47,* 443–449.

36.   Gordon reports that a Kaiser Family Foundation study found 92% of physicians take and distribute these free samples (Gordon, D. [2002]. Dealing with drug reps: Make your time together more productive. Shands Health Care article on the web at http://www .shands.org/professional/ppd/practice_article.asp?ID=142).

37.   It is true that the really extravagant gifts and trips were mostly eliminated after July 1, 2002. These perks did not become illegal, but many drug companies voluntarily agreed to follow guidelines established by their trade organization Pharmaceutical Research and Manufacturers of America. The costs were getting out of hand, and a stricter policy actually benefits the drug companies. The American Medical Association (AMA) policy on gifts from industry emphasizes that gifts should have the same benefit for patients (free samples, textbooks, dinners with an educational speaker all meet the requirement). Drug reps can even pay for a physician's continuing medical education (CME) under the AMA policy as long as the CME payment goes directly to the CME sponsor and not to the physician (ibid).

38. The figure is based on the 90,000 drug reps in America in 2003 as reported by the *Wall Street Journal* (Hensley, S. [June 13, 2003]. Side effects: As drug–sales teams multiply, doctors start to tune them out. *Wall Street Journal*, A–1).

39. In 2002 there were 516,000 office–based physicians (U.S. Bureau of the Census [2004]. *Statistical Abstract of the U.S.*, 124th ed. Washington, D.C., Table 149, Physicians by selected activity: 1980 to 2002).

40. Backer, E. L.; Lebsack, J. A., et al. (2000). The value of pharmaceutical representative visits and medication samples in community–based family practices. *Journal of Family Practice, 49*, 817–819; Gordon, D. (2002). Dealing with drug reps: Make your time together more productive. Shands Health Care article on the web at http://www.shands.org/professional/ppd/practice_article.asp?ID=142.

41. O'Donnell, M. J.; Molloy, D. W., et al. (2004). The self–perceived role and educational needs of pharmaceutical representatives: A survey. *Education for Health* (Abingdon, England), *17*, 339–345.

42. Ibid.

43. Avorn, J. (2004). *Powerful Medicines: The Benefits, Risks, and Costs of Prescription Drugs.* New York: Alfred A. Knopf, p. 292. I have great respect for Dr. Avorn as a man of conviction. As a top drug research authority, he could command over $500/hour by serving as an expert witness in court. He has been an expert witness many times, but he will not accept pay for this work.

44. Bellin, M.; McCarthy, S., et al. (2004). Medical students' exposure to phamaceutical industry marketing: A survey at one U.S. medical school. *Academic Medicine, 79*, 1041–1045.

45. Vainiomake, M.; Helve, O. & Vuorenkoski, L. (2004). A national survey on the effect of pharmaceutical promotion on medical students. *Medical Teacher, 26*, 591–593. This study examined Finnish medical students, but the practice there is similar to the practice in the U.S. For example, see the article by Brodkey referenced in endnote 48 below.

46. Ibid., p. 591.

47. Jerry Avorn addresses this problem in his book *Powerful Medicines*. I'll quote but one sentence from his discussion and provide the quote's page number so his observations can be located quickly. "In many medical schools, clinical pharmacology has lost its curriculum time to more modern fields such as molecular biology" (Avorn, J. [2004]. *Powerful Medicines: The Benefits, Risks, and Costs of Prescription Drugs.* New York: Alfred A. Knopf, p. 272). Also see the following article which argues that the industry does play an important educational role for physicians. (The research studies which determine many drugs' efficacy and adverse events are often so flawed, unbeknownst to the pharmaceutical educators presenting research to physicians, that I cannot agree.) Mohl, P. C. (2005). Psychiatric training program engagement with the pharmaceutical industry: An educational issue, not strictly an ethical one. *Academic Medicine, 29*, 215–221. My position is especially warranted in view of the lack of knowledge physicians have about the impact of drug marketing on their own behavior. For this see Watkins, R. S. & Kimberly, J. (2004). What residents don't know about physician–pharmaceutical industry interactions. *Academic Medicine, 79*, 432–437.

48. Brodkey, A. C. (2005). The role of the pharmaceutical industry in teaching psychopharmacology: A growing problem. *Academic Psychiatry, 29*, 222–229.

49. Ibid., p. 222.

50. Bornstein, R. F. (1989). Exposure and effect: Overview and meta–analysis of research, 1968–1987. *Psychological Bulletin, 106*, 265–289; Zajonc, R. B. (2001). Mere

exposure: A gateway to the subliminal. *Current Directions in Psychological Science, 10,* 224–228.

51.   Mita, T. H.; Dermer, M. & Knight, J. (1977). Reversed facial images and the mere–exposure hypothesis. *Journal of Personality & Social Psychology, 35,* 597–601.

52.   Bornstein, R. F. & D'Agostino, P. R. (1992). Stimulus recognition and the mere exposure effect. *Journal of Personality & Social Psychology, 63,* 545–552.

53.   Abbasi, K. & Smith, R. (2003). No more free lunches. *British Medical Journal, 326,* 1155–1156.

54.   Lohiya, S. (2005). Pharmaceutical advertisements in medical journals received in a medical clinic: Are we having "too much of a good thing"? *Journal of the National Medical Association, 97,* 718–720.

55.   Davidson, J. R. T.; Gadde, K. M., et al. (2002). Effect of Hypericum perforatum (St. John's Wort) in Major Depressive Disorder: A randomized controlled trial. *JAMA, 287,* 1807–1814.

56.   Ibid.

57.   Swartz, C. M. (June 1, 2004). Knowing that we don't know. *Psychiatric Times,* p. 53.

58.   Weight gain is not consistent among the various antipsychotics. 37% of patients on the best–selling Zyprexa experience significant (7% or more) increase in weight during their first 26 weeks on that drug. However, patients typically lose weight while on Abilify. See McQuade, R. D.; Stock, E., et al. (2004). A comparison of weight change during treatment with olanzapine or aripiprazole: Results from a randomized, double–blind study. *Journal of Clinical Psychiatry, 65* (Suppl. 18), 47–56.

59.   The overall increase is 4 to 6 times, but rates vary greatly by antipsychotic. The increased risk is 3.1 times for Zyprexa, 7.44 times for Clozaril, and 3.46 times for Melleril. Several studies have found that taking antipsychotics can lead to hyperglycemia and diabetes and that it often develops within months of initiating the antipsychotic. One study which surveyed the effects of risperidone found effects ranging from mild diabetic symptoms to ketoacidosis and even hyperosmolar coma (Koller, E. A.; Cross, J. T., et al. [2003]. Risperidone–associated diabetes mellitus: A pharmacovigilance study. *Pharmacotherapy, 23,* 735–744). Clozapine and olanzapine are even more hazardous than risperidone, and all pose additional risks if the person is also on an SSRI antidepressant (Hedenmalm, K; Hagg, S., et al. [2002]. Glucose intolerance with atypical antipsychotics. *Drug Safety, 25,* 1107–1116). In 2003 the FDA began requiring drug manufacturers to put warnings on antipsychotics concerning the diabetes risk. Pancreatitis occurs within six months of beginning an atypical antipsychotic typically with the greatest risks coming from Clozaril, Zyprexa, and then Risperdol (Koller, E. A.; Cross, J. T., et al. [2003]. Pancreatitis associated with atypical antipsychotics: From the Food and Drug Administration's MedWatch surveillance system and published reports. *Pharmacotherapy, 23,* 1123–1130).

60.   Newcomer, J. W.; Nasrallah, H. A. & Loebel, A. D. (2004).   The Atypical Antipsychotic Therapy and Metabolic Issues National Survey: Practice patterns and knowledge of psychiatrists. *Journal of Clinical Psychopharmacology, 24,* S1–S6. The authors reported that "the response rate was approximately 30%" (p. S2). Since the questions dealt with their knowledge of antipsychotics, it seems fair to assume that those with the least knowledge would be the least inclined to participate in this survey and that the meager knowledge demonstrated by this sample is representative of the knowledge (on the health effects of antipsychotics) of America's most knowledgeable psychiatrists.

61.   This is a rare event, but all patients taking these drugs need to be appropriately warned of possible health consequences and told to watch for signs that might lead to a fatal event. Many antipsychotic induced diabetic ketoacidosis case studies are now in the litera-

ture; e.g., Ragucci, K. R. & Wells, B. J. (2001). Olanzapine–induced diabetic ketoacidosis. *The Annals of Phamacotherapy, 35*, 1556–1558 as well as small retrospective studies (Jin, H; Meyer, J. M. & Jeste, D. V. [2002]. Phenomenology of and risk factors for new–onset diabetes mellitus and diabetic ketoacidosis associated with atypical antipsychotics: An analysis of 45 published cases. *Annals of Clinical Psychiatry, 14*, 59–64).

62. Dozens of warning letters are issued every year to pharmaceutical companies. These can be found on the web at http://www.fda.gov/cder/warn/.

63. For a copy of the letter go to http://www.fda.gov/cder/warn/warn2004.htm and go to the third warning letter issued in April. Alternatively, go to http://www.fda.gov/foi/warn ing_letters/g4628d.htm. The letter was released on April 19, 2004.

64. Ibid.

65. Ibid.

66. Ibid.

67. Ibid.

68. I refer specifically to the FDA's alert for healthcare professionals issued April 11, 2005, which stated that risk of death is elevated for those patients with dementia–related psychosis treated with Zyprexa versus placebo. (The alert is available on the web at http://www .fda.gov/cder/drug/InfoSheets/HCP/olanzapineHCP.htm.) Of course, it is certainly true that these drugs are shortening lives for millions of other Americans. Just the well–established diabetes link by itself poses the threat of a shortened life.

69. Avorn, J. (2004). *Powerful Medicines: The Benefits, Risks, and Costs of Prescription Drugs.* New York: Alfred A. Knopf, p. 363.

70. Ibid., pp. 71–72.

Chapter 4 — Advertising Works

1. Wilson, E. O. (1975). *Sociobiology: The New Synthesis.* Cambridge, MA: Harvard University Press, p. 562. Harvard entomologist Edward O. Wilson held absurd views, but his book which espoused many of those views was immensely popular—and attacked. He saw most behavior, altruism, creativity and other human traits arising from our genes—genes molded through an evolutionary past. Such conclusions run counter to a view that says the environment (advertising) has a great influence. I believe the quote has validity, yet it is ironic that it came from Wilson's pen.

2. Epstein, E. J. (1982). Have you ever tried to sell a diamond? *Atlantic Monthly, 249*, 23–34.

3. Garfield, B. (1999). Top 100 advertising campaigns. *Advertising Age,* C.20. It reached this status in 1972.

4. Ibid.

5. See the Massachusetts Institute of Technology (MIT) archive of inventions for this and other examples at http://web.mit.edu/invent/iow/hulahoop.html.

6. Latham, M. C. (1977). Infant feeding in national and international perspective: An examination of the decline in human lactation, and the modern crisis in infant and young child feeding practices. *Annals of the New York Academy of Sciences, 300*, 197–209. This switch to formula can lead to a large number of negative health consequences and higher infant mortality, especially in developing nations. Poor women, even in America, are more likely to be influenced by formula marketing efforts (Isenalumhe, T. E. [1984]. Decline of breast–feeding among New York urban poor linked to sources of information on infant feeding practices: A lesson for African countries. *Nigerian Journal of Paediatrics, 11*, 41–45).

7. Burton, B. (2004). New Zealand moves to ban direct advertising of drugs. *British*

Medical Journal, 328, 68.

8. For the fight with the drug manufacturers, see Burton, B. (2004). Drug industry to fight New Zealand's move to ban direct to consumer advertising. *British Medical Journal, 328*, 1026. For the intention to ban DTC advertising altogether in 2006, see Crain Communications (Sept. 5, 2005). Late news; New Zealand to ban DTC advertising by '0. *Advertising Age, 76*, 1.

9. Rosenthal, M. B.; Berndt, E. R., et al. (2002). Promotion of prescription drugs to consumers. *New England Journal of Medicine, 346*, 498–505.

10. The rate was 2.7 billion in 2001 according to the U.S. General Accounting Office (2002). *Prescription Drugs: FDA Oversight of Direct–To–Consumer Advertising Has Limitations.* Washington, D. C. This report is available on the web at http://www.gao.gov/new.items/d03177.pdf.

11. Aikin, J. J.; Swasy, J. L. & Braman, A. C. (2004). Patient and physician attitudes and behaviors associated with DTC Promotion of Prescription Drugs—Summary of FDA Survey Research Results. U.S. Department of Health and Human Services Food and Drug Administration Center for Drug Evaluation and Research. Available on the web at http://www.fda.gov/cder/ddmac/Final%20ReportFRFinalExSu1119042.pdf.

12. Berndt, E. R. (2005). To inform or persuade? Direct–to–consumer advertising of prescription drugs. *New England Journal of Medicine, 352*, 325–328. The graph in this report is based on data published in 2004 by Weissman, J. S.; Blumenthal, D., et al. (April 28, 2004:Wf–219–W4–233). Physicians report on patient encounters involving direct–to–consumer advertising. Bethesda, MD: Health Affairs. (Web exclusive). See this report at http://content.health affairs.org/cgi/reprint/hlthaff.w4.219v1.

13. Ibid.

14. The more exact total was $19.1 billion in 2001 (U.S. General Accounting Office [2002]. *Prescription Drugs: FDA Oversight of Direct–To–Consumer Advertising Has Limitations.* Washington, D. C.). This report is available on the web at http://www.gao.gov/new.items/d03177.pdf and was completed in October of 2002. No other similar report was anticipated as of April 2005. The total promotional spending amount in 2000 was $17.7 billion (Findlay, S. [2002]. Prescription drugs and mass media advertising. *Research Brief, National Institute for Health Care Management*, Washington, D. C.: NICHCM Foundation. The report is available on the web at http://www.nihcm.org/DTCbrief.pdf).

15. GDP rankings of nations can be found at http://aol.countrywatch.com.

16. Rosenthal, M. B.; Berndt, E. R., et. al. (2002). Promotion of prescription drugs to consumers. *New England Journal of Medicine, 346*, 498–505. Total 1999 spending on promotion to physicians and other health care professionals amounts to $985 million. See Table 3.

17. $19.1 billion divided by 52 weeks equals $367 million.

18. U.S. General Accounting Office (2002). *Prescription Drugs: FDA Oversight of Direct–to–Consumer Advertising Has Limitations.* Washington, D.C. Available at http://www.gao.gov/new.items/d03177.pdf.

19. Ibid. See Note 23 on p. 15 of document. This $108 million is just its DTC advertising costs. Total promotional expenditures were likely well in excess of $500 million.

20. Murray, E; Lo, B., et al. (2003). Direct–to–consumer advertising: Physicians' views of its effects on quality of care and the doctor–patient relationship. *Journal of the American Board of Family Practitioners, 16*, 513–524.

21. Ibid. Another study found an even higher (78%) physician compliance rate for DTC advertised drugs (Mintzes, B; Berer, M. L., et al. [2003]. How does direct–to–consumer advertising [DTCA] affect prescribing? A survey in primary care environments with

and without legal DTCA. *Canadian Medical Association Journal, 169,* 405–412).

22. Donohue, J. M.; Berndt, E. R., et al. (2004). Effects of pharmaceutical promotion on adherence to the treatment guidelines for depression. *Medical Care, 42,* 1176–1185.

23. Ibid.

24. Bell, R. A.; Wilkes, M. S. & Kravitz, R. L. (1999). Advertisement–induced prescription drug requests: Patients' anticipated reactions to a physician who refuses. *Journal of Family Practice, 48,* 446–452. This study also found that about 1 in 4 patients will try to get the drug they want from another source.

25. U.S. General Accounting Office (2002). *Prescription Drugs: FDA Oversight of Direct–to–Consumer Advertising Has Limitations.* Washington, D.C., p. 4. This report is available on the web at http://www.gao.gov/new.items/d03177.pdf.

26. Mackler, B. F. (July 28, 2000). Press releases and the internet: FDA regulation of advertising and promotion of drugs, biologics and devices. Palo Alto, CA: Letter of the FDA Legal/Regulatory Group, HellerEhrman Attorneys, p. 2. Accessed online at http://www.hewm.com/news/articles/pressrel.pdf.

27. U.S. General Accounting Office (2002). *Prescription Drugs: FDA Oversight of Direct–to–Consumer Advertising Has Limitations.* Washington, D.C. This report is available on the web at http://www.gao.gov/new.items/d03177.pdf. See p. 17 for this as well as the total number of promotional materials (both DTC and others) submitted in 2001 (c. 34,000 according to footnote 27).

28. Mackler, B. F. (July 28, 2000). Press releases and the internet: FDA regulation of advertising and promotion of drugs, biologics and devices. Palo Alto, CA: Letter of the FDA Legal/Regulatory Group, HellerEhrman Attorneys, p. 1. Accessed online at http://www.hewm.com/news/articles/pressrel.pdf.

29. U.S. General Accounting Office (2002). *Prescription Drugs: FDA Oversight of Direct–to–Consumer Advertising Has Limitations.* Washington, D.C., p. 23. This report is available on the web at http://www.gao.gov/new.items/d03177.pdf.

30. Ibid., Tables 5 and 6. They give duration of DTC advertisements and time (in days) taken to issue warning letters.

31. This quote is found on the Zoloft website available at http://www2.zoloft.com/index.asp?pageid=13.

32. Fernandez, H. (1998). *Heroin.* Center City, MN: Hazelden, p. 25.

33. Consumers Union of U.S. (1992). Miracle drugs or media drugs? *Consumer Reports, 57,* 142–146.

34. Many studies have examined some of these strategies in both the popular and the professional literature. See, for example, two articles done many years ago by *Consumer Reports* (ibid.) as well as Consumers Union of U.S. (Feb. 1992). Pushing drugs to doctors. *Consumer Reports, 57,* 87–94. These strategies remain the same today. The professional literature includes Firlik, A.D. & Lowry, D. W. (2000). Is academic medicine for sale? *New England Journal of Medicine, 343,* 509–510; Tereskerz, P. M. (2003). Research accountability and financial conflicts of interest in industry–sponsored clinical research: A review. *Accountability in Research, 10,* 137–158; Lemmens, T. (2004). Confronting the conflict of interest crisis in medical research. *Monash Bioethics Review, 23,* 19–40; Healy, D. (2004). Conflicting interests: The evolution of an issue. *Monash Bioethics Review, 23,* 8–18.

35. This information is found on the Zoloft website available at http://www2.zoloft.com/index.asp?pageid=52.

36. Ibid.

37. They estimate that more than 16 million Americans have this "disorder." That is over 5% of the nation's population.

38. Waxman, H. A. (2005). The lessons of Vioxx—drug safety and sales. *New England Journal of Medicine, 352*, 2576–2578.

Chapter 5 — Analyzing an Antidepressant Ad — Effexor® XR

1. Lewis, S. cited on the web at http://www.quotationspage.com/subjects/advertising/.
2. Kmietowicz, Z. (2004). Consumer organisations criticise influence of drug companies. *British Medical Journal, 329*, 937.
3. Personal communication with Julia Feliciano, Esq., Deputy Chief Counsel, North America, Wyeth Pharmaceuticals, 500 Arcola Road, Collegeville, PA 19426. No reason was given for denying permission to reproduce the ad or for denying permission to examine the studies.
4. This is the essential purpose for the ECNP and all its related organizations. The quotation from the ECNP's newsletter comes from an article giving a historical overview of the Hungarian College of Neuropsychopharmacology (HCNP) written by Csaba M. Banki, the organization's president (Banki, C. M. [June 2004]. The history of HCNP: Exchanging information and catalysing progress. *ECNP Matters*, No. 7).
5. As part of my interest in this topic, I began a systematic inquiry in October 2004. Many of the organizations would not respond to questions about their funding. It is fair to assume that all the large organizations which sponsor conferences are heavily funded by drug manufacturers. Membership dues could not cover but the smallest portion of a large European College of Neuropsychopharmacology conference, not to mention the hundreds of travel "scholarships" awarded to attend one of these conferences.
6. This statement is based on my own informal examination of medical journals for 2004 and 2005.
7. Angell, M. (2000). Is academic medicine for sale? *New England Journal of Medicine, 342*, 1516–1518.
8. Ibid.

Chapter 6 — Ghostwriting

1. Healy, D. & Cattell, D. (2003). Interface between authorship, industry and science in the domain of therapeutics. *British Journal of Psychiatry, 183*, 22–27.
2. I only counted the number for one article. It had 731 names listed. Thus, there should be approximately 7,310 names listed as authors for the first 10 articles. Obviously, having one's name attached can mean one can boast of more published papers than could be claimed otherwise. However, you should not think that most of the authors ever even saw "their" research paper before it was submitted for publication.
3. Bosely, S. (Feb. 7, 2002). Special Investigation: Scandal of scientists who take money for papers ghostwritten by drug companies. *The Guardian*, p. 4.
4. Abbasi, K. (2004). Transparency and trust. *British Medical Journal, 329*, 0.
5. Healy, D. & Cattell, D. (2003). The interface between authorship, industry and science in the domain of therapeutics. *British Journal of Psychiatry, 182*, 22–27.
6. Healy, D. (2004). *Let Them Eat Prozac*. New York: New York University Press, p. 113. I have changed Healy's spelling of Effexor to avoid confusion. He spells it "Efexor," the European spelling for the same product.
7. Healy notes the article appeared in the *Journal of Psychiatry & Neuroscience, 27*, 241–247 in 2002 under the title "The Prevalence and Outcome of Partial Remission in Depression." He also discusses this example and others at his "Let Them Eat Prozac" website. Go to http://www.healyprozac.com/GhostlyData/default.htm.

8. Healy, D. (2004). *Let Them Eat Prozac*. New York: New York University Press, p. 116f.

9. Kmietowicz, Z. (2004). Consumer organisations criticise influence of drug companies. *British Medical Journal, 329,* 937. Healy's "50%" figure led to a response by the *British Medical Journal* acting editor indicating he felt the figure needed substantiation. In a "Rapid Response," a *British Medical Journal* method of allowing quick commentary on articles and editorials in the journal, Healy emphasized that he did not say "50% of all articles," the figure sometimes appearing in the popular press (see e.g., the article by Antony Barnett in *The Observer*, Dec. 7, 2003), but "50% of the articles dealing with therapeutics." He also noted that some of the evidence for the 50% figure came from research he co–authored and published in the *British Journal of Psychiatry* (Healy, D. & Cattell, D. [2003]. The interface between authorship, industry and science in the domain of therapeutics. *British Journal of Psychiatry, 182,* 22–27).

10. *British Medical Journal* (2003), *326* (issue 7400). This May 31st issue contained editorials, articles, and letters aimed at addressing this concern, and it makes an important contribution to this problem. It is available online at http://bmj.bmjjournals.com/content/vol326/issue7400/. However, though the problem has been discussed, it is far from being overcome. See the rapid response dated June 20, 2003, by Graham P. Beck, "Not Just the Doctors Who Need to Disentangle," available on the web at http://bmj.bmjjournals.com/cgi/eletters/326/7400/1202.

11. Rees, S. T. (June 12, 2003). Who actually wrote the research paper? How to find it out. *British Medical Journal*. Internet rapid response to a May 31 special issue article by the *British Medical Journal's* editor (Smith, R. [2002]. Medical journals and pharmaceutical companies: Uneasy bedfellows. *British Medical Journal, 326,* 1202–1205). To find this "rapid response" easily, I would suggest entering the title (or the first sentence from the title) into the Google search engine. Put quotation marks at the beginning and at the end of the article title.

12. The original article was Shamim, W.; Yousufuddin, M., et al. (2002). Nonsurgical reduction of the interventricular septum in patients with hypertrophic cardiomyopathy. *New England Journal of Medicine, 347,* 1326–1333. The retraction appeared in the *New England Journal of Medicine*, March 6, 2003, *348*, 951.

13. The full statement which must be accepted to submit an article for publication reads, "I hereby certify on behalf of all the authors that we accept responsibility for the conduct of this study and for the analysis and interpretation of the data. I helped write this manuscript and agree with the decisions about it. We all meet the definition of an author as stated by the International Committee of Medical Journal Editors, and I have seen and approved the final manuscript. Neither the article nor any essential part of it, including tables and figures, will be published or submitted elsewhere before appearing in the *Journal*." See the *New England Journal of Medicine's* "Author Center—Instructions For Submitting Your New Manuscript" at http://authors.nejm.org/Manuscripts/mssub1.asp. *JAMA* takes a similar position, and it is likely the standards established by the International Committee of Medical Journal Editors (first published in 1979) will eventually be adopted by most medical journals (ICMJE website. See "About the Uniform Requirements" at http://www.icmje.org/#aboutur.) However, that will not entirely stop the practice. *JAMA* focused on authorship concerns in a July 15, 1998, issue. One of the articles surveyed 809 authors from six peer–reviewed journals and found 30% of the articles had either honorary authors (19%) or ghost authors (11%). Most significantly this 30% was based on a 69% response rate. Obviously, those who did not respond would be even more likely to have their names on articles which were actually ghosted. The article's conclusion was simply, "A substantial proportion of articles in peer–reviewed medical journals demonstrate evidence of honorary

authors or ghost authors" (Flanagin, A.; Carey, L. A., et al. [1998]. Prevalence of articles with honorary authors and ghost authors in peer–reviewed medical journals, *JAMA, 280,* 222–224). I would add that the percentage of mind–drug articles with this problem would be much greater than for any other area of medicine.

14. Kmietowicz, Z. (2004). Consumer organisations criticise influence of drug companies. *British Medical Journal, 329*, 937.

Chapter 7 — Tricks of the Trade

1. Sifakis, C. (1993). *Hoaxes and Scams: A Compendium of Deceptions, Ruses, and Swindles.* New York: Facts On File, Inc.

2. See the statement by the Committee on Safety in Medicines (CSM) Working Group on the web at http://medicines.mhra.gov.uk/ourwork/monitorsafequalmed/safetymessages/urgent.htm#Introduction.

3. *Time* (Feb. 2, 2004). Depression drugs for kids: How safe? *Time, 163*, 78.

4. Emslie, G.; Mann, J. J., et al. (Jan. 21, 2004). Preliminary report on the task force on SSRIs and suicidal behavior in youth. American College of Neuropsychopharmacology. The report is available on the web at http://www.acnp.org/exec_summary.pdf. The task force members are found at the end of the report. Nine of the ten members disclosed financial ties to pharmaceutical companies.

5. Ibid., p. 1.

6. Healy, D. (2004). Conflicting interests: The evolution of an issue. *Monash Bioethics Review, 28*, 8–18.

7. I have no idea which GYMR employees wrote the Task Force's report. I am just speculating when I suggest they are individuals with English degrees. I did contact GYMR and ask about this issue. They were not willing to state who the author really was or what credentials he or she may have had.

8. Okie, S. (2005). What ails the FDA? *New England Journal of Medicine, 352*, 1063–1066.

9. Quote of Representative Peter Deutsch (D–Fla.) as reported by Schneider, M. E. (Oct. 15, 2004). FDA slow to move on antidepressant link with suicide: Safety and efficacy questions handled in "an unscrupulous manner" congressman says. *Family Practice News, 34*, 1–2.

10. Representative Joe Barton (R–TX) as quoted in Ault, A. (Oct. 1, 2004). Congress upset by dearth of antidepressant data. *Family Practice News, 34*, 7.

11. Using the drug companies' own data, the Freedom of Information Act request revealed that 57% of the studies found no significant difference between SSRI–antidepressant drugs and a placebo. See Kirsch, I.; Scoboria, A. & Moore, T. J. (2002). Antidepressant and placebos: Secrets, revelations, and unanswered questions. *Prevention & Treatment, 5*, Article 33. Available on the web at http://www.journals.apa.org/prevention/volume5/pre0050033r.html.

12. This trick has been known for many years. It was reported for nonsteroidal anti–inflammatory drugs in 1994 (Rochon, P. A.; Gurwitz, J. H., et al. [1994]. A study of manufacturer–supported trials of nonsteroidal anti–inflammatory drugs in the treatment of arthritis. *Archives of Internal Medicine, 154*, 157–163). More recently the practice was noted for mind drugs (Safer, D. J. [2002]. Design and reporting modifications in industry–sponsored comparative psychopharmacology trials. *Journal of Nervous & Mental Disease, 190*, 583–592).

13.   Breggin, P. (2001). *The Antidepressant Fact Book: What Your Doctor Won't Tell You About Prozac, Zoloft, Paxil, Celexa, and Luvox.* Cambridge, MA: Perseus, p. 145.

14.   For confirmation look at a *Physician's Desk Reference* (*PDR*) which lists the frequency of various side effects for approved medications. (For example, see Prozac side effects listed in Table 1, *Physicians' Desk Reference* [2004], 58th ed. Montvale, NJ: Thomson PDR, p. 1843.) Chapter 10 (Physical Side Effects of Antidepressants) and Chapter 11 (Psychological Side Effects of Antidepressants) provide a full discussion of side effects.

15.   Kirsch, I.; Moore, T. J., et al. (posted July 15, 2002). The emperor's new drugs: An analysis of antidepressant medication data submitted to the U.S. Food and Drug Administration. *Prevention & Treatment, 5*, Article 23. The quote is found in the 4th paragraph of the "Method" section. Available on the web at http://www.journals.apa.org/prevention/volume5/pre0050023a.html.

16.   The study by Keller, et al. (Keller, M. B.; McCullough, J. P., et al. [2000]. A comparison of nefazodone, the cognitive–behavioral–analysis system of psychotherapy, and their combination for the treatment of chronic depression. *New England Journal of Medicine, 342,* 1462–1470) is not atypical when they note, "Patients were excluded from the study if they had any of the following: a history of seizures, abnormal findings on electroencephalography, severe head trauma, or stroke; evidence suggesting they were at high risk for suicide; a history of psychotic symptoms or schizophrenia; bipolar disorder, an eating disorder (if it had not been in remission for at least one year), obsessive–compulsive disorder, or dementia; antisocial, schizotypal, or severe borderline personality disorder; a principal diagnosis of panic, generalized anxiety, social phobia, or post–traumatic stress disorders or any substance–related abuse or dependence disorder (except those involving nicotine) within six months before the study began; absence to a response to a previous adequate trial of nefazodone or a cognitive behavioral–analysis system of psychotherapy; absence of a response to three previous adequate trials of at least two different classes of antidepressants or electroconvulsive therapy or to two previous adequate trials of empirical psychotherapy in the three years preceding the study...." A former SmithKlineBeecham executive admitted, "Rarely do [patients used in drug trials] reflect the exact clinical profiles, including use of concomitant medications of the patient population to whom the drugs will be administered after marketing" (Graham, G. K. [2002]. Postmarketing surveillance and black box warning [letter]. *JAMA, 288,* 955–956). The following comments which address adverse drug reactions (ADR) have application here.

> In practice, drugs are prescribed to patients with uncountable combinations of other drugs and with an uncountable variety of underlying medical conditions and risk factors. Added to this are other recognized threats to external validity (e.g., placebo run–in trials, volunteer subject characteristics, dropout characteristics) that limit the validity of generalizations to the larger target patient population.

> Thus, representatives of the vast majority of potential consumers frequently are excluded from RCTs. It should therefore be no surprise, however unpleasant the reality, when ADRs begin to appear as use becomes more widespread under conditions that were never encountered during even the most rigorous clinical trials (Greene, P. J. & LaVaque, T. J. [2002]. Postmarketing surveillance and black box warnings [letter]. *JAMA, 288,* 957).

17.   Each of these occurred in the *New England Journal of Medicine* study noted in the previous endnote.

18.   Kirsch, I.; Moore, T. J., et al. (posted July 15, 2002). The emperor's new drugs: An analysis of antidepressant medication data submitted to the U.S. Food and Drug Administration. *Prevention & Treatment, 5*, Article 23.   Available on the web at http://www.journals .apa.org/prevention/volume5/pre0050023a.html.   The authors reported that in analyzing the drug trials submitted to the FDA they discovered that three out of the five Prozac drug trials and all three of the drug trials for Zoloft used this strategy.

19.   Bodenheimer reported that the industry sent only 40% of their outsourced clinical trials money to universities in 1998. In 1991 it was 80% (Bodenheimer, T. [2000]. Uneasy alliance: Clinical investigators and the pharmaceutical industry. *New England Journal of Medicine, 342*, 1539–1544).

20.   Lexchin, J.; Bero, L. A., et al. (2003).   Pharmaceutical industry sponsorship and research outcome and quality: Systematic review. *British Medical Journal, 326*, 1167–1170; Bhandari, M.; Busse, J. W., et al. (2004). Association between industry funding and statistically significant pro–industry findings in medical and surgical randomized trials. *Canadian Medical Association Journal, 170*, 477–480.

21.   Keller, M. B.; McCullough, J. P., et al. (2000).   A comparison of nefazodone, the cognitive–behavioral–analysis system of psychotherapy, and their combination for the treatment of chronic depression. *New England Journal of Medicine, 342*, 1462–1470.

22.   David Barlow, PhD, so identifies it on the web at http://www.biocritique.com/ viewref.cfm?messageid=dd91b596–6e12–11d5–b295–00b40080d29c.

23.   This is the study that led Marcia Angell, then–editor of the *New England Journal of Medicine*, to write her editorial "Is Academic Medicine for Sale?" in the same issue (2000, *New England Journal of Medicine, 342*, 1516–1518). She complained that finding an academic psychiatrist who could write a commentary on the article but was not encumbered with numerous financial ties to the drug manufacturing industry was very difficult. The commentary on the article indicates that the research is very important, and its basic findings and conclusions were accepted (Scott, J. [2000]. Treatment of chronic depression. *New England Journal of Medicine, 342*, 1518–1520). This further indicates the lack of ability found even among physicians writing in our leading medical journals to evaluate research design issues. The study should never have been published. Incidentally, the antidepressant used in the study was removed from the market in 2003 because of drug–caused liver damage resulting in numerous fatalities.

24.   Keller, M. B.; McCullough, J. P., et al. (2000).   A comparison of nefazodone, the cognitive–behavioral–analysis system of psychotherapy, and their combination for the treatment of chronic depression. *New England Journal of Medicine, 342*, 1462–1470, p. 1462.

25.   The study reported that better than either Serzone or psychotherapy was a combination of both. But without placebo groups, the "end point" measures are still meaningless. The authors might object and note they used the Hamilton Scale for Depression and, using that scale, depression did drop. The Hamilton Scale has its own shortcomings. See comments on the Hamilton Rating Scale for Depression at endnote 75 for Chapter 9, The FDA Drug Approval Process.

26.   Hite, S. (1981). *The Hite Report on Male Sexuality*. New York: Knopf.

27.   Hite, S. (1987). *Women and Love, A Cultural Revolution in Progress*. New York: Knopf.

28.   Hite, S. (1976). *The Hite Report: A Nationwide Study on Female Sexuality*. New York: Macmillan.

29.   The Freedom of Information Act request and subsequent report by Kirsch and his colleagues stated that only 4 of 45 trials met the 70% standard. Among placebo subjects, 60% completed the drug trials; 63% of active drug subjects did so (Kirsch, I.; Moore, T. J.,

et al. [posted July 15, 2002]. The emperor's new drugs: An analysis of antidepressant medication data submitted to the U.S. Food and Drug Administration. *Prevention & Treatment, 5*, Article 23. Available on the web at http://www.journals.apa.org/prevention/volume5/pre0050023a.html.

30. Cooper, R. J. & Schriger, D. L. (2005). The availability of references and the sponsorship of original research cited in pharmaceutical advertisements. *CMAJ, 172*, 487–491.

31. Villanueva, P.; Peiró, S., et al. (2003). Accuracy of pharmaceutical advertisements in medical journals. *Lancet, 361*, 27–32.

32. Ibid., p. 28.

33. Smith, R. (2003). Medical journals and pharmaceutical companies: Uneasy bedfellows. *British Medical Journal, 326*, 1202–1205, pp. 1202–1203.

34. Ibid., p. 1202.

35. The AMA's advertising policy reads in part, "As a matter of policy, the AMA will sell advertising space in its publications when the inclusion of advertising does not interfere with the mission or objectives of the AMA or its publications" (p. 2). When large dollar amounts are being paid to advertise in AMA publications, there is not much that would be judged to be an interference with the AMA's mission or objectives. Both *JAMA* and the *BMJ* state their assumption that advertising will comply with all government regulations. That clearly has not been an effective screening standard. Principles Governing Advertising in Publications of the American Medical Association (Revised September 2002) is available on the web at http://pubs.ama–assn.org/misc/adprinciples.pdf.

36. Lankinen, K. S.; Levola, T., et al. (2004). Industry guidelines, laws and regulations ignored: Quality of drug advertising in medical journals. *Pharmacoepidemiology & Drug Safety, 13*, 789–795. This is a Finnish study. The advertised drugs would be virtually the same as those sold in the U.S. and in other European nations. The advertisements and the research they cite would be virtually the same as well. This is a worldwide problem.

Chapter 8 — Do Antidepressants Work?

1. Kirsch, I. (posted July 15, 2002). Yes, there *is* a placebo effect, but is there a powerful antidepressant drug effect? *Prevention & Treatment, 5*, Article 22, p. 5. Available on the web at http://www.journals.apa.org/prevention/volume5/pre00500221.html.

2. Greenwood had a history of very thorough and demanding investigations of the NIH, FDA and pharmaceutical companies. To prepare for the July hearings he sent identical letters to some of the largest drug manufacturers asking them to fully disclose all research data related to their antidepressant drug testing with children. (The letter is available on the web at the House Committee on Energy and Commerce site: http://energycommerce.house .gov/108/letters/02032004_1210.htm.) I do not see Greenwood as ever having been in the pocket of the industry he investigated in any sense. However it is indisputable that Congress is a stepping stone to much higher salaries working in industry or as a lobbyist. Many who go to Congress leave Congress but do not leave Washington. As a congressman, Greenwood earned $158,100 per year. His annual salary at BIO was expected to be several times his annual congressional salary. (Carl Felbaum, the previous president of BIO, earned over $800,000 per year in salary and benefits, according to Knight Ridder/Tribune Business News [July 20, 2004]. Pennsylvania congressman to quit House, join biotechnology lobby. *The Morning Call, Allentown, PA*. Accessed via InfoTrac Newspapers, Item 04202001.) Sidney Wolfe, MD, director of Public Citizen's Healthcare Research Group, contended that "Greenwood's move was another example of blurred lines between the government and industry" (ibid.). The question, then, is how many members of the House or the Senate allow

the knowledge that the big money will come following a career in government to influence them?

3. U.S. Congress. House of Representatives. Committee on Energy and Commerce. *Publication and Disclosure Issues in Antidepressant Pediatric Clinical Trials: Hearing Before the Subcommittee on Oversight and Investigations.* 99th Cong., 2nd sess., Sept. 9, 2004, p. 7. Available on the web at http://www.access.gpo.gov/congress/house.

4. Ibid., p. 6.

5. Since the passage of the Best Pharmaceuticals for Children Act, the FDA has been required by law to publish results of clinical data. Two years after its passage they still had not done so. Congressman Joe Barton addressed this in his opening statement: "In addition to the problem of cooperation, this subcommittee will also review the FDA's spotty record on sharing results from clinical trial data with the public, as required under Section 9 of the Best Pharmaceuticals for Children Act. Although required by law since 2002, the FDA has not published any summaries of the pediatric antidepressants until this year, and almost all of them were just 3 weeks ago after I made a personal phone call to an individual at the FDA" (ibid, p. 3).

6. Wagner, K. D.; Ambrosini, P., et al. (2003). Efficacy of Sertraline in the treatment of children and adolescents with major depressive disorder. *JAMA, 290,* 1033–1041.

7. U.S. Congress. House of Representatives. Committee on Energy and Commerce (Sept. 9, 2004). *Publication and Disclosure Issues in Antidepressant Pediatric Clinical Trials: Hearing Before the Subcommittee on Oversight and Investigations.* 99th Cong., 2nd sess., p. 149. Available on the web at http://www.access.gpo.gov/congress/house.

8. Ibid., p. 150.

9. Ibid., p. 177.

10. The failure of the system to allow anyone but the drug companies and the FDA to examine clinical trials *before* a drug is approved is seen in testimony involving Congressman Joe Barton and the FDA's Janet Woodcock. Barton: "Do you feel there is any reluctance on behalf of the FDA to disclose negative clinical information—clinical trial information?" Ms. Woodcock: "No. I believe that we have legal restraints on the amount of information we can disclose and when we can disclose that information. And we must follow the law as far as it pertains to information disclosure. As I said in my testimony, prior to approval of a drug, it is not possible for FDA to disclose information on clinical trials, clinical trial results and so forth until the drug would be approved for that particular indication" (ibid., p. 35).

11. Ibid.

12. Ibid., p. 2.

13. Ibid., p. 3.

14. Kirsch, I. (posted July 15, 2002). Yes, there *is* a placebo effect, but is there a powerful antidepressant drug effect? *Prevention & Treatment, 5,* Article 22, p. 5. Available on the web at http://www.journals.apa.org/prevention/volume5/pre00500221.html.

15. Ibid.

16. Merlo, J.; Ranstom, J., et al. (1996). Incidence of myocardial infarction in elderly men being treated with anti–hypertensive drugs: Population–based cohort study. *British Medical Journal, 13,* 457–461.

17. Ferry, B.; Bernard, N., et al. (1994). Influence of hepatic impairment on the pharmacokinetics of nefazodone and two of its metabolites after single and multiple oral doses. *Fundamental & Clinical Pharmacology, 8,* 467–473.

18 Schirren, C. A. & Baretton, G. (2000). Nefazodone–induced acute liver failure. *American Journal of Gastroenterology, 95,* 1596–1597.

19. vanBattum, P. L.; van de Vrie, W., et al. (2000). [Acute liver failure ascribed to nefazodone: Importance of "postmarketing surveillance" for recently introduced drugs]. *Nederlands Tijdschrift Geneeskunde, 144*, 1964–1967.

20. Harris, G. (Jan. 9, 2003). Bristol–Myers halts drug in Europe. *Wall Street Journal*, D.2.

21. Associated Press (May 20, 2004). Bristol–Myers will stop selling Serzone in U.S. *Wall Street Journal*, D.4.

22. Martinez, B. (April 20, 2004). Teen death stirs fresh debate about depression medication; Bristol–Myer's Serzone, despite removal elsewhere, is still available in U.S. *Wall Street Journal*, D.5.

23. The first half could also be Pondimin (fenfluramine), of which Redux was a cousin but an improved version.

24. There were approximately 6 million fen–phen users. In 1999 over 4,000 lawsuits had already been filed (Associated Press [Aug. 28, 1999]. Diet drug suit to go to trial. *NY Times*, C.14). Based on a rate of 35 idiopathic cardiac–valve disorders (for those on fen–phen 4 months or more) per 10,000 users, it appears that approximately 21,000 users will experience this life–threatening condition (Jick, H.; Vasilakis, C., et al. [1998]. A population–based study of appetite–suppressant drugs and the risk of cardiac–valve regurgitation. *New England Journal of Medicine, 339*, 765–766). Brain damage and primary pulmonary hypertension would appreciably increase the number who have been harmed. See McCann, U. D.; Seiden, L. S., et al. (1997). Brain serotonin neurotoxicity and primary pulmonary hypertension from fenfluramine and dexfenfluramine. *JAMA, 278*, 666–672.

25. Saul, S. (Feb. 1, 2005). Wyeth lifts estimate on suits. *NY Times*, C.2.

26. The FDA posted an announcement of the committee's vote on November 27, 1995, under the title "Advisory committee votes on dexfenfluramine." The announcement is available on the web at http://www.fda.gov/bbs/topics/ANSWERS/ANS00698.html. The *PDR* stated that one of the side effects of Redux was diarrhea. This side effect alone could explain the small difference between those on Redux versus those on a placebo. Another FDA site noted, "Animal studies have shown long–term brain changes. To determine relevance of these findings to humans, further human studies will be conducted." (See http://www.fda.gov/fdac/ departs/696_upd.html. This quote is under the "New Weight–Loss Drug" heading.) Redux was essentially an antidepressant type of drug in that it affected the brain's serotonin levels.

27. Stolberg, S. G. (Sept. 10, 1999). Questions for drug maker on honesty of test results. *NY Times*, A.18.

28. Rheingold, P. D. (1998). Fen–phen and Redux: A tale of three drugs. *Trial, 34*, 78–82.

29. This is not an unfair characterization of what occurred. The FDA had received the Mayo Clinic data on July 7, 1996, and immediately issued a Public Health Advisory. However, it was only when that same data was published by the *New England Journal of Medicine* seven weeks later (Aug. 28) that it became apparent that lawsuits would follow and Wyeth pulled the drug. See the FDA's own account at http://www.fda.gov/cder/news/phen/fenphenqa2.htm.

30. Two of the studies did not report completion rates. The FDA should have sent these back to the drug companies. Of the 45 remaining studies, only 63% of those given antidepressants participated until the studies were completed.

31. This trick was used with three Prozac and three Zoloft clinical trials. It may have been used by other studies as well, but the reporting of study details was not adequate to know how many studies allowed substitutions. This information is reported in the

"Methods" section of the Kirsch paper (Kirsch, I. Yes, there *is* a placebo effect, but is there a powerful antidepressant drug effect? *Prevention & Treatment, 5,* Article 22, p. 5). Available on the web at http://www.journals.apa.org/prevention/volume5/pre00500221.html.

32. You can find the article by typing the exact web address http://www.journals.apa .org/prevention/volume5/pre0050023a.html or by putting "Prevention and Treatment Emperor's New Drugs" into the Google search engine. When you find the article, go to the "Methods" section. The information on the use of sedatives is in the second half of the fourth paragraph.

33. The difference between the placebo and the active medications was very little (not enough to reach statistical significance) but, nevertheless, the placebo did result in greater measured change in 4 of the 47 clinical trials.

34. Kirsch, I.; Moore, T. J., et al. (posted July 15, 2002). The emperor's new drugs: An analysis of antidepressant medication data submitted to the U.S. Food and Drug Administration. *Prevention & Treatment, 5,* Article 23, p. 6. Available on the web at http://www. journals.apa.org/prevention/volume5/pre0050023a.html.

35. To be exact, "82% of the drug response was duplicated by the placebo response" (ibid.).

36. Laughren, T. P. (March 26, 1998). Recommendations for approvable action for Celexa (citalopram) for the treatment of depression: Memoradum: Department of Health and Human Services, Public Health Service, Food and Drug Administration, Center for Drug Evaluation and Research, Washington, D.C. in ibid., p. 9.

37. Greenberg, R. P.; Bornstein, R., et al. (1994). A meta–analysis of fluoxetine outcome in the treatment of depression. *Journal of Nervous & Mental Disease, 182,* 547–551, p. 549.

38. Even, C.; Siobud–Dorocant, E. & Dardennes, R. M. (2000). Critical approach to antidepressant trials: Blindness protection is necessary, feasible and measurable. *British Journal of Psychiatry, 177,* 47–51; Slack, M. K. & Draugalis, J. R. (2001). Establishing the internal and external validity of experimental studies. *American Journal of Health–System Pharmacy, 58,* 2173–2181.

39. Greenberg, R. P.; Bornstein, R. F., et al. (1992). A meta–analysis of antidepressant outcome under "blinder" conditions. *Journal of Consulting & Clinical Psychology, 60,* 664–669. The antidepressants under scrutiny in this study were the older tricyclic antidepressants. These have consistently been found to work as well as SSRIs (Guaiana, G.; Barbui, C. & Hotopf, M. [2003]. Amytriptyline versus other types of pharmacotherapy for depression. *Cochrane Database of Systematic Reviews* [online]:CD004186; Wilson, K. & Mottram, P. [2004]. A comparison of side effects of selective serotonin reuptake inhibitors and tricyclic antidepressants in older depressed patients: A meta–analysis. *International Journal of Geriatric Psychiatry, 19,* 754–762), but they are known to have more adverse effects including cognitive and cardiovascular effects (Brambilla, P; Cipriani, A., et al. [2005]. Side–effects profile of fluoxetine in comparison with other SSRIs, tricyclic and newer antidepressants: A meta–analysis of clinical trial data. *Pharmacopsychiatry, 38,* 69–77; Nelson, J. C.; Kennedy, J. S., et al. [1999]. Treatment of major depression with nortriptyline and paroxetine in patients with ischemic heart disease. *American Journal of Psychiatry, 156,* 1024–1028; Estebe, J. P. & Myers, R. R. [2004]. Amitriptyline neurotoxicity: Dose–related pathology after topical application to rat sciatic nerve. *Anesthesiology, 100,* 1519–1525; Roose, S. P. & Spatz, E. [1999]. Treatment of depression in patients with heart disease. *Journal of Clinical Psychiatry, 60* [Suppl. 20], 34–37; Podewils, L. J. & Lyketsos, C. G. [2002]. Tricyclic antidepressants and cognitive decline. *Psychosomatics, 43,* 31–35).

40.   Prozac, the first of the SSRI antidepressants, was on the market when this study was published but had yet to gain the popularity it would later receive. The antidepressants studied for this meta–analysis included a number of older antidepressants—imipramine, amitriptyline, amoxapine, maprotiline and trazadone.

41.   Roose, S. P.; Sackeim, H. A., et al. (2004). Antidepressant pharmacotherapy in the treatment of depression in the very old: A randomized, placebo–controlled trial. *American Journal of Psychiatry, 161*, 2050–2059, p. 2050.

42.   Ibid., p. 2051.

43.   Babyak, M.; Blumenthal, J. A., et al. (2000). Exercise treatment for major depression: Maintenance of therapeutic benefit at 10 months. *Psychosomatic Medicine, 62*, 633–638.

44.   Examples of this bias are numerous. *JAMA* published a comparison of Zoloft and St. John's wort (Hypericum perforatum) which found neither performed significantly differently from the placebo. However, the abstract's conclusion reads, "This study fails to support the efficacy of *H perforatum* in moderately severe major depression." Why did they not state, "This study fails to support the efficacy of *Zoloft* in moderately severe major depression"?

45.   Examples include Schneider, L. S.; Nelson, J. C., et al. (2003). An 8–week multicenter, parallel–group, double–blind, placebo–controlled study of sertraline in elderly outpatients with major depression. *American Journal of Psychiatry, 160*, 1277–1285; Brown, E. S.; Vigil, L.; et al. (2005). A randomized trial of citalopram versus placebo in outpatients with asthma and major depressive disorder: A proof of concept study. *Biological Psychiatry* (e–published ahead of print); Moncrieff, J.; Wessely, S. & Hardy, R. (2001). Antidepressants using active placebos. *Cochrane Database of Systematic Reviews (2)*:CD003012; Moncrieff, J.; Wessely, S. & Hardy R. (2004). Active placebos versus antidepressants for depression. *Cochrane Database of Systematic Reviews (1)*:CD003012.

46.   Khan, A.; Warner, H. A. & Brown, W. A. (2000). Symptom reduction and suicide risk in patients treated with placebo in antidepressant clinical trials: An analysis of the Food and Drug Administration database. *Archives of General Psychiatry, 57*, 311–317. The overall difference was 40.7% vs. 30.9%. Even this modest difference was not likely genuine. (See Kirsch's "Article 23" referenced in note 34 for a discussion of this.) The Khan study examined 43 clinical trials and found that in two studies the placebo outperformed the antidepressant. Another major study of FDA clinical trial data found that less than half of the nine antidepressants which gained FDA market approval between 1985 and 2000 worked better than the placebos with which they were compared (Khan, A. & Brown, W. A. [2002]. Are placebo controls necessary to test new antidepressants and anxiolytics? *International Journal of Neuropsychopharmacology, 5*, 193–197).

47.   This is the pattern found in many studies and will be discussed later. If this study were the only one to find such an association, I would not mention it at all as the difference (.4% on placebo, .8% on antidepressant) did not achieve statistical significance because the total number of suicides (34) was small.

48.   There were 30 minutes of relatively strenuous exercise which came after a 10–minute warmup routine. A 5–minute "cool down" followed the exercise.

49.   Blumenthal, J. A.; Babyak, M. A., et al. (1999). Effects of exercise training on older patients with major depression. *Archives of Internal Medicine, 159*, 2345–2356.

50.   Babyak, M.; Blumenthal, J. A., et al. (2000). Exercise treatment for major depression: Maintenance of therapeutic benefit at 10 months. *Psychosomatic Medicine, 62*, 633–638.

51.   Ibid., p. 636.

52. Ibid.

53. Rosenthal, N. E.; Sack, D. A., et al. (1984). Seasonal affective disorder: A description of the syndrome and preliminary findings with light therapy. *Archives of General Psychiatry, 41*, 72–80 in Wirz–Justice, A. (1998). Beginning to see the light. *Archives of General Psychiatry, 55*, 861–862.

54. The *DSM–IV–TR* specifies that official diagnosis is to be Major Depressive Disorder with Seasonal Pattern. See American Psychiatric Association (2000). *Diagnostic Statistical Manual–IV–TR*. Washington, D. C.: APA, p. 747f.

55. Martiny, K. (2004). Adjunctive bright light in non–seasonal major depression. *Acta Psychiatrica Scandinavica* (Suppl.), *425*, 7–28; Martiny, K.; Lunde, M., et al. (2005). Adjunctive bright light in non–seasonal major depression: Results from clinician–rated depression scales. *Acta Psychiatrica Scandinavica, 112*, 117–125; Avery, D. H. & Eder, D. N. (2001). Dawn stimulation and bright light in the treatment of SAD: A controlled study. *Biological Psychiatry, 50*, 205–216; Wehr, T. A. (1992). Seasonal vulnerability to depression: Implications for etiology and treatment. *Encephale, 18*, 479–483; Benedetti, F.; Colombo, C., et al. (2003). Morning light treatment hastens the antidepressant effect of cialopram: A placebo–controlled trial. *Journal of Clinical Psychiatry, 64*, 648–653.

56. Terman, M.; Terman, J. S. & Ross, D. C. (1998). A controlled trial of timed bright light and negative air ionization for treatment of winter depression. *Archives of General Psychiatry, 55*, 875–882, p. 875. The article reported that low–density ionization (the machine could be set to high– or low–ion densities) resulted in the least amount of change in subjects' depression scores. All other conditions (high–density ionization, morning light or evening light) had similar outcomes.

57. Eastman, C. I.; Young, M. A., et al. (1998). Bright light treatment of winter depression: A placebo–controlled trial. *Archives of General Psychiatry, 55*, 883–889.

58. Golden, R. N.; Gaynes, B. N.; et al. (2005). The efficacy of light therapy in the treatment of mood disorders: A review and meta–analysis of the evidence. *American Journal of Psychiatry, 162*, 656–662, p. 656.

59. Sung, J. J. Y. (2002). Acupuncture for gastrointestinal disorders: Myth or magic. *Gut, 51*, 617–619.

60. van Tulder, M. W.; Furlan, A. D. & Gagnier, J. J. (2005). Complementary and alternative therapies for low back pain. *Best Practice & Research: Clinical Rheumatology, 19*, 639–654.

61. Birch, S.; Hesselink, J. K., et al. (2004). Clinical research on acupuncture. Part 1. What have reviews of the efficacy and safety of acupuncture told us so far? *Journal of Alternative & Complementary Medicine* (New York), *10*, 468–480. Also see the National Institutes of Health consensus statement which reaches essentially the same conclusions. Available on the web at http://odp.od.nih.gov/consensus/cons/107/107_statement .htm.

62. Ibid.

63. Ibid.

64. Luo, H; Jia, Y; & Zhan, L. (1985). Electro–acupuncture vs. amitriptyline in the treatment of depressive states. *Journal of Chinese Medicine, 5*, 3–8 in Acupuncture Research Resource Centre (2002). Depression, anxiety and acupuncture. Briefing paper No. 9. British Acupuncture Council. Available on the web at http://www.acupuncture.org.uk/content/Library/pdf/anxiety_bp9.pdf.

65. Smith, C. A. & Hay, P. P. (2005). Acupuncture for depression. *Cochrane Database of Systematic Reviews* (2):CD004046.

66. Streitberger, K.; Diefenbacher, M., et al. (2004). Acupuncture compared to placebo–acupuncture for postoperative nausea and vomiting prophylaxis: A randomised

placebo–controlled patient and observer blind trial. *Anaesthesia, 59,* 142–149. A response and a reply were published in reference to this research (*Anaesthesia, 59,* 730–731) concerning duration of needle placement and the use of additional acupuncture locations. The effectiveness of acupuncture to control postoperative nausea and vomiting was not challenged.

67. Examples include Uebelhack, R.; Gruenwald, J., et al. (2004). Efficacy and tolerability of Hypericum extract STW3–VI in patients with moderate depression: A double–blind, placebo–controlled clinical trial. *Advances in Therapy, 21,* 265–275; Lecrubier, Y.; Clerc, G., et al. (2002). Efficacy of St. John's wort in major depression: A double–blind, placebo–controlled trial. *American Journal of Psychiatry, 159,* 1361–1366; Linde, K.; Ramirez, G., et al. (1996). St. John's wort for depression: An overview and meta–analysis of randomized clinical trials. *British Medical Journal, 313,* 253–258.

68. Szegedi, A.; Kohnen, R., et al. (2005). Acute treatment of moderate to severe depression with hypericum extract WS5570 (St. John's wort): Randomised controlled double blind non–inferiority trial versus paroxetine. *British Medical Journal, 330,* 759.

69. Schulz, V. (2002). Clinical trials with hypericum extracts in patients with depression: Results, comparisons, conclusions for therapy with antidepressant drugs. *Phytomedicine, 9,* 468–474.

70. Gastpar, M; Singer, A. & Zeller, K. (2005). Efficacy and tolerability of hypericum extract STW3 in long–term treatment with once–daily dosage in comparison with sertraline. *Pharmacopsychiatry, 38,* 78–86.

71. Philipp, M.; Kohnen, R. & Hiller, K. O. (1999). Hypericum extract versus imipramine or placebo in patients with moderate depression: Randomized multicentre study of treatment for eight weeks. *British Medical Journal, 319,* 1534–1538; Linde, K.; Mulrow, C. D., et al. (2005). St. John's Wort for depression. *Cochrane Database of Systematic Reviews* (3):CD000448. This article is available on the web at http://www.mrw.interscience .wiley.com/cochrane/clsysrev/articles/CD000448/frame.html.

72. Knuppel, L. & Linde, K. (2004). Adverse effects of St. John's Wort: A systematic review. *Journal of Clinical Psychiatry, 65,* 1470–1479. The Knuppel and Linde study makes it clear that by itself St. John's wort is very safe. However, many concerns about possible drug interactions have been voiced. I have no doubt that some adverse reactions do occur, but only time will make clear what those various drug interactions may be and how serious they are.

73. Linde, K.; Mulrow, C. D., et al. (2005). St. John's Wort for depression. *Cochrane Database of Systematic Reviews* (3):CD000448. This article is available on the web at http://www.mrw.interscience.wiley.com/cochrane/clsysrev/articles/CD000448/frame.html.

74. Lang, A. R.; Goeckner, D. J., et al. (1975). Effects of alcohol on aggression in male social drinkers. *Journal of Abnormal Psychology, 84,* 508–518.

75. Beecher, H. K. (1959). *Measurement of Subjective Responses: Quantitative Effects of Drugs.* New York: Oxford University Press.

76. The Coronary Drug Project Research Group (1980). Influence of adherence to treatment and response of cholesterol on mortality in the Coronary Drug Project. *New England Journal of Medicine, 303,* 1038–1041.

77. Leigh, R.; MacQueen, G., et al. (2003). Change in forced expiratory volume in 1 second after sham bronchoconstrictor in suggestible but not suggestion–resistant asthmatic subjects: A pilot study. *Psychosomatic Medicine, 65,* 791–795; Lemaigre, V.; Van den Bergh, O., et al. (2005). Effects of long–acting bronchodilators and placebo on histamine–induced asthma symptoms and mild bronchusobstruction. *Respiratory Medicine, 99* (e–published ahead of print); DePeuter, S.; Van Diest, I., et al. (2005). Can subjective asthma symptoms be learned? *Psychosomatic Medicine, 67,* 454–461; Adams, N. P.; Bestall, J. C., et al. (2005).

Inhaled fluticasone versus placebo for chronic asthma in adults and children. *Cochrane Database of Systematic Reviews (2)*:CD003135.

78.   Vayssairat, M.; Baudot, N. & Sainte–Beuve, C. (1988). Why does placebo improve severe limb ischemia? *Lancet, 1*, 356.

79.   Cobb, L. A.; Thomas, G. I., et al. (1959). An evaluation of internal–mammary–artery ligation by a double–blind technic. *New England Journal of Medicine, 260*, 1115–1118. By way of explanation I will note that after the incisions were made, the surgeon was handed an envelope which held a printed card instructing him to continue the operation or to sew up the patient. Physicians who followed the patients after the operation did not know who had the completed surgery and who did not. Other examples are shared by Roberts, A. H.; Kewman, D. G., et al. (2001). The power of nonspecific effects in healing: Implications for psychosocial and biological treatments. *Clinical Psychology Review, 13*, 375–391.

80.   Amanzio, M.; Pollo, A., et al. (2001). Response variability to analgesics: A role for non–specific activation of endogenous opioids. *Pain, 90*, 205–215; Leuchter, A. F.; Cook, I. A., et al. (2002). Change in brain function of depressed subjects during treatment with placebo. *American Journal of Psychiatry, 159*, 122–129 (for electroencephalogram); Lieberman, M. D.; Jarcho, J. M., et al. (2004). The neural correlates of placebo effects: A disruption account. *NeuroImage, 22*, 447–455 (for PET measured changes).

81.   Mayberg, H. S.; Silva, J. A., et al. (2002). The functional neuroanatomy of the placebo effect. *American Journal of Psychiatry, 159*, 728–737.

82.   de Craen, A. J.; Tijssen, J. G., et al. (2000). Placebo effect in the acute treatment of migraine: Subcutaneous placebos are better than oral placebos. *Journal of Neurology, 247*, 183–188.

83.   de Craen, A. J.; Moerman, D. E., et al. (1999). Placebo effect in the treatment of duodenal ulcer. *British Journal of Clinical Pharmacology, 48*, 853–860.

84.   Amanzio, M.; Pollo, A., et al. (2001). Response variability to analgesics: A role for non–specific activation of endogenous opioids. *Pain, 90*, 205–215; Benedetti, F.; Maggi, G., et al. (2003). Open versus hidden medical treatments: The patient's knowledge about a therapy affects the therapy outcome. *Prevention & Treatment, 6*, Article 1. Available online at http://www.apa.org/prevention/volume6/pre006000la.html. These articles found that pain–killing drugs do not work as well when they are less openly given. When a doctor enters a room, uses an injection, speaks enthusiastically about the drug, etc., the effects are more dramatic whether an active drug or a placebo is used.

85.   Evans, F. J. (1974). The placebo response in pain reduction. *Advances in Neurology, 4*, 289–296 in Kirsch, I. (posted July 15, 2002). Yes, there *is* a placebo effect, but is there a powerful antidepressant drug effect? *Prevention & Treatment, 5*, Article 22, p. 5. Available on the web at http://www.journals.apa.org/prevention/volume5/pre00500221.html.

86.   Branthwaite, A. & Cooper, P. (1981). Analgesic effects of branding in treatment of headaches. *British Medical Journal* (Clinical Research Edition), *282*, 1576–1578.

87.   Alderman, E. L.; Davies, R. O., et al. (1975). Dose response effectiveness of propranolol for the treatment of angina pectoris. *Circulation, 51*, 964–975.

88.   Roberts, S. S. (2003). The placebo response and you. *Diabetes Forecast, 56*(5), 25–27.

89.   Shapiro, A. K. & Morris, L. A. (1978). The placebo effect in medical and psychological therapies in Garfield, S. L. & Bergin, A. E., eds. *Handbook of Psychotherapy and Behavior Change: An Empirical Analysis*, 2nd ed. New York: Wiley. Therapy, not pills, was the focus of the Shapiro and Morris article.

90.   Lowinger, P. & Dobie, S. (1969). What makes placebos work? A study of placebo response rates. *Archives of General Psychiatry, 20*, 84–88. This study found high doses of

placebo were particularly effective as doctors, though blind to who received the active drugs and who received placebos, were still more enthused and anticipated more change. The review of five studies published by Roberts, et al. (Roberts, A. H.; Kewman, D. G., et al. [1993]. The power of nonspecific effects in healing: Implications for social and biological treatments. *Clinical Psychology Review, 13*, 375–391) found that when placebos are presented with enthusiasm, approximately 70% of the active treatment response can be expected.

91. Walsh, B. T.; Seidman, S. N., et al. (2002). Placebo response in studies of major depression: Variable, substantial, and growing. *JAMA, 287*, 1840–1847.

92. Lowinger, P. & Dobie, S. (1969). What makes placebos work? A study of placebo response rates. *Archives of General Psychiatry, 20*, 84–88.

Chapter 9 — The FDA Drug Approval Process

1. Topol, E. J. (2005). Nesiritide—not verified. *New England Journal of Medicine, 353*, 113–116, p. 113.

2. Ibid. Dr. Topol mentions that physicians are encouraged to establish centers where the drug is given and Medicare is billed; i.e., doctor greed is encouraged. He also discussed the FDA advisory panel problem.

3. Insight Team of the *Sunday Times* of London (1979). *Suffer the Children: The Story of Thalidomide*. New York: Viking Press in Annas, G. J. & Elias, S. (1999). Thalidomide and the Titanic: Reconstructing the technology tragedies of the twentieth century. *American Journal of Public Health, 89*, 98–101.

4. This is the number given by Stephens and Brynner. Others give similar figures. However, I have not seen a number that has been carefully documented. The authors state that 5,000 of these babies survived childhood (Stephens, T. & Brynner, R. [2001]. *Dark Remedy: The Impact of Thalidomide and Its Revival As a Vital Medicine*. Cambridge, MA: Perseus, p. 37). This book is the basis for undocumented details in my brief account of the thalidomide tragedy.

5. Dr. Widukind Lenz states 40% didn't survive one year (Lenz, W. [1992]. The history of thalidomide. Lecture, 1992 UNITH Congress [international thalidomide association]). Available on the web at http://www.thalidomide.ca/en/information/history_of_ thalidomide.html.

6. *BBC News* (June 7, 2002). Thalidomide: 40 years on. Available on the web at http://news.bbc.co.uk/1/hi/uk/2031459.stm.

7. I assembled this list from several sources. See the following for other thalidomide–caused effects including others I have not noted (Newman, C. G. H. [1986]. The thalidomide syndrome: Risk of exposure and spectrum of malformations. *Clinics in Perinatology, 13*, 555–573). Also see Wu, J. J.; Huang, D. B., et al. (2005). Thalidomide: Dermatological indications, mechanisms of action and side–effects. *British Journal of Dermatology, 153*, 254–273; Ghobrial, I. M. & Rajkumar, S. V. (2003). Management of thalidomide toxicity. *The Journal of Supportive Oncology, 1*, 194–205.

8. Stephens, T. & Brynner, R. (2001). *Dark Remedy*. New York: Perseus, p. 19.

9. Ibid., pp. 14–15.

10. Ibid., p. 15.

11. McBride, W. G. (1961). Thalidomide and congenital abnormalities. *Lancet, 1*, 1358.

12. Ibid.

13. Stephens, T. & Brynner, R. (2001). *Dark Remedy*. New York: Perseus, p. 30.

14. Ibid., p. 31.

15. Ibid., p. 32.

16. Ibid., p. 35.

17. Somers, G. F. (1962). Thalidomide and congenital abnormalities. *Lancet, i,* 912–913.

18. Though never approved, the U.S. drug company who gained American distribution rights, Richardson–Merrell, provided free samples to 1,267 physicians. They could do this since it was part of a drug trial—"dramatically larger than any previous drug trial conducted in the United States" (Stephens, T. & Brynner, R. [2001]. *Dark Remedy.* Cambridge, MA: Perseus, p. 43). Numerous children were born with serious birth defects as a result of this "drug trial."

19. Actually, few women who received a thalidomide prescription for morning sickness were ever harmed by the drug. Thalidomide is so safe, except for the very early days of pregnancy, that by the time most women realized they were pregnant and began having morning sickness, they had already passed the critically dangerous period. For a breakdown by day (since achieving pregnancy), see Lenz, W. (1992). The history of thalidomide. Lecture, 1992 UNITH Congress. Available on the web at http://www.thalidomide.ca/en/information/history_of_thalidomide.html.

20. *LA Times* (October 11, 1988). Police arrest AIDS protesters blocking access to FDA offices, p. 2.

21. Center for Drug Education and Research (2001). FDA's drug review and approval times. The Center for Drug Education and Research is an arm of the FDA. This government site is available on the web at http://www.fda.gov/cder/reports/reviewtimes/default.htm# Approval%20time. This 22–month average represented a significant improvement in the time required to get drugs approved. In the 1979–1986 period it took 33.6 months on average (49.9 months for central nervous system drugs). The 1997–2002 period saw approval times cut by more than half to 16.1 months (22.7 months for central nervous system drugs) (Berndt, E. R.; Gottschalk, A. H., et al. [2005]. Industry funding of the FDA: Effects of PDUFA on approval times and withdrawal rates. *Nature Reviews: Drug Discovery, 4,* 545–554).

22. Bodenheimer, T. (2000). Uneasy alliance: Clinical investigators and the pharmaceutical industry. *New England Journal of Medicine, 342,* 1539–1544.

23. Patent laws and FDA approval work hand in hand. While it is true a drug must be patented and then go through what may be a multi–year FDA approval process, Title II of the Drug Price Competition and Patent Term Restoration Act allows for patent extension to compensate for time lost in pursuit of FDA approval (Public Law 98–417). This law allows for up to 5 years of patent restoration time but states that a drug's total marketing time may not exceed 14 years. The FDA's Center for Drug Evaluation and Research has a website which explains these laws at http://www.fda.gov/cder/about/smallbiz/patent_term.htm. (I find it most amusing that they place this "*Small* Business Assistance" site.)

24. *Physicians' Desk Reference* (2004), 58th ed. Montvale, NJ: Thomson PDR.

25. Ibid., Tables 2 & 3, p. 2109.

26. Ibid.

27. See the FDA website at http://www.fda.gov/cder/drug/infopage/vioxx/vioxxQA .htm (item 9).

28. This was a 3–year prospective, randomized, placebo–controlled study called the APPROVE (Adenomatous Polyp Prevention on Vioxx) trial. The risk of having a heart attack or stroke was almost doubled for those on a dosage of 25 mg/day. For a discussion of Vioxx as an FDA blunder see Okie, S. (2005). What ails the FDA? *New England Journal of Medicine, 352,* 1063–1066.

29. The Vioxx–Naproxen comparison trial used a 50 mg/day dosage. Obviously, Merck hoped that the heart attacks and strokes would not occur if they cut the dosage in half. Yet clinical trials should not be allowed to determine a drug's safety profile by using dosages that are below what many patients take each day. It would be better to use higher than recommended doses so unanticipated adverse effects could be found in study subjects who are being closely monitored, not in Americans who are completely unaware that the drug can cause harmful side effects.

30. Four facts make this a very ironic story. (1) Vioxx, Celebrex and Bextra have never been shown to be superior for the control of pain to the older nonsteroidal anti–inflammatory drugs (NSAIDS such as Naproxen) which likely caused fewer heart attacks and strokes (Okie, S. [2005]. Raising the bar: The FDA's Coxib Meeting. *New England Journal of Medicine, 352*, 1283–1285). (2) Of the three COX–2 inhibitors, *only* Vioxx has been found to reduce the occurrence of ulcers and bleeding, the advertised benefit for the entire class of drugs (ibid.). (3) As the FDA advisory panel was discussing what they should recommend, the *New England Journal of Medicine* published the results of a large, randomized clinical trial that found Celebrex carried significant risk of increasing the incidence of congestive heart failure (Solomon, S. D.; McMurray, J. J. V., et al. [2005]. Cardiovascular risk associated with celecoxib use in a large, randomized clinical trial for colorectal adenoma prevention. *New England Journal of Medicine, 352,* 1071–1080). (4) FDA drug safety scientist David Graham was pressured by FDA officials to change his research conclusions when his study revealed the dangers of Vioxx—his conclusions being "inconsistent with the FDA's position on the drug's safety" (Okie, S. [2005]. What ails the FDA? *New England Journal of Medicine, 352*, 1063–1066, p. 1063). Graham complied though "it caused me a great deal of mental anguish" (ibid., p. 1066).

31. The *NY Times* had actually asked the Center for Science in the Public Interest to do this analysis. The *Times* article appeared on Feb. 25, 2005 (Harris, G. & Berenson, A. Ten voters on panel backing pain pills had industry ties. *NY Times*, A.1).

32. Ibid.

33. Steinbrook, R. (2005). Financial conflicts of interest and the Food and Drug Administration's advisory committees. *New England Journal of Medicine, 353*, 116–118. Conflicts of interest issues in the Vioxx case and a breast implant case were discussed by Steinbrook.

34. Cauchon reports the higher number. Steinbrook reports an average of 194 waivers per year were granted in 2003 and 2004. See Cauchon, D. (Sept. 25, 2000). Number of drug experts available is limited; many waivers granted for those who have conflicts of interest. *USA Today*, A.10; Steinbrook, R. (2005). Financial conflicts of interest and the Food and Drug Administration's advisory committees. *New England Journal of Medicine, 353*, 116–118.

35. Steinbrook (ibid.).

36. Cauchon, D. (Sept. 25, 2000). FDA advisers tied to industry. *USA Today*, A.1.

37. Friedberg, M.; Saffran, B., et al. (Oct. 20, 1999). Evaluation of conflict of interest in economic analysis of new drugs used in oncology. *JAMA , 282*, 1453–1457, p. 1455.

38. Ibid.

39. Ibid., p. 1456.

40. Hartmann, M.; Knoth, H., et al. (2003). Industry–sponsored economic studies in oncology vs. studies sponsored by nonprofit organizations. *British Journal of Cancer, 89*, 1405–1408.

41. American Society of Clinical Oncology (2003). American Society of Clinical Oncology: Revised conflict of interest policy. *Journal of Clinical Oncology, 21*, 2394–2396. The policy is available on the web at http://www.jco.org/misc/article.pdf.

42.   The American Society of Clinical Oncology may have done as much as any medical society in trying to address the problem of private industry influence over research results. Their policy recognizes the need for federal oversight of all clinical trials "regardless of the sponsor of the research" (American Society of Clinical Oncology [2003]. *Journal of Clinical Oncology, 21*, 2377–2386, p. 2384).

43.   Stelfox, H. T.; Chua, G., et al. (1998). Conflict of interest in the debate over calcium–channel antagonists. *New England Journal of Medicine, 338*, 101–106.

44.   Meltzer, J. I. (1998). Conflict of interest in the debate over calcium–channel antagonists. *New England Journal Medicine, 338*, 1696.

45.   Opie, L. (1998). Conflict of interest in the debate over calcium–channel antagonists. *New England Journal of Medicine, 338*, p. 1697.

46.   Kuszler, P. C. (2001). Curing COIs in clinical research: Impossible dreams and harsh realities. *Widener Law Symposium Journal, 8*, 115 in Tereskerz, P. M. (2003). Research accountability and financial conflicts of interest in industry–sponsored clinical research: A review. *Accountability in Research, 10*, 137–158.

47.   In an article entitled "In whose best interest? Breaching the academic–industrial wall," Joseph Martin and Dennis Kasper (2000) argue that nowhere on the university campus has industry conquered the academia–industry wall of separation as much as it has in the area of biomedical research. This is where the most money is to be made for both sides (*New England Journal of Medicine, 343*, 2646–2649).

48.   Bekelman, J. E.; Li, Y. & Gross, C. P. (2003). Scope and impact of financial conflicts of interest in biomedical research: A systematic review. *JAMA, 289*, 454–465, p. 463.

49.   FDA (Aug. 2, 2004). Establishment of prescription drug user fee rates for fiscal year 2005. *Federal Register, 69*, 46165.

50.   Willman, D. (Dec. 20, 2000). The new FDA: How a new policy led to seven deadly drugs. *L.A. Times*, A.1.

51.   I base this number on a report coming from the Office of the Inspector General which reviewed the FDA's new drug application process in 2003. They reported a total of 1,021 formal meetings occurred during FY2001 (Office of Inspector General [March 2003]. FDA's review process for new drug applications: A management review. OEI–01–01–00590. Available on the web at http://www.oig.hhs.gov/oei/reports/oei–01–00590.pdf.).

52.   Nordenberg, T. (Sept./Oct. 1997). Why should FDA regulate drugs? *FDA Consumer*. Available on the web at http://www.fda.gov/fdac/features/1997/697_q&a.html.

53.   Willman, D. (Dec. 20, 2000). The new FDA: How a new policy led to seven deadly drugs. *LA Times*, A.1.

54.   Woodcock, J. (March 3, 2005). Ensuring drug safety: Where do we go from here? Hearing before the U.S. Senate Committee on Health, Education, Labor and Pensions. Available on the web at http://help.senate.gov/testimony/t207_tes.html.

55.   Ibid.

56.   Office of Inspector General (March 2003). FDA's review process for new drug applications: A management review. OEI–01–01–00590, p. 2. Available on the web at http://www.oig.hhs.gov/oei/reports/oei–01–00590.pdf.

57.   Ibid.

58.   This paper notes how the PDUFA III fee funds will be spent by the FDA. "64 percent of the fee revenues will be allocated for employee salary and benefit costs" (FDA [July 2003]. PDUFA III: Five–year plan—FY2003). See the executive summary on p. 3 of the online PDF document for this projection. Available on the web at http://www.fda.gov/oc/pdufa3/2003plan/2003%20Plan20%20rev%209–11–03.pdf.

59. Harris, G. (Aug. 27, 2004). Glaxo agrees to post results of drug trials on website. *NY Times,* C.4.

60. The statement was published by *JAMA* (DeAngelis, C. D.; Drazen, J. M., et al. [2004]. Is this clinical trial fully registered? *JAMA, 293,* 2927–2929) as part of a "joint and simultaneous" editorial by each of the editors of 13 journals and the executive editor of Medline.

61. Mangan, K. S. (May 6, 2005). Medical–school group backs trials registry. *Chronicle of Higher Education, 51,* A.30.

62. DeAngelis, C. D.; Drazen, J. M., et al. (2004). Is this clinical trial fully registered? *JAMA, 293,* 2927–2929.

63. WHO will likely be the primary host registration site in time. The WHO International Clinical Trial Registry Platform is being developed in 2005. Much of the work is on the web but will undoubtedly disappear in favor of completed documents later. Entering "International Clinical Trial Registry Platform" into Google's search engine will likely yield the most recent developments.

64. I am referring to Drummond Rennie. Dr. Rennie (2002) co–edited an AMA published book, *Users' Guides to the Medical Literature: A Manual for Evidence–Based Clinical Practice,* which argues that clinical research needs to become more objective and more evidence–based (Chicago: AMA Press).

65. Drummond, R. (2004). Trial registration: A great idea switches from ignored to irresistible. *JAMA, 292,* 1359–1362. Roughly a year before Eliot Spitzer brought suit against Glaxo, Kay Dickersin and Rennie published a *JAMA* article aimed at encouraging the registration of clinical trials (Dickersin, K. & Rennie, D. [2003]. Registering clinical trials. *JAMA, 290,* 516–523). This piece is filled with important information and may have been pivotal in encouraging the NY attorney general's office to take Glaxo to court. Yet, the call to register trials, as noted in the 2003 *JAMA* article, had been proposed 30 years earlier but never became common practice.

66. Kuehn, B. M. (2005). Trials on the record. *JAMA, 294,* 673.

67. This experience involved the antiarrhythmic drugs which were given to patients who had suffered heart attacks to prevent a second heart attack. The study which found these actually to be dangerous drugs was completed in 1980. Because of concerns over a loss of drug sales, the study was not published when it was concluded. Tambocor (flecainide) made by 3M proved especially deadly with approximately 50,000 deaths attributable to its use in just a few years (Moore, T. [1995]. *Deadly Medicine: Why Tens of Thousands of Heart Patients Died in America's Worst Drug Disaster.* New York: Simon & Schuster).

68. The Food and Drug Administration Modernization Act (FCDAMA) became law in 1997. It included funds for the creation of a public registry of clinical trials. The clinical trials.gov database went online in April 2000. Trials for serious and life–threatening conditions must, by law, be posted. Unfortunately, less than half of trials sponsored by private industry have been registered, despite the law (McDonald, D. & Molinari, P. M. [2005]. Breaking the trial result disclosure logjam now. *Applied Clinical Trials, 14,* 28–30.

69. Drummond argues that even the clinical trial registration effort will not succeed unless it includes all clinical trials, "is adequately funded, is made mandatory, is adequately policed, has substantial penalties for noncompliance, and unless all aspects of the enterprise are taken out of the hands of the pharmaceutical industry" (Drummond, R. [2004]. Trial registration: A great idea switches from ignored to irresistible. *JAMA, 292,* 1359–1362, p. 1361).

70. Kendell, R. E.; Cooper, J. E., et al. (1971). Diagnostic criteria of American and British psychiatrists. *Archives of General Psychiatry, 25,* 123–130.

71. This statement is available at http://www.fda.gov/opacom/morechoices/mission .html.

72. Healy, D. (2002). *The Creation of Psychopharmacology*. Cambridge, MA: Harvard University Press, p. 308.

73. Ibid.

74. Ibid.

75. The Hamilton Rating Scale for Depression is a 17–item scale administered by a health care professional to assess the severity of depression (Hamilton, M. [1967]. Development of a rating scale for primary depressive illness. *British Journal of Social & Clinical Psychology, 6*, 278–296). Four additional items are often added to the end of the scale (diurnal variation, depersonalization and derealization, paranoid symptoms, and obsessional and compulsive symptoms), and one form has 24 items. High reliability and validity have been reported, but a multi–center evaluation of antidepressant use for depression which employed a randomized, placebo–controlled design found huge variation in Hamilton scores (Roose, P. R.; Sackeim, H. A. [2004]. Antidepressant pharmacotherapy in the treatment of depression in the very old: A randomized, placebo–controlled trial. *American Journal of Psychiatry, 161*, 2050–2059).

76. In January 2003 after its patent had expired, Eli Lilly did receive approval for Prozac use among 7–17 year olds for Major Depressive Disorder and Obsessive–Compulsive Disorder. Available on the web at http://www.fda.gov/bbs/topics/ANSWERS/2003/ANS01187.html.

77. The FDA mission statement is available on the web at http://www.fda.gov/opacom/morechoices/mission.html.

Chapter 10 — Physical Side Effects of Antidepressants

1. Baldessarini, R. (Oct. 16, 1998). Keynote address, "Psychopharmacology: Where have we been; Where are we; Where are we going?" Massachusetts General Hospital/ Harvard Medical School Conference on psychopharmacology in Glenmullen, J. (2000). *Prozac Backlash*, New York: Simon & Schuster, p. 21.

2. *Physicians' Desk Reference* (2004), 58th ed. Montvale, NJ: Thomson PDR, p. 2298.

3. Extein, I. (1978). Methylphenidate–induced choreoathetosis. *American Journal of Psychiatry, 135*, 252–253 in Heinrich, T. W. (2002). A case report of methylphenidate–induced dyskinesia. *Primary Care Companion to the Journal of Clinical Psychiatry, 4*, 158–159.

4. Weiner, W. J. & Sanchez–Ramos, J. Movement disorders and dopaminomimetic stimulant drugs in Lang, A. E. & Weiner, W. J., eds. (1992). *Drug Induced Movement Disorders*. Mount Kisco, NY: Futura Publishing, pp. 315–337 in Heinrich, T. W. (2002). A case report of methylphenidate–induced dyskinesia. *Primary Care Companion to the Journal of Clinical Psychiatry, 4*, 158–159.

5. Heinrich (ibid.).

6. Klawans, H. L. & Margolin, D. I. (1975). Amphetamine–induced dopaminergic hypersensitivity in guinea pigs: Implications in psychosis and human movement disorders. *Archives of General Psychiatry, 32*, 725–732; Klawans, H. L.; Crossett, P. & Dana, N. (1975). Effect of chronic amphetamine exposure on stereotyped behavior: Implications for pathogenesis of l–dopa–induced dyskinesias. *Advances in Neurology, 9*, 105–112; Costall, B.; Naylor, R. J. & Pinder, R. M. (1975). Dyskinetic phenomena caused by the intrastriatal

injection of phenylethylamine, phenylpiperazine, tetrahydroisoquinoline and tetrahydron-aphthalene derivatives in the guinea pig. *European Journal of Pharmacology, 31*, 94–109. This last study found that it was phenylethylamine, whose pharmacological properties are most similar to amphetamine, which caused "the most conspicuous dyskinesias."

7.   Varley, C. K.; Vincent, J., et al. (2001). Emergence of tics in children with attention deficit hyperactivity disorder treated with stimulant medications. *Comprehensive Psychiatry, 42*, 228–233.

8.   Morgan, J. C.; Winter, W. C. & Wooten, G. F. (2004). Amphetamine–induced chorea in attention deficit–hyperactivity disorder. *Movement Disorders, 19*, 840–842.

9.   A study of sexual dysfunction problems among antidepressant users concluded that "physicians consistently underestimated the prevalence of antidepressant–associated sexual dysfunction. Rates of sexual dysfunction ranged from 36%–43% among users of Remeron and Effexor. Among those identified as least likely to develop sexual dysfunction, 7%–30% developed problems" (Clayton, A. H.; Pradko, J. F., et al. [2002]. Prevalence of sexual dysfunction among newer antidepressants. *Journal of Clinical Psychiatry, 63*, 357–366, p. 357).

10.   Young, A. H. & Currie, A. (1997). Physicians' knowledge of antidepressant withdrawal effects: A survey. *Journal of Clinical Psychiatry, 58* (Suppl. 7), 28–30.

11.   Tinsley, J. A.; Shadid, G. E., et al. (1998). A survey of family physicians and psychiatrists: Psychotropic prescribing practices and educational needs. *General Hospital Psychiatry, 20*, 360–367.

12.   Dording, C. M. & Mischoulon, D. (2002). The pharmacologic management of SSRI–induced side effects: A survey of psychiatrists. *Annals of Clinical Psychiatry, 14*, 143–147.

13.   Hallberg, P. & Sjoblom, V. (2005). The use of selective serotonin reuptake inhibitors during pregnancy and breast–feeding: A review and clinical aspects. *Journal of Clinical Psychopharmacology, 25*, 59–73. Most antidepressants carry warnings against their use if nursing.

14.   Sleath, B. & Shih, Y. C. (2003). Sociological influences on antidepressant prescribing. *Social Science & Medicine, 56*, 1335–1344.

15.   Swartz, C. M. (June 1, 2004). Knowing that we don't know. *Psychiatric Times, 21*, 53–54.

16.   A study comparing prescribing patterns among 174 general practices found some practices prescribe six times as many antidepressants as other practices (Hansen, D. G.; Sondergaard, J., et al. [2003]. Antidepressant drug use in general practice: Inter–practice variation and association with practice characteristics. *European Journal of Clinical Pharmacology, 59*, 143–149). Even greater differences were found for prescribing rates for new drugs in a Canadian study. See Tamblyn, R; McLeod, P., et al. (2003). Physician and practice characteristics associated with the early utilization of new prescription drugs. *Medical Care, 41*, 895–908.

17.   Brambilla, P.; Cipriani, A., et al. (2005). Side–effect profile of fluoxetine in comparison with other SSRIs, tricyclic and newer antidepressants: A meta–analysis of clinical trial data. *Pharmacopsychiatry, 38*, 69–77.

18.   Damsa, C.; Bumb, A., et al. (2004). Dopamine–dependent side effects of selective serotonin reuptake inhibitors: A clinical review. *Journal of Clinical Psychiatry, 65*, 1064–1068; Caley, C. F. (1997). Extrapyramidal reactions and the selective serotonin–reuptake inhibitors. *Annals of Pharmacotherapy, 31*, 1481–1489; DiRocco, A.; Brannan, T., et al. (1998). Sertraline induced parkinsonism: A case report and an in–vivo study of the effect of sertraline on dopamine metabolism. *Journal of Neural Transmission, 105*,

247–251; Arai, M. (2003). Parkinsonism associated with a serotonin and noradrenaline reuptake inhibitor, milnacipran. *Journal of Neurology, Neurosurgery, and Psychiatry, 74,* 137–138; Lambert, M. T.; Trutia, C. & Petty, F. (1998). Extrapyramidal adverse effects associated with sertraline. *Progress in Neuro–psychopharmacology & Biological Psychiatry, 22,* 741–748; Anand, K. S.; Prasad, A., et al. (1999). Fluoxetine–induced tremors. *Journal of the Association of Physicians of India, 47,* 651–652; Bates, G. D. & Khin–Maung–Zaw, F. (1998). Movement disorder with fluoxetine. *Journal of the American Academy of Child & Adolescent Psychiatry, 37,* 14–15.

19. Sackner–Bernstein, J. D.; Kowalski, M., et al. (2005). Short–term risk of death after treatment with nesiritide for decompensated heart failure. *JAMA, 293,* 1900–1905.

20. The tables listing adverse events do not indicate how long the trials lasted. That appears under "CLINICAL TRIALS: Major Depressive Disorder."

21. See the package insert (PI) or the *Physicians' Desk Reference* (*PDR*) for this information. (I used both in order to compare the older *PDR* information with the newest PI information. They are identical.) Three percent of the patients on placebo also developed tremors (*Physicians' Desk Reference* [2004], 58th ed. Montvale, NJ: Thomson PDR, p. 1843).

22. Ibid., p. 2693. As in the Prozac trials, 3% of patients on placebo also developed tremors.

23. Kalia, M; O'Callaghan, J. P., et al. (2000). Comparative study of fluoxetine, sibutramine, sertraline and dexfenfluramine on the morphology of sertonergic nerve terminals using serotonin immunohistochemistry. *Brain Research, 858,* 92–105. The five damaged brain regions were "the frontal and occipital cortex, hippocampus, superior and inferior colliculi" (p. 101) for both Prozac and Zoloft.

24. Linazasoro, G. (2000). Worsening of Parkinson's disease by citalopram. *Parkinsonism & Related Disorders, 6,* 111–113; Steur, E. N. (1993). Increase of Parkinson disability after fluoxetine medication. *Neurology, 43,* 211–213.

25. Bottcher, J. (1975). Morphology of the basal ganglia in Parkinson's disease. *Acta Neurologica Scandinavica Supplementum, 62,* 1–87.

26. Szeszko, P. R.; MacMillan, S., et al. (2004). Amygdala volume reductions in pediatric patients with obsessive–compulsive disorder treated with paroxetine: Preliminary findings. *Neuropsychopharmacology, 29,* 826–832.

27. Actually, the effect of Prozac on dopamine levels was reported before Prozac was even released to the American people. See Kelly, E.; Jenner, P. & Marsden, C. D. (1985). Evidence that [3H] dopamine is taken up and released from nondopaminergic nerve terminals in the rat substantia nigra in vitro. *Journal of Neurochemistry, 45,* 137–144. Also see Porras, G; DeDeurwaerdere, P., et al. (2003). Conditional involvement of striatal serotonin3 receptors in the control of in vivo dopamine outflow in the rat striatum. *European Journal of Neuroscience, 17,* 771–781; DeDeurwaerdere, P; L'hirondel, M., et al. (1997). Serotonin stimulation of 5–HT4 receptors indirectly enhances in vivo dopamine release in the rat striatum. *Journal of Neurochemistry, 68,* 195–203; Dziedzicka–Wasylewska, M. & Solich, J. (2004). Neuronal cell lines transfected with the dopamine D2 receptor gene promoter as a model for studying the effects of antidepressant drugs. *Brain Research.Molecular Brain Research, 128,* 75–82. In theory dopamine release by antidepressants should lessen Parkinson's disease symptoms. (It has been suggested that Parkinson's disease patients take antidepressants in hopes of preventing an increase in symptoms.) See Falkenburger, B. H.; Barstow, K. L. & Mintz, I. M. (2001). Dendrodendritic inhibition through reversal of dopamine transport. *Science, 293,* 2465–2470. However, as already noted, the theory and reality do not seem to match since antidepressants increase symptoms in those with Parkinson's disease.

28. The FDA has a website which describes the drug approval process: http://www.fda.gov/fdac/features/2002/402_drug.html. Their site states that Phase 2 studies use "from a few dozen to about 300" subjects and that a Phase 3 study "usually ranges from several hundred to about 3,000 people." Most trials have sample sizes that are smaller than the high end numbers suggested by the FDA.

29. These provisions are part of the FDA Modernization Acts of 1997. The registry went online in February 2000 and can be seen at http://www.clinicaltrials.gov. The Pharmaceutical Research and Manufacturers of America (PhRMA) which is the industry's lobbying association sent a letter to the National Institutes of Health Data Bank with its recommendations for how the law should be implemented ("PhRMA Recommended Approach to Implementing FDA Modernization Act §113") which suggested that no reporting of trial results be required for Phase 1, 2, and 4 trials. This letter is available on the web at http://www.phrma.org/issues/fda/fdama/5–28–98. cfm.

30. Vedantam, S. (July 6, 2004). Drugmakers prefer silence on test data; Firms violate U.S. law not registering trials. *Washington Post*, A.01. The comments were made by Abbey Meyers, the president of the National Organization of Rare Disorders.

31. Ibid.

32. When the drug company's defiance became publicized, Eliot Spitzer brought a lawsuit against GlaxoSmithKline which makes Paxil and then began an investigation of Forest Laboratories, maker of Celexa and Lexapro, in hopes of forcing "greater industry disclosure of clinical trial findings." See Meier, B. (Aug. 4, 2004). Spitzer asks drug maker for off–label use material. *NY Times*, C.2.

33. Cotterchio, M; Kreiger, N., et al. (2000). Antidepressant medication use and breast cancer risk. *American Journal of Epidemiology, 151*, 951–957.

34. Moorman, P. G.; Grubber, J. M., et al. (2003). Antidepressant medications and their association with invasive breast cancer and carcinoma in situ of the breast. *Epidemiology, 14*, 307–314; Steingart, A.; Cotterchio, M., et al. (2003). Antidepressant medication use and breast cancer risk: A case–control study. *International Journal of Epidemiology, 32*, 961–966; Bahl, S.; Cotterchio, M. & Krieger, N. (2003). Use of antidepressant medication and the possible association with breast cancer risk: A review. *Psychotherapy & Psychosomatics, 72*, 185–194.

35. Wang, P. S.; Walker, A. M., et al. (2001). Antidepressant use and the risk of breast cancer: A non–association. *Journal of Clinical Epidemiology, 54*, 728–734. For a nonsignificant non–Hodgkin's lymphoma risk, see the following: Bahl, S.; Cotterchio, M, et al. (2004). Antidepressant medication use and non–Hodgkin's lymphoma risk: No association. *American Journal of Epidemiology, 160*, 566–575.

36. Steingart, A. B. & Cotterchio, M. (1995). Do antidepressants cause, promote, or inhibit cancers? *Journal of Clinical Epidemiology, 48*, 1407–1412; Sternbach, H. (2003). Are antidepressants carcinogenic? A review of preclinical and clinical studies. *Journal of Clinical Psychiatry, 64*, 1153–1162. Some animal studies also found no link or even protective effects. This is still years away from being fully settled.

37. The Prozac adverse event is listed as "impotence." The Zoloft adverse event is "ejaculation failure."

38. Gregorian, R. S. & Golden, K. A. (2002). Antidepressant–induced sexual dysfunction. *Annals of Pharmacotherapy, 36*, 1577–1589.

39. Survey questions can be phrased in ways to have either high or low affirmative answers. It has often been demonstrated that changing a single word in a question can yield vastly different results. For example, one research team showed two groups of matched subjects a video of two cars involved in a minor accident. One group was asked, "About how

fast were the cars going when they 'smashed into' each other?" The other group was asked the same question, but "smashed into" was replaced with "hit" (or collided, bumped or contacted). A week later they were asked if they saw broken glass. Only 14% of the "hit" subjects thought they did, but 32% of "smashed into" subjects saw broken glass though there was no broken glass (Loftus, E. F. & Palmer, J. C. [1974]. Reconstruction of automobile destruction: An example of the interaction between language and memory. *Journal of Verbal Learning & Verbal Behavior, 13*, 585–589).

40. Labbate, L. A.; Croft, H. A. & Oleshansky, M. A. (2003). Antidepressant–related erectile dysfunction: Management via avoidance, switching antidepressants, antidotes, and adaptation. *Journal of Clinical Psychiatry, 64* (Suppl. 10), 11–19, p. 11. Also see the following study for rates (approximately 32%) in women in a study of 110 women treated with SSRI antidepressants: Shen, W. W. & Hsu, J. H. (1995). Female sexual side effects associated with selective serotonin reuptake inhibitors: A descriptive clinical study of 33 patients. *International Journal of Psychiatry in Medicine, 25*, 239–248.

41. Montejo–Gonzalez, A. L. & Llorca, G. (1997). SSRI–induced sexual dysfunction: Fluoxetine, paroxetine, sertraline, and fluvoxamine in a prospective, multicenter, and descriptive clinical study of 344 patients. *Journal of Sex & Marital Therapy, 23*, 176–194.

42. DeAbajo, F. J.; Rodriguez, L. A. G. & Montero, D. (1999). Association between selective serotonin reuptake inhibitors and upper gastrointestinal bleeding: Population based case–control study. *British Medical Journal, 319*, 1106–1109. Also see Dalton, S. O.; Johansen, C., et al. (2003). Use of selective serotonin reuptake inhibitors and risk of upper gastrointestinal tract bleeding: A population–based cohort study. *Archives of Internal Medicine, 163*, 59–64.

43. The effect is described with other related terms also. These include naproxen–induced acute gastroduodenal injury, naproxen–induced mucosal injury, naproxen–induced gastric mucosal damage, and naproxen–induced blood loss. Non–steroidal anti–inflammatory drugs (NSAIDs) cause inflammation in the small intestine in 40% to 70% of those taking these drugs long term (Davies, N. M. & Saleh, J. Y. [2000]. Detection and prevention of NSAID–induced enteropathy. *Journal of Pharmacy & Pharmaceutical Sciences, 3*, 137–155).

44. Monster, T. B.; Johnsen, S. P., et al. (2004). Antidepressants and risk of first–time hospitalization for myocardial infarction: A population–based case–control study. *American Journal of Medicine, 117*, 732–737.

45. Cohen, H. W.; Gibson, G. & Alderman, M. H. (2000). Excess risk of myocardial infarction in patients treated with antidepressant medications: Association with use of tricyclic agents. *American Journal of Medicine, 108*, 2–8. Another study found if patients are given low doses of the tricyclic, the heart attack risk can be minimized (Ray, W. A.; Meredith, S, et al. [2004]. Cyclic antidepressants and the risk of sudden cardiac death. *Clinical Pharmacology & Therapeutics, 75*, 234–241).

46. Tata, L. J.; West, J., et al. (2005). General population based study of the impact of tricyclic and selective serotonin reuptake inhibitor antidepressants on the risk of acute myocardial infarction. *Heart, 91*, 465–471.

47. van Dijken, J.; von Knorring, A. L., et al. (1981). [Antidepressive agents can cause dental damages in children and adults.] *Lakartidningen, 78*, 4366–4368.

48. Keene, J. J.; Galasko, G. T. & Land, M. F. (2003). Antidepressant use in psychiatry and medicine: Importance for dental practice. *Journal of the American Dental Association, 134*, 71–79.

49. Little, J. W. (2004). Dental implications of mood disorders. *General Dentistry, 52*, 442–450.

50. The statistics come from Rundegren, J.; van Dijken, J., et al. (1985). Oral conditions in patients receiving long–term treatment with cyclic antidepressant drugs. *Swedish Dental Journal, 9*, 55–64. Newer studies which examine SSRI–antidepressants find this same pattern. For example, see Rindal, D. B.; Rush, W. A., et al. (2005). Antidepressant xerogenic medications and restoration rates. *Community Dentistry & Oral Epidemiology, 33*, 74–80.

51. Warden, S. J.; Robling, A. G., et al. (2005). Inhibition of the serotonin (5–hydroxytryptamine) transporter reduces bone accrual during growth. *Endocrinology, 146*, 685–693.

52. Ansorge, M. S.; Zhou, M., et al. (Oct. 29, 2004). Early–life blockage of the 5–HT transporter alters emotional behavior in adult mice. *Science, 306*, 879–881.

53. Price, J. H. (April 3, 2004). Antidepressant use by preschoolers rising. *Washington Times*, A.01. The statistics are for 2002. More boys (2.3/1,000) than girls (1.4/1,000) were on antidepressants.

54. Esaki, T; Cook, M., et al. (2005). Developmental disruption of serotonin transporter function impairs cerebral responses to whisker stimulation in mice. *Proceedings of the National Academy of Sciences of the United States of America, 102*, 5582–5587.

55. Rice, D. & Barone, S. (2000). Critical periods of vulnerability for the developing nervous system: Evidence from human and animal models. *Environmental Health Perspectives, 108* (Suppl. 3), 511–533.

56. Simon, G. E.; Cunningham, M. L. & Davis, R. L. (2002). Outcomes of prenatal antidepressant exposure. *American Journal of Psychiatry, 159*, 2055–2061.

57. Kallen, B. (2004). Neonate characteristics after maternal use of antidepressants in late pregnancy. *Archives of Pediatric & Adolescent Medicine, 158*, 312–316.

58. Casper, R. C.; Fleisher, B. E., et al. (2003). Follow–up of children of depressed mothers exposed or not exposed to antidepressant drugs during pregnancy. *Journal of Pediatrics, 142*, 402–408.

59. Lucena, M. I.; Carvajal, A., et al. (2003). Antidepressant–induced hepatoxicity associated with the new antidepressants. *Expert Opinion on Drug Safety, 2*, 249–262. Also Carvajal, G–P. A.; Garcia del Pozo, J., et al. (2002). Hepatoxicity associated with the new antidepressants. *Journal of Clinical Psychiatry, 63*, 135–137.

60. Drug manufacturers report rates of approximately 10% to 20% typically. See the package inserts or a *Physicians' Desk Reference.*

61. I think it is a somewhat arbitrary decision to separate "agitation" from "akathisia." Both can have a "can't sit still" effect, and both can be extremely distressful.

62. Fava, M. (2000). Weight gain and antidepressants. *Journal of Clinical Psychiatry, 61* (Suppl. 11), 37–41.

Chapter 11 — Psychological Side Effects of Antidepressants

1. FDA Public Health Advisory (June 30, 2005). Available on the web at http://www.fda.gov/cder/drug/advisory/SSRI200507.htm.

2. The data is that supplied to the FDA and used for FDA–approved labeling. It is available not only from package inserts but also on both the FDA's website and the more easily accessed RxList website (www.rxlist.com). Enter a drug name into the drug–search box on the left. On the next page click on the drug name under the RxList Monographs. Then click on the "side effects, drug interactions" tab.

3. The first three definitions come from the *American Heritage Dictionary of the English Language* (2000), 4th ed. Boston: Houghton Mifflin Company. I recognize that all readers know the definition of the first three terms. However, I felt it would be valuable to examine the definitions in order to be more impacted by their meaning.

4.   Other names applied to this syndrome include SSRI–induced apathy syndrome (Barnhart, W. J.; Maekla, E. H. & Latocha, M. J. [2004]. SSRI–induced apathy syndrome: A clinical review. *Journal of Psychiatric Practice, 10*, 196–199) and SSRI treatment– emergent hypomania (Ramasubbu, R. [2001]. Dose–response relationship of selective sero- tonin reuptake inhibitors treatment–emergent hypomania in depressive disorders. *Acta Psychiatrica Scandinavica, 104*, 236–238) among others.

5.   Garland, E. J. (2001). Amotivational Syndrome linked with SSRI use in youth for the first time. *Brown University Child & Adolescence Psychopharmacology Update, 3*(10): 1, 6–8.

6.   Preda, A.; MacLean, R. W., et al. (2001). Antidepressant–associated mania and psychosis resulting in psychiatry admissions. *Journal of Clinical Psychiatry, 62*, 30–33. In a subsequent study the Department of Psychiatry found that those receiving SSRIs experi- enced a change in blood chemistry which they believed caused the mania or psychosis (Fortunati, F.; Preda, A., et al. [2002].   Plasma catecholamine metabolites in antidepressant–exacerbated mania and psychosis. *Journal of Affective Disorders, 68*, 331–334).

7.   It should be recognized that in many of these trials a large number of volunteers choose to stop participating due to the unpleasant drug side effects. If a company chooses to exclude these subjects or start a second study after a "washout" period, the numbers which will be reported as having agitation will be artificially low.

8.   The lawsuit was brought by the grown children of William and June Forsyth. On March 4, 1993, William Forsyth murdered his wife June and then killed himself.

9.   "Eighty–six, the Court's not going to allow that under 402 and 403. That may be, possibly, relevant regarding punitive damages and we'll take that up later. Eighty–seven, the Court will not allow that, 402 and 403. Eighty–eight, the Court will allow that as far as notice and not for the truth. Eighty–nine, the Court will not allow that. Ninety, the Court will allow. It's a memo from Dr. Beasley." The full transcript of the court proceedings as regards exhibits to be admitted as well as a large body of transcripts from the case have been made available on the web at Dr. Healy's *Let Them Eat Prozac* website.   See http:// www.healyprozac.com/Trials/ Forsyth/Transcripts/default.htm.

10.   A photocopy of the actual document is available online at http://www.healy prozac.com/Trials/CriticalDocs/teammeeting230779.htm.   This document is from the Fluoxetine Project Team minutes of July 23, 1979.

11.   Healy, D. (2004). *Let Them Eat Prozac.* New York: New York University Press.

12.   The documents are found at http://www.healyprozac.com/Trials/CriticalDocs.

13.   Ibid. Fluoxetine Project Team Meeting Minutes, 7–31–1978. Minutes #78–2, p. 2.

14.   That lawsuit is the most famous of the Prozac lawsuits. Known as Fentress v Lilly, the suit involved the case of Joseph Wesbecker who was on medical leave in 1989 when he went to the printing plant where he had worked and killed 8 fellow employees and wounded 12 others before killing himself. A brief account of these events is told by Peter Breggin in his book *The Antidepressant Fact Book* (2001, Cambridge, MA: Perseus). Breggin was the expert witness for the plaintiff. The case went to jury for a judgment, but unbeknownst to Breggin or the judge at that time, Lilly had paid the plaintiff and the plaintiff's lawyers to purposely lose the case in favor of Lilly. For a full account, read John Cornwell's *The Power to Harm* (1996). New York: Viking Press.

15.   *The Guardian* (Oct. 30, 1999). They said it was safe. An article devoted to this subject is found on the web at http://www.guardian.co.uk/weekend/story/0,3605,258000,00 .html.

16. Ibid. In Germany Prozac's brand name is Fluctin. It must be noted that the BGA's warning to the German people which was printed on the drug packaging inserts was issued 14 years before the FDA's warning was finally announced to the American public.

17. Ibid.

18. The warning and the increase in suicide risk can be seen on the FDA's website. See http://www.fda.gov/cder/drug/antidepressants/SSRIPHA200410.htm.

19. 5th page, unnumbered, of the section entitled "Our serotonin aftermath" in Tracy, A. B. (2001). *Prozac: Panacea or Pandora?* Salt Lake City: Cassia Publications. Note: The "PZ" numbers she gives are all Eli Lilly & Co. documents released as a result of law-suits brought against Lilly. Vickery and Waldner, a Houston law firm, has put many of these documents on the web at http://www.justiceseekers.com. The easiest way to locate specific documents (e.g., PZ 878 1383) is to enter the document number in Google's search engine.

20. Tracy, p. 55.

21. Ibid.

22. Kessler, D. A. (1993). Introducing MedWatch. *JAMA, 269*, 2765–2768.

23. Teicher, M. H.; Glod, C. & Cole, J. O. (1990). Emergence of intense suicidal pre-occupation during fluoxetine treatment. *American Journal of Psychiatry, 147*, 207–210.

24. Teicher, M. H.; Glod, C. A. & Cole, J. O. (1990). Dr. Teicher and associates reply. *American Journal of Psychiatry, 147*, 1692–1693.

25. Papp, L. A. & Gorman, J. M. (1990). Letters to the editor: Suicidal preoccupation during fluoxetine treatment. *American Journal of Psychiatry, 147*, 1380.

26. Miller, R. A. (1990). Discussion of fluoxetine and suicidal tendencies. *American Journal of Psychiatry, 147*, 1571.

27. Grady, D. (Oct. 1990). Wonder drug/killer drug. *American Health, 9*, 60–65.

28. See, for example, Tollefson, G. D.; Fawcett, J., et al. (1993). Evaluation of suici-dality during pharmacologic treatment of mood and nonmood disorders. *Annals of Clinical Psychiatry, 5*, 209–224. This study was a double–blind, placebo–controlled investigation. How could it come to the opposite conclusion of other double–blind, placebo–controlled investigations? I do not know. All the authors were Eli Lilly employees.

29. Harris, G. (Sept. 14, 2004). FDA links drugs to being suicidal, *NY Times*, A.1.

30. These cases can never be used to prove an antidepressant–murder link. Obviously, those with the most problems are also more likely to have seen a psychiatrist or a physician about those problems and to have a prescription written. Also, in the case of Kip Kinkel, he was off of Prozac when he murdered his parents and classmates. The only way to determine if there is a link is to carry out well–designed experimental studies which measure antide-pressant use and agitation, suicide ideation, confusion, and so forth. Studies have found anti-depressants cause no negative changes in all these. It then involves speculation as to whether or not someone who is emotionally agitated or confused is more apt to commit acts of vio-lence.

31. Breggin writes in simple, clear language. As an expert witness in numerous trials, he has had the advantage of being able to see documents not made public by drug manufac-turers. As regards this subject, his most helpful books include *Toxic Psychiatry* (1991), *Prozac: Panacea or Pandora* (1994), *Talking Back to Prozac* (1994), *Brain–Disabling Treatments in Psychiatry* (1997), and *Your Drug May Be Your Problem* (1999).

32. FDA Public Health Advisory (June 30, 2005). Available on the web at http://www .fda.gov/cder/drug/advisory/SSRI200507.htm.

Chapter 12 — Fooled, Fooled and Fooled Again

1. Baughman, F. (May 24, 2001). Source: Baughman's "adhdfraud" website commenting on David Kaiser article. Available online at http://www.adhdfraud.org/commentary/11–07–00–2.htm.

2. The book was published posthumously in 1553. My source is the excellent collection by Richard Hunter and Ida Macalpine (1963), *Three Hundred Years of Psychiatry, 1535–1860* (London: Oxford University Press, pp. 5–6).

3. My "translation" is not exact. The exact and slightly fuller quote (using the original spellings) is as follows: "I beyng advertysed of these pageauntes, and beynge sent unto and requyred by very devout relygyouse folke, to take some other order wyth hym caused him as he came wanderyng by my dore, to be taken by the constables and bounden to a tre in the strete byfore the whole towne, and there they stryped hym with roddys therfore tyl he waxed wery and somwhat lenger. And it appered well that hys remembraunce was good inough, save yt it wente about in grasynge tyll it was beten home. For he could than very well reherse hys fawtes hym selfe, and speke and trete very well, and promyse to do afterwarde as well. And veryly god be thanked I here none harme of hym now."

4. Cited in Zilboorg, G. (1941). *A History of Medical Psychology.* New York: W. W. Norton & Co., p. 69. The irony of the late Middle Ages is that as the humanists began to reject religious dogma and embrace the scholars of ancient Greece and Rome, it became dangerous even to question the wisdom of the Greek and Roman fathers. As Galileo learned more than once, experimentation was seldom even tolerated—acceptance of the Greek and Roman fathers' ideas was expected. Thus, it should not be surprising to see the medical texts of this period continue to accept and pass on these views.

5. Again, I have "translated" the Middle English. The passage is also found in Hunter and Macalpine's *Three Hundred Years of Psychiatry, 1535–1860* (London: Oxford University Press, p. 15). Andrew Boorde was a physician, monk and bishop of Chichester. His advice appears in his second medical book, *The Seconde Boke of the Brevyary of Health, Named the Extravagantes* published in 1552.

6. Cited in Zilboorg, G. (1941). *A History of Medical Psychology.* New York: W. W. Norton & Co., p. 261.

7. Ibid., p. 287.

8. Reil's work is *Rhapsodieen über die Anwendung der psyuchischen Curmethode auf Geisteszerrüttungen.* See G. Zilboorg's (1941) *A History of Medical Psychology* (Note 5) for an informative treatment of the subject.

9. Bethlehem (Bethlem) is reported by Zilboorg (ibid.) to be the oldest hospital in Europe which has been in continuous service. Daniel Hack Tuke reports one penny was charged for any members of the public who desired to visit and be so amused. The "Act for Regulating Madhouses" was approved by Parliament in 1774. The practice did not extend beyond that date. Though Bethlehem is the origin of the institution's name, in time Bethlem was the proper noun used even on official documents. The proper noun "Bedlam" was never made official though it was the name by which the institution became known to the people of London in time.

10. O'Donoghue, E. G. (1913). *The Story of Bethlehem Hospital From Its Foundation in 1247*, p. 237 in Jones, K. (1972). *A History of the Mental Health Services.* London: Routledge & Kegan Paul, pp. 14–15.

11. The words are those of Dr. William Cullen who was also Benjamin Rush's instructor at Edinburgh. See Deutsch, A. (1949) *The Mentally Ill in America*, 2nd ed. New York: Columbia University Press, p. 81.

12. Select Committee on Madhouse (1815), pp. 93 & 95 in Scull, A.; MacKenzie, C. & Hervey, N. (1996). *Masters of Bedlam.* Princeton, NJ: Princeton University Press, p. 3.

13. For a good discussion of Hippocrates' views see Zilboorg, G. (1941). *A History of Medical Psychology.* New York: W. W. Norton & Co., especially pp. 41–51. For the fact that Hippocrates recognized the influence of purely mental or emotional states on the mind, see p. 46.

14. Ducey, C. & Simon, B. (1975). Ancient Greece and Rome (pp. 1–38) in Howells, J. G., ed. *World History of Psychiatry.* New York: Brunner/Mazel.

15. Burton, Robert (1821). *The Anatomy of Melancholy.* Faulkner, T. C.; Kessling, N. K. & Blair, R. L., eds. (1989–94), 3 vols. Oxford: Clarendon Press.

16. Cotton was not the first to advocate the removal of infected teeth. As he noted in a 1923 article, recovery from mental disorders following extraction of infected teeth was reported as early as 1875 by a British psychiatrist named Savage. "The full significance of this report, of course, was not realised [*sic*] at the time, for it had been recognised [*sic*], an entirely different history of the care and treatment of mental disorders during the last century would have been written" (p. 434). He further noted that a British doctor, William Hunter, published papers on the relationship of chronic sepsis and mental disorders in 1900 and 1910 and an American doctor, Henry Upson, published "Nervous disorders due to the teeth" and "Dementia Praecox caused by dental infection" in 1907 and 1909, respectively (Cotton, H. A. [1923]. The relation of chronic sepsis to the so–called functional mental disorders. *Journal of Mental Science, 69,* 434–462). In a 1910 paper Henry Upson discussed his experience in studying dental infections, especially decay occurring under fillings, in relation to mental health and declared without equivocation, "A study of their relations with various nervous and mental conditions extending over almost four years has shown me that they are often disastrous to nervous and mental health" (Upson, H. S. [1910]. Serious mental disturbances caused by painless dental lesions. *American Quarterly of Roentgenology, 2,* 223–243, p. 223).

17. Cotton, H. A. (1922). The etiology and treatment of the so–called functional psychoses: Summary of results upon the experience of four years. *American Journal of Psychiatry,* 157–194, p. 183.

18. Ibid., p. 184.

19. Ibid., p. 185.

20. Cotton, H. A. (1923). The relation of chronic sepsis to the so–called functional mental disorders. *Journal of Mental Science, 69,* 434–462, p. 455.

21. Dr. Cotton reported that over a two–year period full colectomies were done in 133 cases and resulted in 33 recoveries and 44 deaths. Partial resection of the colon "was done in 148 cases, with 44 recoveries and 59 deaths" (ibid., p. 457).

22. Cotton, H. A. (1921; 1980 reprint). *The Defective, Delinquent, and Insane: The Relation of Focal Infection to Their Causation, Treatment, and Prevention.* Princeton, NJ: Princeton University Press, p. v.

23. Cotton, H. A. (1923). The relation of chronic sepsis to the so–called functional mental disorders. *Journal of Mental Science, 69,* 434–462, p. 461.

24. Cotton, H. A. (1922). The etiology and treatment of the so–called functional psychoses. *American Journal of Psychiatry, 2,* 157–210 in Valenstein, E. S. (1986). *Great and Desperate Cures.* New York: Basic Books, p. 41.

25. Kopeloff, N. & Kirby, G. H. (1923). Focal infection and mental disease. *American Journal of Psychiatry, 3,* 149–197 in ibid., p. 42.

26. A typical patient would be treated for about 40 days. Some of the notes taken by Sakel from days 14 and 15 of the treatment are enlightening. "November 23, 1934

(Fourteenth day of treatment.).... He received 115 units of insulin at 6:30 a.m. At 11 a.m. the patient was perspiring profusely and grimacing. He appeared to be completely unresponsive to his surroundings. He had a fixed, vacant gaze and did not respond to questions or commands. Soon afterwards, the patient grew quite disturbed, threw himself about the bed, and tossed his head from side to side, crying, 'Where's Dr. S?'.... Finally, he grew comatose and somnolent. He lay perfectly quiet in bed, bathed completely in perspiration, with half–closed eyes. His eyes moved slowly from side to side, but more often turned upward. His pupils were somewhat contracted and fixed. The corneal reflex was absent on both sides. He showed a left facial weakness.... His extremities were limp and flaccid to passive movement.... The patient was left in this condition until 1 p.m. His breathing at this time had become labored and stertorous. At 1 p.m. the shock was terminated by tube feeding.... November 24, 1934. (Fifteenth day of treatment.) The patient was given 120 units of insulin at 7:30 a.m. He perspired mildly at 10 a.m. and showed a tremor of the outstretched fingers. When questioned he said that he was sleepy. Soon after he grew more somnolent and finally went into coma. He was tube–fed at 2 p.m. Soon afterwards, the patient began to talk in a definitely childish way. 'I'd like some milk and some sugar and some applesauce,' he said. 'Then my head will be clear again.' Half an hour later the patient talked quite normally. He laughed and said it was all a funny business and he only wished he could remember what he had been talking about. He added that he was still 'in a bit of a fog.' When the patient was conducted to another bed, his gait was unsteady and atactic. 'I'm still a bit shaky,' the patient remarked. Later the patient said he still felt rather tired, but that he felt better than yesterday. The patient was quiet and cooperative all day" (Sakel, M. [1937]. A new treatment of schizophrenia. *American Journal of Psychiatry, 93*, 829–841, pp. 837–838).

27. Ibid., p. 829.

28. Sakel, M. (1958). *Schizophrenia*. New York: Philosophical Library, pp. 317–318.

29. Accornero, F. (1938). Experimental histopathological researches on insulin shock. *American Journal of Psychiatry, 94* (Suppl.), 130–133; Katzenelbogen, S. (1940). A critical appraisal of the "shock therapies" in the major psychoses, II—insulin. *Psychiatry, 3*, 211–228.

30. Sakel, M. (1958). *Schizophrenia*, New York: Philosophical Library, p. 334.

31. Bourne, H. (1953). The insulin myth. *Lancet, 2*, 964–968, p. 968.

32. Hoff, H. (1958). Foreword in Sakel, M. *Schizophrenia*. New York: Philosophical Library, pp. v, vii.

33. Bourne, H. (1953). The insulin myth. *Lancet, 2, 964–968*. Bourne argued that the extra attention given insulin therapy patients might explain the success reported with this treatment by some studies. He noted a study using sulphosine therapy that had a recovery rate of 35–40% in 1932 but a recovery rate of only 15–20% in 1939. The fact that the same therapy in the same hospital saw a recovery rate drop by half suggests a diminishing of staff enthusiasm. The same principle might explain a degree of the success for any treatment strategy.

34. Mowbray, R.M. (1959). Historical aspects of electric convulsive therapy. *Scottish Medical Journal, 4*, 373–378.

35. Burrow, S. G. (1828). *Commentaries on the Causes, Forms, Symptoms and Treatment, Moral and Medical, of Insanity.* London: T & G Underwood, pp. 656–657. Cited by Abrams, R. (2002). *Electroconvulsive Therapy*, 4th ed. Oxford University Press, who cites Sandford, J. L. (1966). Electric and convulsive treatments in psychology. *Diseases of the Nervous System, 27*, 333–338.

36. Meduna, L. (1985). Autobiography, Part 1. *Convulsive Therapy, 1*, 43–57 cited in Abrams, R. (2002). *Electroconvulsive Therapy*, 4th ed. Oxford University Press, p. 5.

37. Kalinowsky, L. B. & Hippius, H. *Pharmacological, Convulsive and Other Somatic Treatments in Psychiatry.* New York: Grune & Stratton, 1969, p. 161.

38. Ibid.

39. Reports on how quickly the patient responds to metrazol vary. The 3 to 30 seconds is reported by Kalinowsky and Hippius though they note "quick injection is necessary to provoke a convulsion with a minimal amount" (ibid., p. 161).

40. Katzenelbogen, S. (1940). A critical appraisal of the "shock therapies" in the major psychoses and psychoneuroses, III—convulsive therapy. *Psychiatry, 3,* 409–420, p. 414.

41. Polatin, Friedman, Harris, et al. in ibid., p. 414.

42. Ibid., p. 412.

43. Ibid., p. 419.

44. Ibid., p. 420.

45. Freeman, W. (1940). Brain–damaging therapeutics. *Diseases of the Nervous System, 2,* 83 in Whitaker, R. (2002). *Mad in America.* New York: Perseus, p. 96.

46. As pointed out by virtually all histories of ECT, electric shock to the brain has been advocated and practiced for at least 2,000 years. The Roman Emperor Claudius (10 B.C.–A.D. 54) suffered headaches which were treated by placing an electric eel against his head. Galan (130?–200?), the "second father of medicine," used electric fish for treating gout and other ills. But the heyday of electrical stimulation for health came in the 18th century. Concerning its use for treating mental problems John Wesley wrote in his 1760 work *The Desideratum,* "I doubt not but more nervous disorders would be cured in one year by this single remedy than the whole English Materia Medica will cure by the end of the century" (Wesley, J. [1760]. *The Desideratum: Or, Electricity Made Plain and Useful by a Lover of Mankind and of Common Sense.* London: W. Flexney. Reprinted [1992] by The United Methodist Publishing House: Nashville, TN. Quote cited in Bradon, S. The history of shock treatment in Palmer, R. L, ed. [1981]. *Electroconvulsive Therapy: An Appraisal.* New York: Oxford University Press, pp. 3–10, p. 3).

47. Brandon, S. The history of shock treatment in Palmer, R. L., ed. (1981). *Electroconvulsive Therapy: An Appraisal.* New York: Oxford University Press, pp. 3–10.

48. Cerletti, U. (1950). Old and new information about electroshock. *American Journal of Psychiatry, 107,* 87–94, p. 88.

49. Minor details differ slightly according to the source used. I am using Cerletti's own account (ibid.) as well as that of ECT's leading proponent, Dr. Richard Abrams whose book *Electroconvulsive Therapy* is currently in its fourth edition. Several other sources were also consulted. Cerletti's own account is generally relied upon where minor details differ.

50. Brandon, S. The history of shock therapy. In Palmer, R. L., ed. (1981). *Electroconvulsive Therapy: An Appraisal.* New York: Oxford University Press, p. 9.

51. Ibid.

52. Ibid.

53. Ibid.

54. The article, A new method of shock therapy "The electroshock," appeared in Italian. Cerletti, U. & Bini, L. (1938). Un nuevo metodo di shockterapie, *Bollettino Accademia Medica Roma, 64,* 136–138.

55. Ibid.

56. Shorter, E. (1997). *A History of Psychiatry: From the Era of the Asylum to the Age of Prozac.* New York: John Wiley & Sons. Cited by Shorter, E. (2004). The history of ECT: Unsolved mysteries. *Psychiatric Times, 21,* 93, 95–96.

57. Ibid.

58. Ibid.

59. Ibid., p. 95.

60. Many reasons have been cited. Shorter (May 2004) considers this decline a reflection of a combination of the counter–culture sentiments of the 1960s, the popularity of Ken
Kesey's *One Flew Over the Cuckoo's Nest* (1962), and the efforts against psychiatry led by
the Church of Scientology. It was the film version of Kesey's book (released in 1975) which
had the most dramatic effect on the public's views about ECT. (Every semester when discussing ECT students ask, "Have you seen the movie 'One Flew Over the Cuckoo's Nest?'"
It is likely my students' primary source of prior information about ECT.) In 1982 the Board
of Supervisors for Berkeley, CA, passed an ordinance making the use of ECT in city hospitals a crime punishable by fine or imprisonment or both. The citizens of Berkeley voted to
approve the ordinance in November 1982. The courts later overturned the ordinance.

61. The full report is available on the web at http://consensus.nih.gov/cons/
051/051_statement.htm. The quote is found in the statement's introduction.

62. The 2001 report like the 1990 report encourages right unilateral electrode placement (placing both electrodes on the right side of the head) rather than bilateral electrode
placement as the former has been reported to cause fewer cognitive losses, less confusion following treatment and less effect on the patient's speech. However, Max Fink, a leading ECT
proponent, has criticized this since it requires raising the electrical charge to a level that is
six times that required of bilateral ECT. "Neither the safety nor the merits of this procedure
compel its use" (Fink, M. [2002]. The practice of electroconvulsive therapy:
Recommendations for treatment, training, and privileging, 2nd ed., book review. *Psychiatric
Services, 53*, 1040–1041, p. 1041).

63. Glass, R. M. (2001). Electroconvulsive therapy: Time to bring it out of the shadows. *Journal of the American Medical Association, 285*, 1346–1348.

64. The 1986 number comes from a National Institutes of Mental Health survey. The
total number of patients receiving ECT in 1986 was found to be 36,558, hugely lower than
58,667 patients found to have received this treatment in 1975. The 1995 treatment estimate
is based on 8.2 treatments per patient, the number of patients being the estimate provided by
Hermann, et al. For Hermann's data or more on these estimates see Abrams, R. (2002).
Electroconvulsive Therapy, 4th ed. Oxford: Oxford University Press, pp. 13–14.

65. Dodge, M. M. (1943). *Hans Brinker or The Silver Skates*. New York: Charles
Scribner's Sons, pp. 220–221.

66. Ibid., p. vii.

67. As a matter of interest I will note that damaging one frontal lobe had no effect on
post–surgical results. However, if both lobes were damaged, the chimps manifested a "complete inability to respond even after delays as short as five seconds" (Jacobsen, C. F.; Wolfe,
J. B. & Jackson, T. A. [1935]. An experimental analysis of the functions of the frontal association areas in primates. *Journal of Nervous & Mental Disease, 82*, 1–14, p. 9).

68. Ibid.

69. Ibid., p. 10.

70. The question is as it was remembered by John Fulton in his book on frontal lobotomy (Fulton, J. F. [1949]. *Functional Localization in Relation to Frontal Lobotomy*. New
York: Oxford University Press, pp. 63–64).

71. Macdonald Tow surveyed the research on brain injuries resulting from war (ch. 4),
tumors (ch. 5), experimental studies with animals (ch. 7), as well as lobotomy. See Tow, P.
M. (1955). *Personality Changes Following Frontal Leucotomy*. London: Oxford University
Press.

72. Ibid. See especially chapters 10–25 (part 2 of the book) which are a careful study of a number of intellectual (psychological) aspects of lobotomies.

73. I am not overlooking Dr. Richard Brickner's papers discussing the function of the frontal lobes. One of his papers was referenced by Jacobsen in his Jan. 8, 1935, presentation to the New York Neurological Society covering the same work presented at the London conference which Egas Moniz attended later that year. Dr. Brickner's work involved frontal lobe removal due to a tumor. See Brickner, R. M. (1932). An interpretation of frontal lobe function based on the study of a case of partial frontal lobectomy. *Proceedings of the Association for Research in Nervous & Mental Disease, 13*, 259–351.

74. Stone, J. L. (2001). Dr. Gottlieb Burckhardt—the pioneer of psychosurgery. *Journal of the History of Neurosciences, 10*, 79–92.

75. The basic facts of Egas Moniz's life can be found on the web at http://nobel prize.org/medicine/laureates/1949/moniz–bio.html as well as in standard encyclopedias. More detail can be found in Elliot Valenstein's (1986) *Great and Desperate Cures: The Rise and Fall of Psychosurgery and Other Radical Treatments for Mental Illness*. New York: Basic Books, especially ch. 4.

76. Ibid., p. 103.

77. Egas Moniz did not actually perform the surgery. He had suffered from gout for many years, and his hands were swollen. Neurologist Almeida Lima performed this operation just as he did many others as Egas Moniz's disciple. The best researched accounts of these events are found in Valenstein's *Great and Desperate Cures* (endnote 75) and *Brain Control* (endnote 89). Except for the original sources which are cited, these two works are the basis of the Moniz story. (Many sources contain inaccuracies, including published books by academic researchers. Discrepancies, when investigated, always matched Valenstein's accounts.)

78. Valenstein, E. S. (1986). *Great and Desperate Cures*, New York: Basic Books, p. 107.

79. See the official site for the Nobel Prize from which this phrase is taken at http://nobelprize.org/medicine/laureates/1949/. Also see the article linked to that site by Bengty Jansson, "Controversial Psychosurgery Resulted in Nobel Prize," in which justification for the award is suggested. "I see no reason for indignation at what was done in the 1940s as at that time there were no other alternatives!"

80. Valenstein, E. S. (1986). *Great and Desperate Cures*. New York: Basic Books, p. 112.

81. This statement is based on the fact that the Paris lectures, when published, revealed that the summary of the first 20 cases on which Egas Moniz was reporting was already "in press" (ibid., p. 113).

82. Ibid.

83. Freeman, W. (1936). Book review: Tentatives opératories dans le traitement de certaines psychoses. *Archives of Neurology & Psychiatry, 36*, 1413.

84. Freeman, W. (n.d.). History of psychosurgery. Unpublished manuscript in Valenstein, E. S. (1986). *Great and Desperate Cures*. New York: Basic Books, p. 142.

85. Freeman, W. & Watts, J. (1936–1937). Prefrontal lobotomy in agitated depression: Report of a case. *Medical Annals of the District of Columbia, 5–6*, 326–328 in ibid. The conversation was recorded differently by Freeman and Watts in a report they published ten months later: (Jan. 1937). Prefrontal lobotomy in the treatment of mental disorders. *Southern Medical Journal, 30*, 23–31. There the conversation seems to be between the patient and her physician, not Freeman (p. 25).

Doctor: "Do you have any of your old fears?"
Patient: "No."
Doctor: "What were you afraid of?"
Patient: "I don't know. I seem to forget."
Doctor: "Do you remember being upset when you came here?"
Patient: "Yes, I was quite upset, wasn't I?"
Doctor: "What was it all about?"
Patient: "I don't know. I seem to have forgotten. It doesn't seem important now."

86. Freeman, W. & Watts, J. W. (1937). Prefrontal lobotomy in the treatment of mental disorders. *Southern Medical Journal, 30*, 23–31, pp. 23 & 24.

87. Ibid., pp. 30–31.

88. Ibid.

89. Though crude on its surface, this procedure undoubtedly caused less damage than Moniz's six holes injected with alcohol. This is the procedure most associated with lobotomies although it was not popularized until 1948. The method originated in Italy, but it was Freeman who promoted it in America. See "The evolution of psychosurgical operations," pp. 277–293 in Valenstein, E. S. (1973). *Brain Control.* New York: John Wiley & Sons.

90. *Time* reported on the presentation (*Time* [Nov. 30, 1936]. Southern doctors. *28*, 66 & 68), referring to the procedure as a "lobotomy," not Moniz's term "leucotomy."

91. Ibid., p. 68.

92. *Time* (Nov. 30, 1942). Psychosurgery. *40*, 48 & 50, p. 48.

93. Ibid.

94. Ibid.

95. Ibid., p. 50. Drs. Freeman and Watts reported that of 136 cases, 98 were greatly improved and 23 were somewhat improved. That means 89% of all lobotomies resulted in very successful or somewhat successful outcomes. It is immediately obvious that success was in the eye of the beholder; in this case, a very biased beholder. It is also clear that Sigmund Freud's theories were influencing how the mind was being viewed by this time. Rees was so bold as to declare the frontal lobes the location of the superego (Rees, T. P. [1943]. The indications for prefrontal leucotomy. *Journal of Mental Science, 89*, 161 in Tow, P. M. [1955]. *Personality Changes Following Frontal Leucotomy.* London: Oxford University Press, p. 43).

96. Ibid., p. 223.

97. Ibid., p. 225.

98. Ibid., p. 225

99. Ibid., p. 229.

100. Röper, E. (1917). Zur prognose der hirnschüsse. *Münchener Medizinische Wochenschrift, 64*, 121 in ibid., p. 11.

101. Forster, E. (1919). Die psychischen störungen der hirnverletzten. *Monatsschrift für Psychiatrie und Neurologie, 46*, 61 in ibid., p. 11.

102. Feuchtwanger, F. (1926). *Die Funktionen des Sitrnhirnes.* Berlin: J Springer in ibid., p. 11.

103. *Time* (Nov. 30, 1942). Psychosurgery, *40*, 48 &50, p. 50.

104. Jones, C. H. (1949). Social adjustment following transorbital lobotomy. *Postgraduate Medicine, 6*, 392–397; Koskoff, Y. D. & Weniger, F. L. (1949). The adverse effect upon a family resulting from a radical change of personality in one member after

frontal lobotomy. *Research Publications–Association for Research in Nervous & Mental Disease, 29*, 148–154; Grassi, J. R. (1950). Impairment of abstract behavior following bilateral prefrontal lobotomy. *Psychiatric Quarterly, 24*, 74–88; Goldstein, K. (1950). Prefrontal lobotomy: An analysis and warning. *Scientific American, 182*, 44–47.

105.   Valenstein, E. S. (1980). Extent of psychosurgery worldwide in Valenstein, E. S. ed., *The Psychosurgery Debate*. San Francisco: W. H. Freeman, pp. 76–86 in Valenstein, E. S. (1986). *Great and Desperate Cures*. New York: Basic Books, p. 280.

106.   *Time* (Nov. 30, 1942). Psychosurgery, *40*, 48 & 50, p. 50.

107.   Examples include the following: *Newsweek* (Dec. 12, 1949). Lobotomy disappointment, *34*, 51; Goldstein, K. (1950). Prefrontal lobotomy: Analysis and warning. *Scientific American, 182*, 44–47; *Newsweek* (Sept. 18, 1950). Twenty years in a snake pit, *36*, 40; Williams, S. (1957). Lobotomy is a dangerous weapon. *American Mercury, 85*, 141–144.

108.   The quote is from the *Life* article "Return to Sanity in 12 Weeks: Reserpine, Chlorpromazine Restore Two Mental Victims to Normal Life." The fuller quote is "after the first mass trial of the drugs they are proving to be one of the most spectacular triumphs in the history of medicine" (Hodgins, E. [Oct. 15, 1956]. *Life, 41*, 149+). The article was part of a series. The following week (Oct. 22) the magazine declared, "The search has only started: in the next 10 years doctors may learn as much about the mind as in the past 2,000" (from the table of contents). The article itself placed mental diseases parallel to polio which had recently been cured. "But what particularly tantalizes the scientists is the hope that mental sickness, since it sometimes yields to pills, may involve measuring body chemistry as much as it does elusive psychic phenomena. If this should turn out to be true, the prospect would be opened up that mental diseases in the distant future might actually be curable like pneumonia or preventable like polio" (Hodgins, E. [Oct. 22, 1956]. New avenues into sick minds. *Life, 41*, 119+).

109.   See Giuseppe Roccatagliata's excellent *A History of Ancient Psychiatry* (New York: Greenwood Press, 1986) for a thorough discussion of the various ancient approaches used to heal the mind.

110.   Laborit, H. (1949). Sur l'utilisation de certaines agents pharmacodynamiques à action neuro–végétative en periode per–et postopératoire" in *Acta Chirurgica Belgica, 48*, 485–492 as quoted and translated in Swazey, J. P. (1974). *Chlorpromazine in Psychiatry: A Study of Therapeutic Innovation*. Cambridge: The MIT Press, p. 78.

111.   The company's designation was Compound 4560RP, the "RP" being the company's initials. The designation I have used (RP4560) is Anglicized.

112.   Swazey, J. P. (1974). *Chlorpromazine in Psychiatry: A Study of Therapeutic Innovation*. Cambridge: The MIT Press, p. 81.

113.   Laborit, H. & Huguenard, P. (1951). L'hibernation artificielle par moyens pharmacodynamiques et phyusiques. *Press Médicale, 59*, 1329 and Laborit, H.; Huguenard, P. & Alluame, R. (1952). Un nouveau stabilisateur végétatif (le4560RP). *Press Médicale, 60*, 206–208 in Healy, D. (2002). *The Creation of Psychopharmacology*. Cambridge: Harvard University Press, p. 82.

114.   Swazey, J. P. (1974). *Chlorpromazine in Psychiatry: A Study of Therapeutic Innovation*. Cambridge: The MIT Press, p. 93.

115.   Swazey's personal interview with Koetschet in ibid., p. 96.

116.   RP4560 was known as a drug that would potentiate (increase the effect of) barbiturates and other drugs. However, the sleep brought about with RP4560 was unlike the sleep induced by barbiturates alone. Drug–induced sleep puts the person into a state of deep sleep

in which arousal is gradual. They find it difficult to get fully awake. RP4560 led to sleep that appeared deep, but the patient could be easily aroused and be fully aware of his/her environment immediately. The drug allows the person to become so indifferent to the world that sleep occurs easily, but the sleep is truly unique (Healy, D. [2002]. *The Creation of Psychopharmacology*. Cambridge: Harvard University Press p. 91).

117. Ibid., p. 89.

118. Thuillier, J. (1999). *Ten Years That Changed the Face of Mental Illness*. New York: Taylor & Francis Group, p. 111.

119. Ibid., p. 113. In addition to the general beneficial calm Thorazine brought to mental hospitals, it was reported to bring sudden and complete cures to some patients. This is in line with sudden recoveries in numerous historical records. Such recoveries typically involved some type of emotional shock. Pinel reports that a man with suicidal mania was attacked by robbers as he was enroute to drown himself in a river. He fought off the robbers and immediately regained his senses. Cure of insanity following a fever has been often noted. See Ray, I. (1837). "Medical Jurisprudence of Insanity" in Goshen, C. E. (1967). *Documentary History of Psychiatry*. New York: Philosophical Library, pp. 419–420 for these and additional examples.

120. These papers were rushed to press. Dr. David Healy, likely the world's foremost authority on the history of mind drugs, refers to their efforts as "academic gamesmanship of the highest order" (ibid., p. 92.) In fact, another research team had been studying the same effects and had been doing so for a longer period of time. But, the fact that Delay and Deniker were at the University of Paris, published first, and immediately sought numerous speaking opportunities to share their findings has caused their names to be more closely associated with the discovery of RP4560's effects than others. However, determining who should receive the bulk of the credit is difficult to impossible to assess. See Chapter 3, "Explorations in a new world" for an overview of the RP4560 story and some valuable insights into this issue.

121. Lehmann, H. E. & Hanrahan, G. E. (1954). Chlorpromazine: New inhibiting agent for psychomotor excitement and manic states. *AMA Archives of Neurology & Psychiatry, 71*, 227–237, p. 230.

122. Ibid., p. 232.

123. Final approval came on March 26, 1954. Although SmithKline & French originally planned to seek approval for Thorazine as an anti–nausea and anti–vomiting drug, they recognized in 1953 that Thorazine's even larger potential market was in psychiatry. They had received a prepublication copy of the Canadian study by Lehmann and Hanrahan. A SmithKline & French memo stated, "The paper will be tremendously useful when we reach the FDA" (Swazey, J. P. [1974]. *Chlorpromazine in Psychiatry*. Cambridge: The MIT Press, p. 186). However, they felt the studies showing Thorazine to be a relatively safe "neuropsychiatry" drug might not be assembled in time for the FDA application submission. But six studies were in hand and were submitted with the application on March 4, 1954. The agency approved the drug 22 days later on March 26, 1954, as a treatment for nausea, vomiting and for use in psychiatry.

124. Healy D. (2002). *The Creation of Psychopharmacology*. Cambridge: Harvard University Press, p. 97.

125. Table 82, Estimated average annual salary of instructional staff in public elementary and secondary schools and the average annual earnings of full–time employees in all industries: to 1997–98. National Center for Educational Statistics, Digest of Education, Statistics, Tables & Figures, 1999. Available on the web at http://www.nces.ed.gov/programs/digest/d99/d99t082.asp.

126. Swazey reports that there were at least 25 different mind drugs (what she terms "tranquilizing agents") noted in the literature by 1956 (Swazey, J. P. [1974]. *Chlorpromazine in Psychiatry*. Cambridge: MIT Press, p. 192).

127. Kassin, S. (2004). *Psychology*, 4th ed. Upper Saddle River, NJ: Pearson Education, p. 700.

128. Lehmann said it was a comment in a Delay and Deniker paper "in which they compared the effects of CPZ [Thorazine] to those of a prefrontal lobotomy" that excited him and prompted his first use of the new drug (Swazey, J. P. [1974]. *Chlorpromazine in Psychiatry*. Cambridge: MIT Press, p. 155).

129. Ibid., p. 105.

130. Lehmann administered massive doses of up to 800 mg of Thorazine "and that took courage, because it was many times the dosage reported in the French literature" (ibid., p. 156).

131. Valenstein, E. S. (1998). *Blaming the Brain: The Truth About Drugs and Mental Health*. New York: The Free Press, p. 171. However, he gives no citation for this.

132. Odegard, O. (1964). Pattern discharge from Norwegian psychiatric hospitals before and after the introduction of the psychotropic drugs. *American Journal of Psychiatry*, *120*, 772–778, p. 774. This study is particularly valuable since the Norwegian government maintained good records and because, according to Odegard, "psychotropic drugs were introduced with an explosive suddenness…and there was hardly a patient who had not for some time received one or other of the new drugs" (p. 772). This made a study comparing the "pre-drug" period and the "drug period" possible. It is also significant that, in examining the 17 mental hospitals whose statistics were compiled and analyzed, wide variation was found in their individual discharge rates following the introduction of mind drugs.

133. Swazey states, "In the United States, by late 1953, trials with CPZ (Thorazine) and reserpine had begun coextensively in many mental hospitals" (Swazey, J. P. [1974]. *Chlorpromazine in Psychiatry*. Cambridge: The MIT Press, p. 192).

134. Jablensky, A.; Sartorius, N., et al. (1992). Schizophrenia: Manifestations, incidence and course in different cultures, a World Health Organization ten–country study. *Psychological Medicine Monogram, 20* (Suppl.), 1–97.

135. Discussions of the effectiveness of moral treatment are found in various sources: Bucknill, J. C. & Tuke, D. H. (1858). *A Manual of Psychological Medicine: The History, Nosology, Description, Statistics, Diagnosis, Pathology, and Treatment of Insanity*. Philadelphia: Blanchard & Lea, pp. 260–264; Laffey, P. (2003). Psychiatric therapy in Georgian Britain. *Psychological Medicine, 33*, 1285–1297. For Pinel's statistics, see endnote 149. Isaac Ray ("Medical Jurisprudence of Insanity," 1837) discussed the "duration and curability of madness." He surveys the English and French institutions during that time period when moral therapy was spreading rapidly. Citing Esquirol he noted that "the absolute number of recoveries from madness is about one in three" (p. 418). See his comments in Goshen, C. E. (1967). *Documentary History of Psychiatry*. New York: Philosophical Library, pp. 418–423. Samuel Tuke's account and statistics (discussed later in this chapter) I believe to be very plausible (Tuke, S. [1813]. *Description of the Retreat*. Philadelphia: Isaac Peirce, esp. pp. 118–144). Bockoven notes that the State Lunatic Hospital located in Worcester, MA, kept very careful records on each patient. Those records indicate that betwen 1833 and 1845 recovery rates ranged from 82 to 91 percent (Bockoven, J. S. [1976]. Moral treatment in America's asylums. *Hospital & Community Psychiatry, 27*, 468–470). For the threat this approach posed for the medical profession, see Scull, A. (1993). *The Most Solitary of Afflictions*. New Haven, CT: Yale University Press, pp. 188–198.

136. When the study responsible for the first fact was released, psychiatry repeatedly discredited it despite the fact that it was a massive 8–year study and was sponsored by the World Health Organization. This was a follow–up of earlier studies which also found those in developing nations were more likely to recover from schizophrenia than were those in the wealthier, developed nations. This finding continues to be reported. See the two following examples of the several reports now published. The second study calls the finding "provocative" but, even after controlling for "six potential sources of bias," concluded that none could explain why those with schizophrenia receiving treatment in the U.S. and Europe had worse outcomes than those treated in developing countries where mind drugs are not as likely to be available (Sartorius, N.; Jablensky, A., et al. [1986]. Early manifestations and first–contact incidence of schizophrenia in different cultures: A preliminary report on the initial evaluation phase of the WHO Collaborative Study on determinants of outcome of severe mental disorders. *Psychological Medicine, 16*, 909–928; Hopper, K. & Wanderling, J. [2000]. Revisiting the developed versus developing country distinction in course and outcome in schizophrenia: Results from ISoS, the WHO collaborative followup project. International Study of Schizophrenia. *Schizophrenia Bulletin, 26*, 835–846). When the World Health Organization next launched a multination study of mental disorders, they chose to report on the percentage of those suffering various disorders, but excluded schizophrenia and also chose not to report recovery rates. See Kessler, R.C., et al. (2004). Prevalence, severity and unmet need for treatment of mental disorders in the World Health Organization World Mental Health Surveys. *JAMA, 291*, 2581–2590. It was a smart move if modern psychiatry with its arsenal of drugs is truly ineffective or worse. But even this last study, published in 2004, found Nigerians had a rate of mental illness that was nearly six times less than the rate of Americans. In the press release announcing the results, the study's principle investigator, Ronald Kessler of the Harvard Medical School, immediately sought to discredit his own study's findings. "In some countries there is just not this tradition of public opinion and speaking your mind" (Tanner, L. [June 1, 2004]. Study of 14 countries finds mental illness is prevalent. *AP Worldstream*. Available on the web at http://static.highbeam.com/a/apworldstream/june012004/studyof14countriesfindsmentalhealthillnessisprevalent/index .html).

137. Scull, A. (1993). *The Most Solitary of Afflictions: Madness and Society in Britain, 1700–1900*. New Haven, CT: Yale University Press. Scull notes that "the annual mortality rate while fluctuating, usually amounted to about a third of annual admissions" (p. 344). Those living in the worst conditions would have had even higher death rates.

138. Tuke, S. (1813). *Description of The Retreat: An Institution Near York for Insane Persons of the Society of Friends*. York: Thomas Wilson & Sons, Printers. Reprinted 1964, London: Dawson of Pall Mall, chapter 1.

139. Ibid., p. 156

140. Ibid.

141. Ibid., p. 158.

142. Ibid., p. 161.

143. Ibid., p. 178.

144. Ibid., pp. 190–220. Tuke gives detailed statistics and notes that the statistics would likely be even more impressive if some of those who were released after one year had been kept at The Retreat just a little longer. The statistics also reveal that many of the "incurables" (those who had been insane for over 1 year when admitted) were also cured of insanity.

145. In 1847 Dr. Amariah Brigham, an advocate of moral treatment and the superintendent of the New York State Lunatic Asylum, described moral treatment as "the removal of the insane from home and former associations, with respectful and kind treatment under all

circumstances, and in most cases manual labor, attendance on [*sic*] religious worship on Sunday, the establishment of regular habits and of self–control, [and] diversion of the mind from morbid trains of thought" (Brigham, A. [1847]. The moral treatment of insanity. Reprinted in *American Journal of Psychiatry* [1994, June Suppl.], *151*, 11–15).

146. Butler, J. S. (1887). *The Curability of Insanity and the Individualized Treatment of the Insane*. New York: G. P. Putnam's Sons, p. 17.

147. Ibid., p. 45.

148. Bockoven, J. S. (1972). *Moral Treatment in Community Mental Health*. New York: Springer Publishing.

149. Ibid., based on Table 1, p. 15.

150. Pinel's statistics for the hospital de la Salpêtriere were reported in the *Journal de Physique*, Tome lxvii, Sept. 1808. Of 1,002 patients over a 3–year and 9–month span, 473 were cured and discharged. Many if not a majority of the patients had been insane for over one year; some for many years. Cited by Tuke, S. (1813). *Description of The Retreat: An Institution Near York for Insane Persons of the Society of Friends*. York: Thomas Wilson & Sons, Printers. Reprinted 1964, London: Dawson of Pall Mall, p. 205.

151. In 1813 the grandson of William Tuke, The Retreat's primary founder, published a description of The Retreat (now generally called the "York Retreat" as it was located near York, England). Samuel Tuke began his description by noting that the Retreat "has demonstrated, beyond all contradiction, the superior efficacy, both in respect of cure and security, of a mild system of treatment in all cases of mental disorder..." (Tuke, S. [1813]. *Description of The Retreat: An Institution Near York for Insane Persons of the Society of Friends*. York: Thomas Wilson & Sons, Printers. Reprinted 1964, London: Dawson of Pall Mall).

152. Hunter, R. & Macalpine, I. (1964). Introduction in ibid., p. 4.

153. Pinel, P. (1806). A treatise on insanity. Translated from the French by D. D. Davis. London: Cadell & Davies in Bockoven, J. S. (1972). *Moral Treatment in Community Mental Health*. New York: Springer Publishing, p. 33f.

Chapter 13 — Side Effects of Antipsychotics

1. This advertisement was placed on the web by the Benton County Historical Museum in Philomath, OR. It is available at http://www.bentoncountymuseum.org/history minutes/hm011.htm. The *Union–Gazette* was published in Corvallis, OR, located in Benton County.

2. Dorph–Petersen, K. A.; Pierri, J. N., et al. (Mar. 9, 2005). The influence of chronic exposure to antipsychotic medications on brain size before and after tissue fixation: A comparison of haloperidol and olanzapine in macaque monkeys. *Neuropsychopharmacology* (epublished ahead of print).

3. The Society for Neuroscience's *Brain Facts: A Primer on the Brain and Nervous System*, 4th ed. (2002). Washington, D. C.: Society for Neuroscience gives an excellent overview of the brain. Page 39 of this publication addresses the reduction in brain size seen in schizophrenics. This is also available on the web in both PDF and HTML forms. See http://www.vanderbilt.edu/virtualschool/pdf/brain facts.pdf for the PDF version. Also see Pol, H. D. H.; Schnack, H. G., et al. (2001). Focal gray matter density changes in schizophrenia. *Archives of General Psychiatry, 58*, 1118–1125.

4. Stockmeier, C. A.; Mahajan, G. J., et al. (2004). Cellular changes in the postmortem hippocampus in major depression. *Biological Psychiatry, 56*, 640–650.

5.   Goff, D. C.; Cather, C., et al. (2005). Medical morbidity and mortality in schizophrenia: Guidelines for psychiatrists. *Journal of Clinical Psychiatry, 66*, 147, 183–194, 273–274.

6.   See the FDA health advisory at http://www.fda.gov/bbs/topics/ANSWERS/2005/ANS01350.html.

7.   Ray, W. A.; Meredith, S., et al. (2001). Antipsychotics and the risk of sudden cardiac death. *Archives of General Psychiatry, 58*, 1161–1167.

8.   Zarate, C. A. & Patel, J. (2001). Sudden cardiac death and antipsychotic drugs: Do we know enough? *Archives of General Psychiatry, 58*, 1168–1171.

9.   Straus, S. M. J. M.; Bleumink, G. S., et al. (2004). Antipsychotics and the risk of sudden cardiac death. *Archives of Internal Medicine, 164*, 1293–1297.

10.   See either a current package insert or see the *Physician's Desk Reference* (*PDR*) which is a collection of drug packaging inserts. The *PDR* quote can be found in *Physicians' Desk Reference* (2005), 59th ed. Montvale, NJ: Thomson PDR.

11.   Burgyone, K; Audri, K., et al. (2004). The use of antiparkinsonian agents in the management of drug–induced extrapyramidal symptoms. *Current Pharmaceutical Design, 10*, 2239–2248.

12.   Remington, G. & Kapur, S. (2000). Atypical antipsychotics: Are some more atypical than others? *Psychopharmacology* (Berlin), *148*, 3–15.

13.   Leucht, S.; Wahlbeck, K., et al. (2003). New generation antipsychotics versus low–potency conventional antipsychotics: A systematic review and meta–analysis. *Lancet, 361*, 1581–1589.

14.   Smith, J. M. & Baldessarini, R. J. (1980). Changes in prevalence, severity and recovery in tardive dyskinesia with age. *Archives of General Psychiatry, 37*, 1368–1373; Caligiuri, M. P.; Lacro, J. P., et al. (1997). Incidence and risk factors for severe tardive dyskinesia in older patients. *British Journal of Psychiatry, 171*, 148–153.

15.   Woerner, M. G.; Alvir, J. M., et al. (1998). Prospective study of tardive dyskinesia in the elderly: Rates and risk factors. *American Journal of Psychiatry, 155*, 1521–1528.

16.   Morgenstern, H. & Glazer, W. M. (1993). Identifying risk factors for tardive dyskinesia among long–term outpatients maintained with neuroleptic medications: Results of the Yale Tardive Dyskinesia Study. *Archives of General Psychiatry, 50*, 723–733.

17.   Kinon, B. J.; Jeste, D. V., et al. (2004). Olazapine treatment for tardive dyskinesia in schizophrenia patients: A prospective clinical trial with patients randomized to blinded dose reduction periods. *Progress in Neuro–psychopharmacology & Biological Psychiatry, 28*, 985–996.

18.   *Physicians' Desk Reference* (2005), 59th ed. Montvale, NJ: Thomson PDR.

19.   Ibid.

20.   Healy, D. (2004). *Let Them Eat Prozac: The Unhealthy Relationship Between the Pharmaceutical Industry and Depression*. New York: New York University Press, p. 82.

21.   Many examples of a media attack on new research that could hurt drug sales occur each year. However, historical perspective is always of value, so consider again the estrogen debacle. Two paragraphs from a 1995 *Wall Street Journal* article make it plain that Wyeth (at that time the corporate name was American Home Products) was not about to let a large, Harvard study which found that taking estrogen increased breast cancer go unanswered. (Remember that we now know estrogen increases the risk of breast cancer, heart disease and strokes.)

American Home says many studies have looked at the breast–cancer risk but haven't found a link with estrogen use. "The medical community has long recognized the long–term benefits of [estrogen replacement therapy], including the prevention of osteoporosis, a reduction in the incidence of associated hip and wrist fractures by 60% and the potential reduction of coronary heart disease by 50%," the company says.... American Home is lining up a prestigious crew of scientists to counter the Harvard results in the news media. One, Prof. Leon Speroff of Oregon Health Sciences University in Portland, sent a letter by overnight mail urging caution in interpreting the study. "As a physician/researcher who treats and studies menopausal women, I've witnessed first hand the hysteria that can be generated as a result of unbalanced study data—particularly data related to breast cancer," writes Dr. Speroff, who says he is speaking independently and wasn't paid by American Home, although he has done clinical–trial work for the company. American Home also disseminated a National Institutes of Health statement regarding the Harvard study saying that more than 30 studies have examined the possible link between hormones and breast cancer, with conflicting results. "When all the studies are combined, it appears that there is very little or no overall risk of breast cancer associated with use of hormone replacement therapy," although some studies suggest a risk associated with prolonged use, the N.I.H. says. (Source: Taouye, E. [June 15, 1995]. Delicate balance: Estrogen study shifts ground for women—and for drug firms—breast–cancer data may give boost to alternative way to treat osteoporosis—tough decision gets harder. *Wall Street Journal*, A.1)

An interesting case involving Zoloft can be read on the internet. David Healy who had been paid by Pfizer as an expert consultant until he became convinced Zoloft was causing harm was attacked by Pfizer as unqualified and incompetent on an FDA website. Dr. Healy, in response, sent a letter to the FDA's Anuja Patel which stated, "The attack on me by Pfizer on your website is extraordinary, perhaps unprecedented." The address for this group of letters and documents is long, but it can be easily found by going to http://www.google.com and entering "PDAC 13 Pfizer Healy." The entry is listed as "PDAC Sept. 13 Pfizer Response–Healy.doc."

22. Pare, C. M. (1976). Unwanted effects of long–term medication in schizophrenia and depression. *Pharmakopsychiatrie, Neuro–psychopharmakologie, 9*, 187–192; Brambilla, F.; Penati, G., et al. (1979). Failure of pyridoxine to effect neuroleptic–induced hyperprolactinemia in psychotic patients. *Journal of Endocrinological Investigation, 2*, 299–302; Marken, P. A.; Haykal, R. F. & Fisher, J. N. (1992). Management of psychotropic–induced hyperprolactinemia. *Clinical Pharmacy, 11*, 851–856.

23. Malarkey, W. B. & Johnson, J. C. (1976). Pituitary tumors and hyperprolactinemia. *Archives of Internal Medicine, 136*, 40–44.

24. Yamazawa, K.; Matsui, H., et al. (2003). A case–control study of endometrial cancer after antipsychotic exposure in premenopausal women. *Oncology, 64*, 116–123.

25. Personal correspondence received April 13, 2005, and April 17, 2005.

Chapter 14 — What Really Causes Severe Mental Problems (Schizophrenia)?

1. Zyprexa ad from Eli Lilly & Co. Available on the web at http://www.zyprexa.com/managing/index.jsp.

2.   Jablensky, A.; Sartorius, N., et al. (1992).   Schizophrenia: Manifestations, incidence, and course in different cultures: A World Health Organization ten–country study. *Psychological Medicine* (Monograph Suppl. 20), 1–97. Also see endnotes 135 and 136 for Chapter 12.   Endnote 135 deals with moral therapy which was therapy without drugs. Endnote 136 involves a discussion of WHO's large international study which found that those in developing nations who are less likely to get medication recover at higher rates.

3.   American Psychiatric Association (1980). *Diagnostic Statistical Manual–III*. Washington, D. C.: APA, p. 185.

4.   American Psychiatric Association (2000). *Diagnostic Statistical Manual–IV–TR*. Washington, D. C.: APA, p. 309.

5.   Dorph–Petersen, K. A.; Pierri, J. N., et al. (2005).   The influence of chronic exposure to antipsychotic medications on brain size before and after tissue fixation: A comparison of holperidol and olanzapine in macaque monkeys. *Neuropsychopharmacology* [epublished ahead of print, March 9, 2005).

6.   Gilbert, A. R.; Moore, G. J., et al. (2000).   Decrease in thalamic volumes of pediatric patients with obsessive–compulsive disorder who are taking paroxetine. *Archives of General Psychiatry, 57*, 459–466.; Szeszko, P. R.; MacMillan, S., et al. (2004).   Amygdala volume reductions in pediatric patients with obsessive–compulsive disorder treated with paroxetine: Preliminary findings. *Neuropsychopharmacology, 29*, 826–832.

7.   See Chapters 10 and 15 for a full discussion of this issue.

8.   Robins, L. N. & Regier, D. A. (eds.) (1991). *Psychiatric Disorders in America: The Epidemiologic Catchment Area Study*. New York: The Free Press; American Psychiatric Association (2000). *Diagnostic and Statistical Manual of Mental Disorders: DSM–IV–TR*. Washington, D.C.: APA, pp. 307–308. Most of the factors I have listed have dozens of studies which have found a relationship to schizophrenia—some would have over one hundred. I will generally provide only two or three references unless each study adds something of particular significance. Some of the older references are, despite their age, particularly good studies. I include a newer study if the study is very old. Much could be said about most of these factors, but space does not permit full discussions of the cited studies. For example, an elaboration of this first factor would include the fact that schizophrenia most commonly develops in males in their late teens and early 20s—approximately 75% of all cases developing between the ages of 17 and 25 (Torrey, E. F. [1995]. *Surviving Schizophrenia: A Manual for Families, Consumers and Providers*, 3rd ed. New York: Perennial, 121). For females the most common time is between the mid–20s and early 30s. Only about 3% to 10% of women have onset after age 40 and "late onset is much less common in men" (American Psychiatric Association [2000]. *Diagnostic and Statistical Manual of Mental Disorders: DSM–IV–TR*. Washington, D.C.: APA, p. 307). I will make an exception for a couple of factors (divorce and urban setting) where there is frequent debate over the directional issue.

9.   Pert, L.; Ferriter, M. & Saul, C. (2004).   Parental loss before the age of 16 years: A comparative study of patients with personality disorder and patients with schizophrenia in a high secure hospital's population. *Psychology & Psychotherapy, 77* (Part 3), 403–407.

10.   Lewis, J. M.; Rodnick, E. H. & Goldstein, M. J. (1981).   Interfamilial interactive behavior, parental communication deviance, and risk for schizophrenia. *Journal of Abnormal Psychiatry, 90*, 448–457.

11.   Vaughn, C. E. & Leff, J. P. (1976).   The influence of family and social factors on the course of psychiatric illness. *British Journal of Psychiatry, 129*, 125–137; Butzlaff, R. L. & Hooley, J. M. (1998).   Expressed emotion and psychiatric relapse: A meta–analysis. *Archives of General Psychiatry, 55*, 547–552. Also Brown, G. W. & Birley, J. L. T. (1968).

Crisis and life changes and the onset of schizophrenia. *Journal of Health & Social Behavior, 9*, 203–214.

12.   David, A. S.; Malmberg, A., et al. (1997).   IQ and risk for schizophrenia: A population–based cohort study.   *Psychological Medicine, 27*, 1311–1323; Aylward, E.; Walker, E. & Bettes, B. (1984).   Intelligence and schizophrenia: Meta–analysis of the research. *Schizophrenia Bulletin, 10*, 430–459; Munro, J. C.; Russell, A. J., et al. (2002).   IQ in childhood psychiatric attendees predicts outcome of later schizophrenia at 21 year follow–up. *Acta Psychiatrica Scandinavica, 106*, 139–142.

13.   Clark. R. E. (1948).   The relationship of schizophrenia to occupational income and occupational prestige. *American Sociological Review, 13*, 325–330; Jarbin, H. & Hansson, L. (2004).   Adult quality of life associated factors in adolescent onset schizophrenia and affective psychotic disorders. *Social Psychiatry & Psychiatric Epidemiology, 39*, 725–729.

14. Brown, A. S.; Susser, E. S., et al. (2000).   Social class of origin and cardinal symptoms of schizophrenic disorders over the early illness course.   *Social Psychiatry & Psychiatric Epidemiology, 35*, 53–60; Faris, R. E. L. & Dunham, H. W. (1939).   *Mental Disorders in Urban Areas*.   Chicago: University of Chicago Press.

15.   Lewis, G.; David, A., et al. (1992).   Schizophrenia and city life. *Lancet, 340*, 137–140; van Os, J.; Hanssen, M., et al. (2001).   Prevalence of psychotic disorder and community level of psychotic symptoms: An urban–rural comparison. *Archives of General Psychiatry, 58*, 663–668.   It has long been argued that the relationship between urban living and schizophrenia may not have anything to do with actually living in the city but that those with mental illness drift to cities.   This "direction" issue can never be proven either way.   The problem gets more complicated in that debate exists as to whether it is urban birth or urban living (both are associated with schizophrenia) which contributes the most to mental problems.   We also know that the larger the city, the greater the incidence of schizophrenia and that the closer one lives to a city center, the greater the odds become of developing schizophrenia.   The evidence suggests that it is the characteristics of large urban areas that have the most impact on the individual.

16.   de Leon, J.; Diaz, F. J., et al. (2002).   Initiation of daily smoking and nicotine dependence in schizophrenia and mood disorders. *Schizophrenia Research, 56*, 47–54.   An interesting and unexpected finding was reported by Stan Zammitt and his colleagues in 2003. Contrary to a consistent set of previous studies, they did not find smoking rates to be higher for those with schizophrenia.   Moreover, when drug users and those with lower IQs were, in effect, removed from the sample, the smokers were actually less likely to develop schizophrenia.   This could be due to some protective effects of nicotine (e.g., nicotine can reduce the incidence of Parkinson's disease which might reduce life stress and, thus, schizophrenia), or it may be that IQ is such an important variable (it predicts academic success, occupational success, frequency of teasing, self–image, etc.) that adjusting the data for IQs (smokers as a group have lower IQs) masked what may be a stronger variable (IQ) than yet realized. Riala and colleagues suggest that initiation of smoking might actually trigger schizophrenia (Riala, K.; Hakko, H., et al. [2005].   Is initiation of smoking associated with the prodromal phase of schizophrenia? *Journal of Psychiatry & Neuroscience, 30*, 26–32).   We are still only able to speculate at this point.

17.   Soyka, M.; Albus, M., et al. (1993).   Prevalence of alcohol and drug abuse in schizophrenic inpatients. *European Archives of Clinical Neuroscience, 242*, 362–372; Cassano, G. B.; Pini, S., et al. (1998).   Occurrence and clinical correlates of psychiatric comorbidity in patients with psychotic disorders. *Journal of Clinical Psychiatry, 59*, 60–68.

18.   There are numerous examples.   Accutane (used for controlling acne) has a package insert (PI) which reads, "Accutane may cause depression, psychosis and, rarely, suicidal

ideation, suicide attempts, and suicide" (*Physicians' Desk Reference* [2004], 58th ed. Montvale, NJ: Thomson PDR, p. 2879). The PI for Larium (an anti–malarial drug) includes this warning, "People taking Larium occasionally experience severe anxiety, feelings that people are against them, hallucinations (seeing or hearing things that are not there, for example), depression, unusual behavior, or feeling disoriented. There have been reports that in some patients these side effects continue after Larium is stopped" (ibid., p. 2930). Concerta (an ADHD drug) and other similar products were the focus of an FDA document (issued June 29, 2005) which stated, "Post–marketing reports received by the FDA regarding Concerta and other methylphenidate products include psychiatric events such as visual hallucinations, suicidal ideation, psychotic behavior, as well as aggression or violent behavior." Available at http://www.fda.gov/ohrms/dockets/ac/05/briefing/2005–415261_00_05_Statement%20for%20June%2030.pdf. Various steroids, anticonvulsants and chemotherapy drugs also report adverse psychiatric events associated with their use.

19. Watt, N. F.; Stolorow, R. D., et al. (1970). School adjustment and behavior of children hospitalized for schizophrenia as adults. *American Journal of Orthopsychiatry, 40*, 637–657; Olin, S. C.; Mednick, S. A., et al. (198). School teacher ratings predictive of psychiatric outcome 25 years later. *British Journal of Psychiatry Supplement, 172*, 7–13.

20. Tolsdorf, C. C. (1976). Social networks, support and coping: An exploratory study. *Family Process, 15*, 407–418. Also Wallace, C. W. (1984). Community and interpersonal functioning in the course of schizophrenic disorders. *Schizophrenia Bulletin, 10*, 233–257.

21. Done, D. J.; Crow, T. J., et al. (1994). Childhood antecedents of schizophrenia and affective illness: Social adjustment at ages 7 and 11. *British Medical Journal, 309*, 699–703. Also Malmberg, A.; Lewis, G., et al. (1998). Premorbid adjustment and personality in people with schizophrenia. *British Journal of Psychiatry, 172*, 308–313; Gureje, O.; Herrman, H., et al. (2002). The Australian National Survey of psychotic disorders: Profile of psychosocial disability and its risk factors. *Psychological Medicine, 32*, 639–647.

22. Janssen, I; Krabbendam, L., et al. (2004). Childhood abuse as a risk factor for psychotic experiences. *Acta Psychiatrica Scandinavica, 109*, 38–45; Goff, D. C.; Brotman, A. W., et al. (1991). Self–reports of childhood abuse in chronically psychotic patients. *Psychiatry Research, 37*, 73–80; Greenfield, S. F.; Strakowski, S. M., et al. (1994). Childhood abuse in first–episode psychosis. *British Journal of Psychiatry, 164*, 831–834; Schenkel, L. S.; Spaulding, W. D., et al. (2005). Histories of childhood maltreatment in schizophrenia: Relationships with premorbid functioning, symptomatology, and cognitive deficits. *Schizophrenia Research, 76*, 273–286.

23. Sigal, J. J.; Perry, J. C., et al. (2003). Unwanted infants: Psychological and physical consequences of inadequate orphanage care 50 years later. *American Journal of Orthopsychiatry, 73*, 3–12.

24. Johnson, J. G.; Smailes, E. M., et al. (2000). Associations between four types of childhood neglect and personality disorder symptoms during adolescence and early adulthood: Findings of a community–based longitudinal study. *Journal of Personality Disorders, 14*, 171–187. This study considers schizotypal personality disorder rather than schizophrenia. It is one of literally hundreds of studies that consider a child's emotional environment and its effect on development. It should be noted that other studies have found those with personality disorders are more likely to develop schizophrenia in time. See, e.g., Gheorge, M. D.; Baloescu, A. & Grigorescu, G. (2004). Premorbid cognitive and behavioral functioning in military recruits experiencing the first episode of psychosis. *Clinical Nurse Specialist, 9*, 604–606.

25. Thewissen, V.; Myin–Germeys, I., et al. (2005). Hearing impairment and psychosis revisited. *Schizophrenia Research, 76*, 99–103. This is a prospective study. The researchers

found that deafness or hearing impairment (which can cause social isolation, an educational handicap and an occupational barrier) resulted in more than 3 times the incidence of psychotic experiences compared with the general population.

26.   Kelley, M. L. & Fals–Stewart, W. (2004).   Psychiatric disorders of children living with drug–abusing, alcohol–abusing, and non–substance–abusing fathers. *Journal of the American Academy of Adolescent Psychiatry, 43*(5), 621–628.

27.   El–Saadi, O.; Pedersen, C. B., et al. (2004).   Paternal and maternal age as risk factors for psychosis: Findings from Denmark, Sweden and Australia. *Schizophrenia Research, 67*, 227–236;   Byrne, M.; Agerbo; E., et al. (2003).   Parental age and risk of schizophrenia: A case–control study. *Archives of General Psychiatry, 60*, 673–678.   Also Zammit, S.; Allebeck, P., et al. (2003).   Paternal age and risk for schizophrenia. *British Journal of Psychiatry, 183*, 405–408.

28.   Dalman, C.; Thomas, H. V., et al. (2001).   Signs of asphyxia at birth and risk of schizophrenia: Population–based case–control study. *British Journal of Psychiatry, 179*, 403–408;   Rosso, I. M.; Cannon, T. D., et al. (2000).   Obstetric risk factors for early–onset schizophrenia in a Finnish birth cohort. *American Journal of Psychiatry, 157*, 801–807;   Buka, S. L.; Tsuang, M. T. & Lipsett, L. P. (1993).   Pregnancy/delivery complications and psychiatric diagnosis: A prospective study. *Archives of General Psychiatry, 50*, 151–156.

29.   Indrekavik, M. S.; Vik, T., et al. (2004).   Psychiatric symptoms and disorders in adolescents with low birthweight. *Archives of Diseases in Childhood. Fetal & Neonatal Edition, 89*, F445–F450;   Elgen, I; Sommerflet, K. & Markestad, T. (2002).   Population based, controlled study of behavioural problems and psychiatric disorders in low birthweight children at 11 years of age. *Archives of Diseases in Childhood. Fetal & Neonatal Edition, 87*, F128–F132.

30.   Leff, J. P. (1976).   Schizophrenia and sensitivity to the family environment. *Schizophrenia Bulletin, 2*, 566–574; Cantor–Graae, E. & Selton, J. P. (2005).   Schizophrenia and migration: A meta–analysis and review. *American Journal of Psychiatry, 162*, 12–24; Jacobs, S. & Myers, J. (1976).   Recent life events and acute schizophrenic psychosis: A controlled study. *Journal of Nervous & Mental Disease, 162*, 75–87.

31.   Siegel, R. K. (1984).   Hostage hallucinations: Visual imagery induced by isolation and life–threatening stress. *Journal of Nervous & Mental Disease, 171*, 264–272.

32.   Perhaps no factor in this listing is more susceptible to directional problems than is divorce. Do mental problems cause divorce, or does divorce cause mental problems? Many studies have tried to settle the issue using research designs that are more sophisticated than simple correlational studies of the past, though simple correlational studies continue to be published (Jenkins, R.; Lewis, G., et al. [2003]. The National Psychiatric Morbidity Surveys of Great Britain—initial findings from the household survey. *International Review of Psychiatry, 15*, 29–42). Time sensitive studies are suggestive though obviously not definitive. in other words, do mental problems *followed* by divorce occur often, or does divorce precede mental problems? Some better studies found huge increases in state and county mental hospital admissions *following* separations and divorces—5,144 admissions for divorced and separated men (a small percentage of all men in 1970) compared with 133 for married men (Redick, R. W. & Johnson, C. [1974]. *Marital Status, Living Arrangements and Family Characteristics of Admissions to State and County Mental Hospitals and Outpatient Psychiatric Clinics, United States, 1970.* Rockville, MD: National Institute of Mental Health, Statistical Note 100). Also, many more cases of psychosis (out of touch with reality) occur among *first admissions* to a mental hospital for the divorced and separated men and women (281.8) than for married men and women (41.9) (Blom, B. L. [1975]. *Changing Patterns of Psychiatric Care.* New York: Human Services Press). Other studies have examined never divorced individuals and those who have divorced or separated at least once and

490

found strong correlations (Richards, M.; Hardy, R. & Wadsworth, M. [1997]. The effects of divorce and separation on mental health in a national UK birth cohort. *Psychological Medicine, 27*, 1121–1128). Newer studies have focused on panel studies in hopes of answering the directional question more satisfactorily (Simon, R. W. & Marcussen, K. [1999]. Marital transitions, marital beliefs, and mental health. *Journal of Health & Social Behavior, 40*, 111–125). Also Wade, T. J. & Pevalin, D. J. (2004). Marital transitions and mental health. *Journal of Health & Social Behavior, 45*, 155–170.

33.   Brugha, T.; Singleton, N., et al. (2005). Psychosis in the community and in prisons: A report from the British Survey of Psychiatric Morbidity. *American Journal of Psychiatry, 162*, 774–780; Weller, M.; Tobiansky, R. I., et al. (1989). Psychosis and destitution at Christmas, 1985–1988. *Lancet, 2*, 1509–1511.

34.   Li, J.; Laursen, T. M., et al. (2005). Hospitalization for mental illness among parents after the death of a child. *New England Journal of Medicine, 352*, 1190–1196.

35.   Schofield, W. & Baliean, L. (1959). A comparative study of the personal histories of schizophrenic and non–psychiatric patients. *Journal of Abnormal & Social Psychology, 59*, 216–225.

36.   Minato, M. & Zemke, R. (2004). Time use of people with schizophrenia living in the community. *Occupational Therapy International, 11*, 177–191. Though schizophrenics spend more time in bed, they do not sleep as well as most people. See Hofstetter, J. R.; Lysaker, P. H. & Mayeda, A. R. (2005). Quality of sleep in patients with schizophrenia is associated with quality of life and coping. *BMC Psychiatry, 5*, 13.

37.   Goodwin, R. D.; Fergusson, D. M. & Horwood, L. J. (2003). Neuroticism in adolescence and psychotic symptoms in adulthood. *Psychological Medicine, 33*, 1089–1097; Krabbendam, L.; Janssen, I., et al. (2002). Neuroticism and low self–esteem as risk factors for psychosis. *Social Psychiatry & Psychiatric Epidemiology, 37*, 1–6.

38.   He wrote these words (in French) in his *A Treatise on Insanity*, a work over 200 years old but filled with scientific observations that are, unfortunately, ignored today. See Hunter, R. & Macalpine, I. (1963). *Three Hundred Years of Psychiatry, 1535–1860*. London: Oxford University Press, p. 608.

39.   I am not actually using Pinel's terms here as he wrote in French. These terms come from the translation of Pinel's work provided by Dr. David D. Davis. Pinel, P. (1806). *A Treatise on Insanity*, trans. Davis, D. D. London: Sheffield, Cadell & Davies in ibid. The first edition of Pinel's book came out in 1801, and the second edition came out in 1809. The Davis translation is a translation of the first edition.

40.   van Os, J.; Bak, M., et al. (2002). Cannabis use and psychosis: A longitudinal population–based study. *American Journal of Epidemiology, 156*, 319–327; Henquet, C.; Krabbendam, L., et al. (2005). Prospective cohort study of cannabis use, predisposition for psychosis, and psychotic symptoms in young people. *British Medical Journal, 330*, 11.

41.   Andreasson, S.; Allebeck, P., et al. (1987). Cannabis and schizophrenia: A longitudinal study of Swedish conscripts. *Lancet, 2*, 1483–1486.

42.   Zammit, S.; Allebeck, P., et al. (2002). Self–reported cannabis use as a risk factor for schizophrenia in Swedish conscripts of 1969: Historical cohort study. *British Medical Journal, 325*, 1199–1201.

43.   Ibid., p. 1199.

44.   An 1845 article may be the first to report the cannabis (hashish)–psychosis relationship. See D'Souza, D. C. (2004). 'Gone to pot': Pharmacological evidence supporting the contribution of cannabinoid receptor function to psychosis (Ch. 15) in McDonald, C.; Schulze, K., et al. (eds.). *Schizophrenia: Challenging the Orthodox*. London: Taylor & Francis, pp. 127–136. "Schizophrenia" was coined in 1911.

45.   In addition to those referenced in endnotes 40–44 above, see Buhler, B.; Hambrecht, M., et al. (2002). Precipitation and retrospective and prospective study of 232 population–based first illness episodes. *Schizophrenia Research, 54*, 243–251; Fowler, I. L.; Carr, V. J., et al. (1998). Patterns of current and lifetime substance use in schizophrenia. *Schizophrenia Bulletin, 24*, 443–455; Farrell, M; Howes, S., et al. (1998). Substance misuse and psychiatric comorbidity: An overview of the OPCS National Psychiatric Morbidity Survey. *Addictive Behaviors, 23*, 909–918.

46.   Dettling, A. C.; Feldon, J. & Pryce, C. R. (2002). Early deprivation and behavioral and physiological responses to social separation/novelty in the marmoset. *Pharmacology, Biochemistry, & Behavior, 73*, 259–269; Meaney, M. J.; Aitken, D. H., et al. (1991). Postnatal handling attenuates certain neuroendocrine, anatomical, and cognitive dysfunctions associated with aging in female rats. *Neurobiology of Aging, 12*, 31–38; Laplante, F.; Stevenson, C. W., et al. (2004). Effects of neonatal ventral hippocampal lesion in rats on stress–induced acetylcholoine release in the prefrontal cortex. *Journal of Neurochemistry, 91*, 1473–1482; Bethea, C. L.; Streicher, J. M., et al. (2005). Serotonin–related gene expression in female monkeys with individual sensitivity to stress. *Neuroscience, 132*, 151–166; Smotherman, W. P.; Hunt, L. E., et al. (1979). Mother–infant separation in group–living rhesus macaques: A hormonal analysis. *Developmental Psychobiology, 12*, 211–217.

47.   Selye, H. (1956). *The Stress of Life*. Toronto: McGraw–Hill; Finamore, T. L. & Port, R. L. (2000). Developmental stress disrupts habituation but spares prepulse inhibition in young rats. *Physiology & Behavior, 69*, 527–530; Lin, K–N.; Barela, A. J., et al. (1998). Prenatal stress generates adult rats with behavioral and neuroanatomical similarities to human schizophrenics. *Society for Neuroscience Abstracts, 24*, 796.

48.   Hinde, R. A. & McGinnis, L. (1977). Some factors influencing the effect of temporary mother–infant separation: Some experiments with rhesus monkeys. *Psychological Medicine, 7*, 197–212.

49.   Schanberg, S. (1995). The genetic basis for touch effects in Field, T. M. (ed.). *Touch in Early Development*. Mahway, NJ: Lawrence Erlbaum Associates, p. 67.

50.   Tiffany Field's research and books are particularly good as her research tends to be very well designed and yet written in ways that nonprofessionals can understand. See Field, T. (2001). *Touch*. Cambridge, MA: MIT Press and Field, T., ed. (1995). *Touch in Early Development*. Mahway, NJ: Lawrence Erlbaum.

51.   Field, T. M.; Schanberg, S. M., et al. (1986). Tactile/Kinesthetic stimulation effects on preterm neonates. *Pediatrics, 77*, 654–658.

52.   Ross, C. A. & Joshi, S. (1992). Schneiderian symptoms and childhood trauma in the general population. *Comprehensive Psychiatry, 33*, 269–273; Cardena, E. & Spiegel, D. (1993). Dissociative reactions to the San Francisco Bay earthquake of 1989. *American Journal of Psychiatry, 150*, 474–478; Mueser, K. T. & Butler, R. W. (1987). Auditory hallucinations in combat–related chronic posttraumatic stress disorder. *American Journal of Psychiatry, 144*, 299–302.

53.   Brown, G. W.; Harris, T. O. & Peto, J. (1973). Life events and psychiatric disorders Part 2: Nature of causal link. *Psychological Medicine, 3*, 159–176. This study actually established a mathematical model aimed at determining whether or not events are "triggers" for mental problems.

54.   Brown, G. W. & Birley, J. L. T. (1968). Crises and life changes and the onset of schizophrenia. *Journal of Health & Social Behavior, 9*, 203–214. Also see Hocking, F. (1965). Human reactions to extreme environmental stress. *Medical Journal of Australia, 18*, 477–483.

55.   Birley, J. L. T. & Brown, G. W. (1970). Crises and life changes preceding the onset or relapse of acute schizophrenia: Clinical aspects. *British Journal of Psychiatry, 116*, 327–333. The numbers may be even higher than these studies report. Schless and Mendels wanted to determine the accuracy of self–reporting among those who had experienced a psychotic breakdown. Their strategy was to interview family members and friends. The result was that they discovered an even higher number of major stressors had entered the lives of schizophrenics than had been previously reported (Schless, A. P. & Mendels, J. [1978]. The value of interviewing family and friends in assessing life stressors. *Archives of General Psychiatry, 35*, 565–567). Uhlenhuth, Balter and Lipman found an even greater decline in the ability to recall stressful events. They reported that the decline amounted to approximately 5% per month during the first 18 months (Uhlenhuth, E. H.; Balter, M. & Lipman, R. [1977]. Remembering life events in Strauss, J.; Babigian, H. & Roff, M. (eds.). *The Origins and Course of Psychopathology.* New York: Plenum Press, pp. 117–132).

56.   Fritz, C. E. & Marks, E. S. (1954). The NORC studies of human behavior in disaster. *Journal of Social Issues, 10*, 26–41. See Tables 2 and 3.

57.   Siegel, R. K. (1984). Hostage hallucinations: Visual imagery induced by isolation and life–threatening stress. *Journal of Nervous & Mental Disease, 172*, 264–272. The degree of stress experienced was also found to be the key to mental collapse in R. L. Swank's study (see endnote 62).

58.   The quote is found on the web at http://old.wolkorea.org/english/syme/messages/d108.htm. A discussion and examples of wartime amnesia are noted by van der Kolk, B. (Mar. 1997). Posttraumatic stress disorder and memory. *Psychiatric Times, 14*(3). Available on the web at http://www.psychiatrictimes.com/p970354.html.

59.   Sargent, W. & Slater, E. (1941). Amnesic syndromes in war. *Proceedings of the Royal Society of Medicine, 34*, 757–764.

60.   Paster, S. (1948). Psychotic reactions among soldiers of WWII. *Journal of Nervous & Mental Disorders, 108*, 54–66. Another research team came up with similar findings. Those with severe schizophrenia had numerous stressful events during the 12 weeks prior to their breakdown (Harder, D.; Strauss, J., et al. [1980]. Life events and psychopathology severity among first psychiatric admissions. *Journal of Abnormal Psychology, 89*, 165–180).

61.   Steinberg, H. R. & Durell, J. (1968). A stressful social situation as a precipitant of schizophrenic symptoms: An epidemiological study. *British Journal of Psychiatry, 114*, 1097–1105.

62.   Swank, R. (1949). Combat exhaustion. *Journal of Nervous & Mental Disease, 109*, 475–508.

63.   Rivers, W. H. R. (1918). The repression of war experience. *Lancet, 1*, 173–177.

64.   Ibid., p. 174.

65.   Ibid.

Chapter 15 — The Continuum Model

1.   Tuke, S. (c. 1813) as quoted by Butler, J. S. (1887). *The Curability of Insanity and the Individualized Treatment of the Insane.* New York: G. P. Putnam's Sons, p. 27.

2.   I firmly believe counseling can be effective if the focus is not on the counselee's dreams, feelings, unmet needs, and communication skills. Communication skills are important but are not likely to experience rapid change because 50 minutes per week is devoted to psychological counseling. However, if a person's words are unkind, if he or she is always talking about themselves, or if they are not complimentary or encouraging to others, they

need to change. Unfortunately, change is not likely to occur unless there is a change of heart. Values control our behavior and our tongue far more than our mind does. Yet, many therapy programs argue for "value–free" therapy. The most famous debate here was between Albert Ellis and Allen Bergin—a debate much discussed by psychology texts and other authors in the years which followed. The original exchange led to debates between the two in other publications. See Bergin, A. E. (1980). Psychotherapy and religious values. *Journal of Consulting & Clinical Psychology, 48,* 75–105 and Ellis, A. (1980). Psychotherapy and atheistic values: A reply to A. E. Bergin's 'Psychotherapy and Religious Values.' *Journal of Consulting & Clinical Psychology, 48,* 635–639). The best known books on therapy not being effective (or more effective when conducted by someone who is highly trained) are Tana Dineen's *Manufacturing Victims* (3rd ed., 2001, Montreal: Robert Davies Publishing) and Robyn M. Dawes' *House of Cards* (1994, New York: The Free Press). Many studies (including the famous meta–analysis of Mary Lee Smith) have found counseling effective, but the RCTs have been hard on the profession. See, for example, the following: Suzanna, R. O.; Jonathan, B. I. & Simon, W. E. (2002). Psychological debriefing for preventing post traumatic stress disorder (PTSD). *Cochrane Database Systematic Review, 2,* CD000560; Priest, S. R.; Henderson, J., et al. (2003). Stress debriefing after childbirth: A randomised controlled trial. *Medical Journal of Australia, 178,* 542–545. At present we cannot argue that professionals are even superior to paraprofessionals (volunteers). See den Boer, P. C.; Wiersma, D., et al. (2005). Paraprofessionals for anxiety and depressive disorders. *Cochrane Database Systematic Reviews, 2,* CD004688.

    3.   A letter to a friend admitted, "Our second boy, a promising bright creature of four years, we were called upon to part with several years ago, and I grieve to say that even at this day I do not feel sufficiently submissive to our loss" (Mary Lincoln to Margaret Preston, July 23, 1853, Wickcliffe–Preston Papers in Baker, J. H. [1987]. *Mary Todd Lincoln: A Biography.* New York: W. W. Norton, p. 128).

    4.   Pinsker, M. (2003). *Lincoln's Sanctuary.* New York: Oxford University Press, p. 30.

    5.   Keckley, E. (1868). *Behind the Scenes.* Repr., New York: Oxford University Press, 1988, p. 105.

    6.   Glyndon, H. (Aug. 10, 1882). The truth about Ms. Lincoln. *The Independent* in Pinsker, M. (2003). *Lincoln's Sanctuary.* New York: Oxford University Press, p. 30.

    7.   Ibid., p. 12.

    8.   Keckley, E. (1868). *Behind the Scenes.* Repr., New York: Oxford University Press, 1988, pp. 104–105. Lincoln historian Matthew Pinsker informed me that the authenticity of this account has been questioned. (The asylum to which Lincoln supposedly pointed could not be seen from the White House.) However, whether or not the words were spoken by Lincoln, they point to an awareness by either Lincoln or by Elizabeth Keckley of how a mind can deteriorate.

    9.   Instructions are given for using the PubMed (Medline) search engine at endnote 32.

    10.   Fava, M.; Alpert, J. E., et al. (2004). Clinical correlates and symptom patterns of anxious depression among patients with major depressive disorder in STAR*D. *Psychological Medicine, 34,* 1299–1308.

    11.   Sim, K.; Mahendran, R., et al. (2004). Subjective quality of life in first episode schizophrenia spectrum disorders with comorbid depression. *Psychiatry Research, 129,* 141–147.

    12.   Lancon, C.; Auquier, P., et al. (2001). Relationships between depression and psychotic symptoms of schizophrenia during an acute episode and stable period. *Schizophrenia Research, 47,* 135–140.

13. Moran, P. & Hodgins, S. (2004). The correlates of comorbid antisocial personality disorder in schizophrenia. *Schizophrenia Bulletin, 30*, 791–802.

14. Braga, R. J.; Petrides, G. & Figueira, I. (2004). Anxiety disorders in schizophrenia. *Comprehensive Psychiatry, 45*, 460–468.

15. Farabaugh, A.; Fava, M., et al. (2005). Relationships between major depressive disorder and comorbid anxiety and personality disorders. *Comprehensive Psychiatry, 46*, 266–271.

16. Bellino, S.; Patria, L., et al. (2005). Major depression in patients with borderline personality disorder: A clinical investigation. *Canadian Journal of Psychiatry, 50*, 234–238.

17. Miller, F. T. & Abrams, T. (1993). Psychotic symptoms in patients with borderline personality disorder and concurrent axis I disorder. *Hospital & Community Psychiatry, 44*, 59–61.

18. Binford, R. B. & leGrange, D. (2005). Adolescents with bulimia nervosa and eating disorder not otherwise specified—purging only. *International Journal of Eating Disorders, 38*, 157–161.

19. Keel, P. K.; Klump, K. L., et al. (2005). Shared transmission of eating disorders and anxiety disorders. *International Journal of Eating Disorders, 38*, 99–105.

20. Yerevanian, B. I.; Koek, R. J. & Ramdev, S. (2001). Anxiety disorders comorbidity in mood disorder subgroups: Data from a mood disorders clinic. *Journal of Affective Disorders, 67*, 167–173.

21. Freud's stages of psychosexual development, including the oral stages, are described in standard reference works, psychology textbooks, and the countless books about Freud and his ideas. For severe but scholarly criticism, see Crews, F. C., ed. (1998). *Unauthorized Freud: Doubters Confront A Legend.* New York: Viking.

22. This is related to Freud's "penis envy" concept and may be a primary reason for Freud's decline. With the rise of feminism, Freud's ideas began to be more boldly challenged.

23. Dember, W. N. & Jenkins, J. J. (1970). *General Psychology: Modeling Behavior and Experience.* Englewood Cliffs, NJ: Prentice–Hall, p. 122. By the 1990s (despite Freud's decline in popularity following the 1960s) 28% of clinical psychology faculty in the U.S. aligned themselves with psychoanalysis, the dominant theoretical orientation among counseling programs (PsyD and practice–oriented PhD programs), though not dominant in programs with a greater research emphasis (Mayne, T. J.; Norcross, J. C. & Sayette, M. A. [1994]. Admission requirements, acceptance rates, and financial assistance in clinical psychology programs. *American Psychologist, 49*, 806–811, Table 3, p. 809). I remember well when I first realized one of my colleagues accepted Freudian ideas. "You mean you don't," he asked in surprise. I held my ground, and he responded, "Well, Freud was a genius, and almost everyone else accepts his ideas." (That was not true by then, but that was my friend's perception.)

24. Skinner, B. F. (1948). *Walden Two.* New York: Macmillan. This book by Skinner is sometimes seen as being the primary force behind the "hippie communes" of the 1960s. A valuable analysis of Skinner's book (and his failure to live his ideals) is Hilke Kuhlmann's *Living Walden Two: B. F. Skinner's Behaviorist Utopia and Experimental Communities* (2005, Urbana, IL: University of Illinois Press).

25. Buss, D. M. (1994). The strategies of human mating: People worldwide are attracted to the same qualities in the opposite sex. *American Scientists, 82*, 238–249; Buss, D. M. (2003). *The Evolution of Desire* (rev. ed.). New York: Basic Books. Buss has even published a psychology textbook devoted to viewing all human behavior through these evolutionary eyes (*Evolutionary Psychology: The New Science of the Mind*, 1998, New York:

Allyn & Bacon). There are many others who have this same orientation. (See Box #11, Biological Thinking Can Get Silly on p. 91 for other examples from this school of thought.)

26. Wyss, J. (1971). *Swiss Family Robinson.* San Rafael, CA: Classic Publishing Corporation, pp. 159–160.

27. Butler, J. S. (1887). *The Curability of Insanity and the Individualized Treatment of the Insane.* New York: G. P. Putnam's Sons, p. 35.

28. This statement is found in the first paragraph of Eli Lilly's Zyprexa website under "Understanding Mental Ilness," available on the web at http://www.zyprexa.com/managing/index.jsp.

29. National Alliance for the Mentally Ill (nd). *Understanding Schizophrenia.* Arlington, VA: National Alliance for the Mentally Ill, p. 2. This booklet's argument against one's background being significantly influential is in stark contrast with Butler's comments. "In my report of the Retreat for 1860, I remarked that over three thousand cases of insanity have now come under my direct care and observation. In a large proportion of those cases whose history I could obtain, I have found that the remote and predisposing causes of insanity could be plainly traced to the malign influences of childhood" (Butler, J. S. [1887]. *The Curability of Insanity and the Individualized Treatment of the Insane.* New York: G. P. Putnam's Sons, p. 33).

30. National Alliance for Research on Schizophrenia and Depression (2003). *Understanding Schizophrenia.* Great Neck, NY: National Alliance for Research on Schizophrenia and Depression. This booklet (unlike the NAMI booklet) acknowledges its printing was funded by "an unrestricted educational grant from AstraZeneca Pharmaceuticals." Pfizer's Geodon website declares, "While there is no cure for schizophrenia, it can be treated." This statement is found under "What causes schizophrenia?" on their "Facts About Schizophrenia" page. It is available on the web at http://www.geodon.com/Geo Pat_Facts.asp.

31. Source: Bristol–Myers Squibb Abilify website available at http://www.abilify.com. Go to the section entitled "The Brain, Schizophrenia, and ABILIFY" for the quote.

32. Patten, S. B. (2004). The impact of antidepressant treatment on population health: Synthesis of data from two national data sources in Canada. *Population Health Metrics, 2,* 9. This is but one more of the numerous studies already cited which have found these facts. I note this study here in part because the full text of this article is available without cost through the PubMed (Medline) website. Enter the article title in PubMed's search engine. The easiest way to find the PubMed site is to enter "PubMed" in the Google search engine at http://www.google.com.

33. This fact has already been documented repeatedly as well. See Preface endnotes 17–19 for several references.

Chapter 16 — Avoiding and Overcoming Depression

1. Williams, P. & Nichols, R. (Recorded 1971). "Rainy Days and Mondays." The lyrics can be found at dozens of sites on the web including http://www.theguitarguy.com/rainyday.htm.

2. Horne, J. A. (1988). *Why We Sleep: The Functions of Sleep in Humans and Other Mammals.* New York: Oxford University Press. See especially pp. 30–31.

3. Lieberman, H. R.; Bathalon, G. P., et al. (2005). Severe decrements in cognitive function and mood induced by sleep loss, heat, dehydration, and undernutrition during simulated combat. *Biological Psychiatry, 57,* 422–429; Leonard, C.; Fannin, N., et al. (1998).

The effect of fatigue and onerous working hours on the physical and mental wellbeing of pre–registration house officers. *Irish Journal of Medical Science, 167,* 22–25; Voelker, R. (2004). Stress, sleep loss, and substance abuse create potent recipe for college depression. *JAMA, 291,* 2177–2179.

4. Marschall–Kehrel, D. (2004). Update on nocturia: The best of rest is sleep. *Urology, 64* (6 Suppl. 1), 21–24; Vgontzas, A. N.; Zoumakis, E., et al. (2004). Adverse effects of modest sleep restriction on sleepiness, performance, and inflammatory cytokines. *Journal of Clinical Endocrinology & Metabolism, 89,* 2119–2126.

5. Spiegel, K.; Leproult, R. & Van Cauter, E. (2003). [Impact of sleep debt on physiological rhythms.] *Revue Neurologique, 159,* 6S11–6S20. This article is in French though an English language abstract is available on Medline.

6. McDermott, C. M.; LaHoste, G. J., et al. (2003). Sleep deprivation causes behavioral, synaptic, and membrane excitability alterations in hippocampal neurons. *Journal of Neuroscience, 23,* 9687–9695.

7. Pilcher, J. J. & Huffcutt, A. I. (1996). Effects of sleep deprivation on performance: A meta–analysis. *Sleep, 19,* 318–326; Dinges, D. F.; Pack, F., et al. (1997). Cumulative sleepiness, mood disturbance, and psychomotor vigilance performance decrements during a week of sleep restricted to 4–5 hours per night. *Sleep, 20,* 267–277.

8. Von Dongen, H. P.; Maislin, G., et al. (2003). The cumulative cost of additional wakefulness: Dose–response effects on neurobehavioral functions and sleep physiology from chronic sleep restriction and total sleep deprivation. *Sleep, 2,* 117–126.

9. Marshall, L. & Born, J. (2002). Brain–immune interactions in sleep. *International Review of Neurobiology, 52,* 93–131; Krueger, J. M.; Toth, L. A., et al. (1994). Sleep, microbes and cytokines. *Neuroimmunomodulation, 1,* 100–109; Irwin, M. (2002). Effects of sleep and sleep loss on immunity and cytokines. *Brain, Behavior & Immunity, 16,* 503–512; Rogers, N. L.; Szuba, M. P., et al. (2001). Neuroimmunologic aspects of sleep and sleep loss. *Seminars in Clinical Neuropsychiatry, 6,* 295–307; Gomez–Merino, D.; Drogou, C., et al. (2005). Effects of combined stress during intense training on cellular immunity, hormones and respiratory infections. *Neuroimmunomodulation, 12,* 164–172.

10. Gottlieb, D. J.; Punjabi, N. M., et al. (2005). Association of sleep time with diabetes mellitus and impaired glucose tolerance. *Archives of Internal Medicine, 165,* 863–867. Insulin resistance, a major factor in the eventual development of Type 2 diabetes, has also been reported to occur when less than 6.5 hours of sleep is averaged (D'Arrigo–Kordella, T. [2001]. Short sleep and risk for Type 2. *Diabetes Forecast, 54*[12], 89–90).

11. Everson, C. A. & Toth, L. A. (2000). Systemic bacterial invasion induced by sleep deprivation. *American Journal of Physiology: Regulatory, Integrative & Comparative Physiology, 278,* R905–R916.

12. Landis, C. A. & Whitney, J. D. (1997). Effects of 72 hours sleep deprivation on wound healing in the rat. *Research in Nursing & Health, 20,* 259–267.

13. Alvarez, G. G. & Ayas, N. T. (2004). The impact of daily sleep duration on health: A review of the literature. *Progress in Cardiovascular Nursing, 19,* 56–59.

14. Ayas, N. T.; White, D. P., et al. (2003). A prospective study of sleep duration and coronary heart disease in women. *Archives of Internal Medicine, 163,* 205–209.

15. Tapert, S. F.; Granholm, E., et al. (2002). Substance use and withdrawal: Neuropsychological functioning over 8 years in youth. *Journal of the International Neuropsychological Society, 8,* 873–883. Another study has shown it is the alcohol causing intellectual declines, not the depression and anxiety which are more common and which are increased by alcohol abuse. See Rosenbloom, M. J.; O'Reilly, A., et al. (2005). Persistent cognitive deficits in community–treated alcoholic men and women volunteering for research:

Limited contribution from psychiatric comorbidity. *Journal of Studies on Alcohol, 66,* 254–265.

16. Hasin, D. S. & Grant, B. F. (2002). Major depression in 6050 former drinkers. *Archives of General Psychiatry, 59,* 794–800.

17. Swendsen, J. D. & Merikangas, K. R. (2000). The comorbidity of depression and substance use disorder. *Clinical Psychology Review, 20,* 173–189; Swendsen, J. D.; Merikangas, K. R., et al. (1998). The comorbidity of substance use disorders with anxiety and depressive disorders in four geographic communities. *Comprehensive Psychiatry, 39,* 176–184; Burns, L.; Teesson, M. & O'Neill, K. (2005). The impact of comorbid anxiety and depression on alcohol treatment outcomes. *Addiction, 100,* 787–796; Dawson, D. A.; Grant, B. F., et al. (2005). Psychopathology associated with drinking and alcohol use disorders in college and general adult populations. *Drug & Alcohol Dependence, 77,* 139–150.

18. Roizen, J. (1993). Issues in the epidemiology of alcohol and violence in Martin, S. E., ed. *Alcohol and Interpersonal Violence: Fostering Multidisciplinary Perspectives.* Rickville, MD: National Institutes of Health.

19. *Physicians' Desk Reference* (2004), 58th ed. Montvale, NJ: Thomson PDR, p. 2879.

20. Other drugs known to cause depression in some people include Symmetrel (amantadine), Adderall (amphetamine), Tegretol (carbamazepine), and Catapres (clonidine). I cite these four only as examples. (This group includes only drugs whose generic name begins with "a" or "c.") A full listing of all drugs known to sometimes cause depression would be quite long.

21. Klesges, R. C.; Shelton, M. L. & Klesges, L. M. (1993). Effects of television on metabolic rate: Potential implications for childhood obesity. *Pediatrics, 91,* 281–286.

22. Hark, W. T.; Thompson, W. M., et al. (2005). Spontaneous sigh rates during sedentary activity: Watching television vs. reading. *Annals of Allergy, Asthma & Immunology, 94,* 247–250.

23. Salbe, A. D.; Weyer, C., et al. (2002). Assessing risk factors for obesity between childhood and adolescence: II. Energy metabolism and physical activity. *Pediatrics, 110,* 307–314.

24. Hu, F. B.; Leitzmann, M. F., et al. (2001). Physical activity and television watching in relation to risk for Type 2 diabetes mellitus in men. *Archives of Internal Medicine, 161,* 1542–1548.

25. Fung, T. T.; Hu, F. B., et al. (2000). Leisure–time physical activity, television watching, and plasma biomarkers of obesity and cardiovascular disease risk. *American Journal of Epidemiology, 152,* 1171–1178.

26. Schwimmer, J. B.; Burwinkle, T. M. & Varni, J. W. (2003). Health–related quality of life of severely obese children and adolescents. *JAMA, 289,* 1813–1819; Carpenter, K. M.; Hasin, D. S., et al. (2000). Relationships between obesity and *DSM–IV* major depressive disorder, suicide ideation, and suicide attempts: Results from a general population study. *American Journal of Public Health, 90,* 251–257.

27. Erickson, S. J.; Robinson, T. N., et al. (2000). Are overweight children unhappy? *Archives of Pediatrics & Adolescent Medicine, 154,* 931–935.

28. Most studies find links between several different diseases and depression. For example, the diabetes–depression link was reported by Anderson, et al. (Anderson, R. J.; Freedland, K. E., et al. [2001]. The prevalence of comorbid depression in adults with diabetes: A meta–analysis. *Diabetes Care, 24,* 1069–1078). However, there are sometimes exceptions to this pattern. An example of this for diabetes is Engum, A.; Mykletun, A., et al. (2005). Depression and diabetes: A large population–based study of sociodemographic,

lifestyle and clinical factors associated with depression in Type 1 and Type 2 diabetes. *Diabetes Care, 28*, 1904–1909.

29.   For children, see Strauss, R. S. & Pollack, H. A. (2003). Social marginalization of overweight children. *Archives of Pediatrics & Adolescent Medicine, 157*, 746–752. For adolescents, see Sanders, C. E.; Field, T. M., et al. (2000). The relationship of Internet use to depression and social isolation among adolescents. *Adolescence, 35*, 237–242. For adults, see Kraut, R.; Patterson, M., et al. (1998). Internet paradox: A social technology that reduces social involvement and psychological well–being? *American Psychologist, 53*, 1017–1031 and Moody, E. J. (2001). Internet use and its relationship to loneliness. *Cyberpsychology & Behavior, 4*, 393–401.

30.   Markoff, J. (Dec. 30, 2004). Internet use said to cut into tv viewing and socializing. *NY Times*, C.5.

31.   Comstock, G.; Chaffee, S., et al. (1978). *Television and Human Behavior.* New York: Columbia University Press.

32.   One journal, *Cyberpsychology & Behavior*, is dedicated to research which reports on the internet's impact on society and personal behavior.

33.   Zimmerman, F. J. & Christakis, D. A. (2005). Children's television viewing and cognitive outcomes: A longitudinal analysis of national data. *Archives of Pediatrics & Adolescent Medicine, 159*, 619–625.

34.   Hancox, R. J.; Milne, B. J. & Poulton, R. (2005). Association of television viewing during childhood with poor educational achievement. *Archives of Pediatrics & Adolescent Medicine, 159*, 614–618.

35.   Ibid.

36.   Ibid.

37.   Collins, R. L.; Elliott, M. N., et al. (2004). Watching sex on television predicts adolescent initiation of sexual behavior. *Pediatrics, 114*, e280–289.

38   Tiggemann, M. & Slater, A. (2004). Thin ideals in music television: A source of social comparison and body dissatisfaction. *International Journal of Eating Disorders, 35*, 48–58.

39.   Wakefield, M.; Flay, B., et al. (2003). Role of the media influencing trajectories of youth smoking. *Addiction, 98* (Suppl. 1), 79–103; Coon, K. A. & Tucker, K. L. (2002). Television and children's consumption patterns: A review of the literature. *Minerva Pediatrica, 54*, 423–436.

40.   Robinson, T. N.; Chen, H. L. & Killen, J. D. (1998). Television and music video exposure and risk of adolescent alcohol use. *Pediatrics, 102*, e54. Available on the web at http://pediatrics.aappublications.org/content/vol102/issue5/index.shtml#ELECTRONIC_ ARTICLE.

41.   Viscott, D. (1974). *How To Live With Another Person.* New York: Pocket Books, p. 73.

42.   Ibid., pp. 72–73.

43.   Smith, J. C.; Mercy, J. A. & Conn, J. M. (1988). Marital status and risk of suicide. *American Journal of Public Health, 78*, 78–80; Kposowa, A. J.; Breault, K. D. & Singh, G. K. (1995). White male suicide in the United States: A multivariate individual–level analysis. *Social Forces, 74*, 315–323; Kposowa, A. J. & Adams, M. (1998). Motor vehicle crash fatalities: The effects of race and marital status. *Applied Behavioral Science Review, 6*, 69–91; Kposowa, A. J. (2003). Divorce and suicide risk. *Journal of Epidemiology & Community Health, 57*, 993; Matthews, K. A. & Gump, B. B. (2002). Chronic work stress and marital dissolution increase risk of posttrial mortality in men from the Multiple Risk Factor Intervention Trial. *Archives of Internal Medicine, 162*, 309–315; Hemminki, K. & Li, X.

(2003). Lifestyle and cancer: Effects of widowhood and divorce. *Cancer Epidemiology, Biomarkers & Prevention, 12*, 899–904; Lillberg, K.; Verkasalo, P. K., et al. (2003). Stressful life events and risk of breast cancer in 10,808 women: A cohort study. *American Journal of Epidemiology, 157*, 415–423; Kessing, L. V.; Agerbo, E. & Mortensen, P. B. (2003). Does the impact of major stressful life events on the risk of developing depression change throughout life? *Psychological Medicine, 33*, 1177–1184.

44. Adapted from Stuart, R. B. (1980). *Helping Couples Change.* New York: The Guilford Press, Table 3, p. 12. The statistics come from several sources. Each is referenced by Stuart in his book.

45. Adapted from Stuart, R. B. (1980). *Helping Couples Change.* New York: The Guilford Press, Table 2, p. 10. The statistics come from several sources. Each is referenced by Stuart in his book.

46. Hendin, H.; Maltsberger, J. T. & Haas, A. P. (2003). A physician's suicide. *American Journal of Psychiatry, 160*, 2094–2097, p. 2095.

47. Ibid.

48. Beach, S. R.; Jouriles, E. N. & O'Leary, K. D. (1985). Extramarital sex: Impact on depression and commitment in couples seeking marital therapy. *Journal of Sexual & Marital Therapy, 11*, 99–108.

49. Hendin, H.; Maltsberger, J. T. & Haas, A. P. (2003). A physician's suicide. *American Journal of Psychiatry, 160*, 2094–2097, p. 2094.

50. Ibid.

51. The scientifically sound report of American sexual behavior issued by the University of Chicago's National Opinion Research Center correctly stated, "There are probably more scientifically worthless 'facts' on extra–marital relations than on any other facet of human behavior" (Smith, T. W. [1993]. American sexual behavior: Trends, socio–demographic differences, and risk behavior. *General Social Survey Topical Report No. 25*, p. 4). Despite clear medical ethics codes in all areas of medicine disallowing any physician–patient sexual contact and severe penalties historically for such contact (see Doctors and adultery [1970]. *British Medical Journal, 2*, 620). Among the 19% willing to respond to a questionnaire on the subject, 9% acknowledged having sexual contact with one or more of their patients (Gartrell, N. K.; Milliken, N., et al. [1992]. Physician–patient sexual contact: Prevalence and problems. *Western Journal of Medicine, 157*, 139–143). Adultery would undoubtedly occur much more commonly with non–patients. The University of Chicago's important sexual behavior study found adultery occurred most frequently "during the last 12 months" among those with graduate degrees (1.8% for individuals with bachelor's degrees vs. 5.4% for graduate degree individuals. Those who did not complete high school also had a high adultery rate—5.2%). Those with a graduate degree also were most likely to have *ever* committed adultery, 10.7% for those with a bachelors vs. 19.1% for graduate degree individuals (Smith, T. W. [1993]. American sexual behavior: Trends, socio–demographic differences, and risk behavior. *General Social Survey Topical Report No. 25*, Table 7, pp. 31–32). Yet physicians have a low divorce rate (Stack, S. [2004]. Suicide risk among physicians: A multivariate analysis. *Archives of Suicide Research, 8*, 287–292). My own experience in counseling wives of physicians is that they are much more willing to put up with their husbands' infidelity, perhaps because they do not want to lose the income and prestige that is often associated with marriage to a physician.

52. Frank, E.; Biola, H. & Burnett, C. A. (2000). Mortality rates and causes among U.S. physicians. *American Journal of Preventive Medicine, 19*, 155–159; Stack, S. (2004). Suicide risk among physicians: A multivariate analysis. *Archives of Suicide Research, 8*, 287–292.

53. Maimonides, M. *Diseases of the Soul* in Goshen, C. E. (1967). *Documentary History of Psychiatry*. New York: Vision Press, p. 34.

54. Leon Festinger is the originator of cognitive dissonance theory (1957, *A Theory of Cognitive Dissonance*. Stanford: Stanford University Press). Literally hundreds of experimental studies have demonstrated the validity of what Festinger originally called a "theory."

55. McCown, W. & Johnson, J. (1989a). Validation of an adult inventory of procrastination. Paper presented at the annual meeting of the Society for Personal Adjustment, New York in Fee, R. L. & Tangney, J. P. (2000). Procrastination: A means of avoiding shame and guilt? *Journal of Social Behavior & Personality, 15*, 167–184.

56. Harris and Rosenthal noted that over 400 studies had been published by 1985 on interpersonal expectation effects (Harris, M. J. & Rosenthal, R. [1985]. Mediation of interpersonal expectancy effects: 31 meta–analyses. *Psychological Bulletin, 97*, 363–386). Fewer studies analyze the effects of either positive or negative expectations based on one's own performance—likely because effects would naturally be anticipated. See the following studies: Wasch, H. H. (1995). Negative mood regulation expectancy and the prediction of changes in mood and health. *Dissertation Abstracts International: Section B. The Sciences & Engineering, 56*, 1124; Roseman, I. J. & Evdokas, A. (2004). Appraisals cause experienced emotions: Experimental evidence. *Cognition & Emotion, 18*, 1–28; Anderson, S. M. & Lyon, J. E. (1987). Anticipating desired outcomes: The role of outcome certainty in the onset of depressive effect. *Journal of Experimental Social Psychology, 23*, 428–443; Cunningham, M. R. (1988). What do you do when you're happy or blue? Mood, expectancies, and behavioral interest. *Motivation and Emotion, 12*, 309–331.

57. American Obesity Association Fact Sheet. Available on the web at http://www .obesity.org/subs/fastfacts/obesity_what2.shtml.

58. Steinbrook, R. (2004). Surgery for severe obesity. *New England Journal of Medicine, 350*, 1075–1079. An estimated total of 103,200 operations for severe obesity were performed in 2003.

59. Rutner, I. T. & Bugle, C. (1969). An experimental procedure for the modification of psychotic behavior. *Journal of Consulting & Clinical Psychology, 33*, 651–653.

60. O'Brien, J. S. (1978). The behavioral treatment of acute reactive depression involving psychotic manifestations. *Journal of Behavior Therapy & Experimental Psychiatry, 9*, 259–264; Fichter, M. M.; Wallace, C. J. & Liberman, R. P. (1976). Improving social interaction in a chronic psychotic using discriminated avoidance ("nagging"): Experimental analysis and generalization. *Journal of Applied Behavior Analysis, 9*, 377–386; Miltenberger, R. G. & Fuqua, R. W. (1985). A comparison of contingent vs. non–contingent competing response practice in the treatment of nervous habits. *Journal of Behavior Therapy & Experimental Psychiatry, 16*, 195–200; Ayllon, T. & Azrin, N. H. (1964). Reinforcement and instructions with mental patients. *Journal of the Experimental Analysis of Behavior, 7*, 327–331; O'Brien, J. S. (1978). The behavioral treatment of a thirty year smallpox obsession and hand washing compulsion. *Journal of Behavior Therapy & Experimental Psychiatry, 9*, 365–368.

61. Fisher, W.; Piazza, C. C. & Page, T. J. (1989). Assessing independent and interactive effects of behavioral and pharmacologic interventions for a client with dual diagnoses. *Journal of Behavior Therapy & Experimental Psychiatry, 20*, 241–250.

62. An older but still very valuable book which covers each of these issues (the topics were taken from its table of contents) is K. Daniel O'Leary and G. Terence Wilson's *Behavior Therapy: Application and Outcome* (1975, Englewood Cliffs, NJ: Prentice–Hall).

63. Rohde, T. (2000). Cross–validation of measures of self–control and behavioral inhibition in young adults. Unpublished thesis in Tangney, J. P.; Baumeister, R. F. & Boone,

A. L. (2004). High self–control predicts good social adjustment, less pathology, better grades, and interpersonal success. *Journal of Personality, 72*, 271–324.

64. Malecki, C. K. & Elliott, S. (2002). Children's social behaviors as predictors of academic achievement: A longitudinal analysis. *Social Psychology Quarterly, 17*, 1–23; Feldman, S. C.; Martinez–Pons, M. & Shaham, D. (1995). The relationship of self–efficacy, self–regulation, and collaborative verbal behavior with grades: Preliminary findings. *Psychological Reports, 77*, 971–978.

65. Parker, J. D. A.; Creque, R. E., Sr., et al. (2004). Academic achievement in high school: Does emotional intelligence matter? *Personality & Individual Differences, 37*, 1321–1330.

66. Wolfe, R. N. & Johnson, S. D. (1995). Personality as a predictor of college performance. *Educational & Psychological Measurement, 55*, 177–185. A measure of self–control was more predictive of college GPA than were SAT scores or any other personality variable.

67. Lievens, F.; Coetsier, P., et al. (2002). Medical students' personality characteristics and academic performance: A five–factor model perspective. *Medical Education, 36*, 1050–1056.

68. Eisenberg, N.; Fabes, R. A., et al. (1997). Contemporaneous and longitudinal prediction of children's social functioning from regulation and emotionality. *Child Development, 68*, 642–664; Elliott, S. N. & Gresham, F. M. (1989). Teacher and self–ratings of popular and rejected adolescent boys' behavior. *Journal of Psychoeducational Assessment, 7*, 323–334.

69. Hughes, J. N.; Cavell, T. A. & Willson, V. (2001). Further support for the developmental significance of the quality of the teacher–student relationship. *Journal of School Psychology, 35*, 289–301; Wentzel, K. R. Does being good make the grade? Social behavior and academic competence in middle school. *Journal of Educational Psychology, 85*, 357–364.

70. Tangney, J. P.; Baumeister, R. F. & Boone, A. L. (2004). High self–control predicts good adjustment, less pathology, better grades, and interpersonal success. *Journal of Personality, 72*, 271. Grade point average, like virtually every factor which I will share in the following paragraphs that correlates with self–discipline, is also related to depression (Lee, R. S.; Staten, R. R. & Danner, F. W. [2005]. Smoking and depressive symptoms in a college population. *Journal of School Nursing, 21*, 229–235).

71. Schouwenburg, H. C. (2004). Counseling the procrastinator in academic settings in Schouwenburg, H. C.; Lay, C., et. al., eds. *Procrastination in Academic Settings: General Introduction*. Washington, D. C.: American Psychological Association, pp. 3–17.

72. Cochran, J. K.; Wood, P. B., et al. (1998). Academic dishonesty and low self–control: An empirical test of a general theory of crime. *Deviant Behavior, 19*, 227–255.

73. Weir, R. E.; Zaidi, F. H. & Whitehead, D. E. J. (2004). School exam results matter in medical job applications. *British Medical Journal, 328*, 585; Monk–Turner, E. (1990). The occupational achievements of community and four–year college entrants. *American Sociological Review, 55*, 719–725. The relationship between grade point average and earnings is relatively meager. See Cohen, P. A. (1984). College grades and adult achievement: A research synthesis. *Research in Higher Education, 20*, 281–293. (This study reported that overall financial and other postgraduate successes were positive but relatively weak.) Donhardt, G. L. (2004). In search of the effects of academic achievement in postgraduate earnings. *Research in Higher Education, 45*, 271–284. (Donhardt found no significant relationship between high and low achieving baccalaureate recipients, but high achievers were

defined as grade point averages above 3.15316 and low achievers as below 3.06150 in one portion of the study.)

74. Romal, J. B. & Kaplan, B. J. (1995). Difference in self–control among spenders and savers. *Psychology—A Quarterly Journal of Human Behavior, 32*, 8–17.

75. Verplanken, B.; Herabadi, A. G., et al. (2005). Consumer style and health: The role of impulsive buying in unhealthy eating. *Psychology & Health, 20*, 429–441.

76. Kokko, K.; Pulkkinen, L. & Puustinen, M. (2000). Selection into long–term unemployment and its psychological consequences. *International Journal of Behavioral Development, 24*, 310–320.

77. Ibid.

78. Terracciano, A. & Costa, P. T., Jr. (2004). Smoking and the Five–Factor Model of personality. *Addiction, 99*, 472–481.

79. Wills, T. A.; DuHamel, K. & Vaccaro, D. (1995). Activity and mood temperament as predictors of adolescent substance use: Test of a self–regulation mediational model. *Journal of Personality & Social Psychology, 68*, 901–916.

80. Neal, D. J. (2005). The relationship between alcohol consumption and alcohol–related problems: An event–level analysis. *Dissertation Abstracts International: Section B. The Sciences & Engineering, 65*, 4842; Hull, J. G. & Sloane, L. B. (2004). Alcohol and self–regulation (pp. 466–491) in Baumeister, R. F. & Vohs, K. D., eds. *Handbook of Self–Regulation: Research Theory and Applications.* New York: Guilford Press.

81. Trobst, K. K.; Herbst, J. H., et al. (2002). Personality pathways to unsafe sex: Personality, condom use, and HIV risk behaviors. *Journal of Research in Personality, 36*, 117–133.

82. Tremblay, R. E.; Boulerice, B., et al. (1995). Does low self–control during childhood explain the association between delinquency and accidents in early adolescence? *Criminal Behaviour & Mental Health, 5*, 439–451; Krueger, R. F.; Caspi, A., et al. (1996). Delay of gratification, psychopathology and personality: Is low self–control specific to externalizing problems? *Journal of Personality, 64*, 107–129.

83. Avakame, E. F. (1998). Intergenerational transmission of violence, self–control, and conjugal violence: A comparative analysis of physical violence and psychological aggression. *Violence & Victims, 13*, 301–316.

84. Chapple, C. L. & Hope, T. L. (2003). An analysis of the self–control and criminal versatility of gang and dating violence offenders. *Violence & Victims, 18*, 671–690.

85. Burton, V. S.; Cullen, F. T., et al. (1998). Gender, self–control, and crime. *Journal of Research in Crime & Delinquency, 35*, 123–147.

86. Tangney, J. P.; Baumeister, R. F. & Boone, A. L. (2004). High self–control predicts good adjustment, less pathology, better grades and interpersonal success. *Journal of Personality, 72*, 271–324.

87. Ibid.

88. Nigg, J. T.; Quamma, J. P., et al. (1999). A two–year longitudinal study of neuropsychological and cognitive performance in relation to behavioral problems and competencies in elementary school children. *Journal of Abnormal Child Psychology, 27*, 51–63. "Inhibitory control" had modest but significant effects on behavior in this study.

89. Murphy, B. C. & Eisenberg, N. (1997). Young children's emotionality, regulation and social functioning and their responses when they are a target of a peer's anger. *Social Development, 6*, 18–36.

90. Mischel, W.; Shoda, Y. & Peake, P. K. (1988). The nature of adolescent competencies predicted by preschool delay of gratification. *Journal of Personality & Social Psychology, 54,* 687–696.

91. Tangney, J. P.; Baumeister, R. F. & Boone, A. L. (2004). High self–control predicts good adjustment, less pathology, better grades, and interpersonal success. *Journal of Personality, 72,* 271–324. Each of the noted mental problems are reported in this first article. Also see Bienvenu, O. J.; Nestadt, G., et al. (2001). Phobic, panic, and major depressive disorders and the five–factor model of personality. *Journal of Nervous & Mental Disease, 189,* 154–161; Bienvenu, O. J.; Samuels, J. F., et al. (2004). Anxiety and depressive disorders and the five–factor model of personality: A higher–and lower–order personality trait investigation in a community sample. *Depression & Anxiety, 20,* 92–97.

92. Beckmann, J. & Kellmann, M. (2004). Self–regulation and recovery: Approaching an understanding of the process of recovery from stress. *Psychological Reports, 95,* 1135–1153; Gramzow, R. H.; Sedikides, C., et al. (2000). Aspects of self–regulation and self–structure as predictors of perceived emotional distress. *Personality & Social Psychology Bulletin, 26,* 188–205.

93. The Brief Self Control Scale developed by June Tangney and her colleagues has 13 items that can literally be completed by a patient in less than two minutes. See endnote 91 above.

94. Karraker, K. H. (1986). Adult attention to infants in a newborn nursery. *Nursing Research, 35,* 358–363.

95. Stephan, C. W. & Langlois, J. H. (1984). Baby beautiful: Adult attributions of infant competence as a function of attractiveness. *Child Development, 55,* 576–585.

96. Samuels, C. A.; Butterworth, G., et al. (1994). Facial aesthetics: Babies prefer attractiveness to symmetry. *Perception, 23,* 823–831; Rubenstein, A. J.; Kalakanis, L. & Langlois, J. H. (1999). Infant preferences for attractive faces: A cognitive explanation. *Developmental Psychology, 35,* 848–855.

97. Salvia, J.; Sheare, J. B. & Algozzine, B. (1975). Facial attractiveness and personal–social development. *Journal of Abnormal Child Psychology, 3,* 171–178.

98. Shaw, W. C. (1981). The influence of children's dentofacial appearance on their social attractiveness as judged by peers and lay adults. *American Journal of Orthodontics, 79,* 399–415.

99. Dion, K. K. (1972). Physical attractiveness and evaluations of children's transgressions. *Journal of Personality & Social Psychology, 24,* 207–213.

100. Berkowitz, L. & Frodi, A. (1979). Reaction to a child's mistakes as affected by her/his looks and speech. *Social Psychology Quarterly, 42,* 420–425.

101. Reis, H. T.; Nezlek, J. & Wheeler, L. (1980). Physical attractiveness in social interaction. *Journal of Personality & Social Psychology, 38,* 604–617.

102. Pashos, A. & Niemitz, C. (2003). Results of an explorative empirical study on human mating in Germany: Handsome men, not high–status men, succeed in courtship. *Anthropologischer Anzeiger, 61,* 331–341.

103. Dollinger, S. J. (2002). Physical attractiveness, social connectedness, and individuality: An autophotographic study. *Journal of Social Psychology, 142,* 25–32.

104. Landy, D. & Sigall, H. (1974). Beauty is talent: Task evaluation as a function of the performer's physical attractiveness. *Journal of Personality & Social Psychology, 30,* 299–304.

105. Ibid.

106. Efran, M. G. (1974). The effect of physical appearance on the judgment of guilt, interpersonal attraction, and severity of recommended punishment in a simulated jury task.

Journal of Research in Personality, 8, 45–54. Not all studies find physical attractiveness results in an advantage for the perpetrator of a crime. See Villemur, N. K. & Hyde, J. S. (1983). Effects of sex of defense attorney, sex of juror, and age and attractiveness of the victim on mock juror decision making in a rape case. *Sex Roles, 9*, 879–889.

107. Mazzella, R. & Feingold, A. (1994). The effects of physical attractiveness, race, socioeconomic status, and gender on defendants and victims on judgments of mock jurors: A meta–analysis. *Journal of Applied Social Psychology, 24*, 1315–1344.

108. Lusnar, M. P. (1999). Job applicant stereotypes: Effects of eyeglasses and job type in a simulated interview. *Dissertation Abstracts International: Section B. The Sciences & Engineering, 60*, 0862. Interestingly, eyeglasses actually increased hiring for managerial positions.

109. Jawahar, I. M. & Mattsson, J. (2005). Sexism and beautyism effects in selection as a function of self–monitoring level of decision maker. *Journal of Applied Psychology, 90*, 563–573; Dubois, M. & Pansu, P. (2004). Facial attractiveness, applicants' qualifications, and judges' expertise about decisions in preselective recruitment. *Psychological Reports, 95*, 1129–1134.

110. Dipboye, R. L.; Fromkin, H. L. & Wilback, K. (1975). Relative importance of applicant sex, attractiveness, and scholastic standing in evaluation of job applicant resumes. *Journal of Applied Psychology, 60*, 39–43.

111. Dipboye, R. L.; Arvey, R. D. & Terpstra, D. E. (1977). Sex and physical attractiveness of raters and applicants as determinants of resume evaluations. *Journal of Applied Psychology, 62*, 288–294.

112. Frieze, I. H.; Olson, J. E. & Russell, J. (1991). Attractiveness and income for men and women in management. *Journal of Applied Social Psychology, 21*, 1039–1057.

113. Walling, A.; Montello, M., et al. (2004). Which patients are the most challenging for second–year medical students? *Family Medicine, 36*, 710–714.

114. Harris, S. M. & Busby, D. M. (1998). Therapist physical attractiveness: An unexplored influence on client disclosure. *Journal of Marital & Family Therapy, 24*, 251–257.

115. Dion, K. L & Dion, K. K. (1987). Belief in a just world and physical attractiveness stereotyping. *Journal of Personality & Social Psychology, 52*, 775–780.

116. Dion, K.; Berscheid, E. & Walster (Hatfield), E. (1972). What is beautiful is good. *Journal of Personality & Social Psychology, 24*, 285–290.

117. Schumacher, M.; Corrigan, P. W. & Dejong, T. (2003). Examining cues that signal mental illness stigma. *Journal of Social & Clinical Psychology, 22*, 467–476; Feignold, A. (1992). Good–looking people are not what we think. *Psychological Bulletin, 111*, 304–341.

118. Diener, E; Wolsic, B. & Fujita, F. (1995). Physical attractiveness and subjective well–being. *Journal of Personality & Social Psychology, 69*, 120–129. In this study the benefit of attractiveness on subjective well–being was surprisingly small, perhaps because of the study's design (a problem noted by the authors). Also see the following study which found 23 mental hospital patients were decidedly less attractive than 30 university employees and 29 shoppers (Farina, A.; Fischer, E. H., et al. [1977]. Physical attractiveness and mental illness. *Journal of Abnormal Psychology, 86*, 510–517). A replication and extension of the study yielded a clear pattern: Unattractive people are more likely to have a mental illness (Napolean, T.; Chassin, L. & Young, R. D. [1980]. A replication and extension of "Physical attractiveness and mental illness." *Journal of Abnormal Psychology, 89*, 250–253).

119. Langlois, J.; Kalakanis, L., et al. (2000). Maxims or myths of beauty? A meta–analytic and theoretical review. *Psychological Bulletin, 126*, 390–423; Shaffer, D. R.; Crepaz, N. & Sun, C. R. (2000). Physical attractiveness in cross–cultural perspective:

Similarities and differences between Americans and Taiwanese. *Journal of Cross–Cultural Psychology, 31*, 557–582.

120. Heinberg, L. J. & Thompson, J. K. (1995). Body image and televised images of thinness and attractiveness: A controlled laboratory investigation. *Journal of Social & Clinical Psychology, 14*, 325–338. The effect in this study was found in those with higher concerns about their body image and sociocultural attitudes concerning appearance. For a similar study see Cattarin, J. A.; Thompson, J. K., et al. (2000). Body image, mood, and televised images of attractiveness: The role of social comparison. *Journal of Social & Clinical Psychology, 19*, 220–239.

121. I suspect that men would also be affected though this effect would likely be less for men. Unfortunately, I know of no equivalent study that used men instead of women.

122. Cattarin, J. A. (1997). The impact of televised images of thinness and attractiveness in body image: The role of social comparison. *Dissertation Abstracts International: Section B. The Sciences & Engineering, 57*, 4697.

123. Brennan, T. (1982). Loneliness at adolescence in Peplau, L. A. & Perlman, D., eds. *Loneliness: A Sourcebook of Current Theory*. New York: Wiley, pp. 269–290.

124. The overall difference between males and females appears to be about 2 per 100,000 for males versus 18 per 100,000 for females. However, teenage girls have been found to have a rate of 50.82 per 100,000 (Pawluck, D. E. & Gorey, K. M. [1998]. Secular trends in the incidence of anorexia nervosa: Integrative review of population–based studies. *International Journal of Eating Disorders, 23*, 347–352). A rate of 269.9 per 100,000 per lifetime has been reported by Lucas, et al. (Lucas, A. R.; Beard, C. M., et al. [1991]. 50–year trends in the incidence of anorexia nervosa in Rochester, Minnesota: A population–based study. *American Journal of Psychiatry, 148*, 917–922). An even higher rate for a sample of urban Swedish 16–year–olds was reported, 700 per 100,000 for girls and 100 per 100,000 for boys (Rastam, M.; Gillberg, C. & Garton, M. [1989]. Anorexia nervosa in a Swedish urban region: A population–based study. *British Journal of Psychiatry, 155*, 642–646). Western countries have higher rates, but as media images are increasingly common in non–Western countries, the incidence is increasing there as well (Makino, M; Tsuboi, K. & Dennerstein, L. [2004]. Prevalence of eating disorders: A comparison of Western and non–Western countries. *Medscape General Medicine, 6*, 49).

125. See, for example, Klump, K. L. & Gobrogge, K. L. (2005). A review and primer of molecular genetic studies of anorexia nervosa. *International Journal of Eating Disorders, 37* (Suppl.), S43–S48.

126. Hoek, H. W. & van Hoeken, D. (2003). Review of the prevalence and incidence of eating disorders. *International Journal of Eating Disorders, 34*, 383–396; Eagles, J. M.; Easton, E. A., et al. (1999). Changes in the presenting features of females with anorexia nervosa in northeast Scotland, 1965–1991. *International Journal of Eating Disorders, 26*, 289–294; Milos, G.; Spindler, A., et al. (2004). Incidence of severe anorexia nervosa in Switzerland: 40 years of development. *International Journal of Eating Disorders, 35*, 250–258. This third study indicates the rise reached a plateau about 1980. Also see Lucas, A. R.; Crowson, C. S., et al. (1999). The ups and downs of anorexia nervosa. *International Journal of Eating Disorders, 26*, 397–405 and Feingold, A. & Mazzella, R. (1998). Gender differences in body image are increasing. *Psychological Science, 9*, 190–195.

127. Stice, E.; Spangler, D. & Agras, W. S. (2001). Exposure to media–portrayed thin–ideal images adversely affects vulnerable girls: A longitudinal experiment. *Journal of Social & Clinical Psychology, 20*, 270–288. Also see Stice, E. & Shaw, H. E. (1994). Adverse effects of the media portrayed thin–ideal on women and linkages to bulimic symptomatology. *Journal of Social & Clinical Psychology, 13*, 288–308.

128.   Irving showed slides of thin, average or heavy models to three different experiment groups of women. He also included a no exposure control group (Irving, L. M. [1990]. Mirror images: Effects of the standard of beauty on the self– and body–esteem of women exhibiting varying levels of bulimic symptoms. *Journal of Social & Clinical Psychology, 9*, 230–242.

129.   Cash, T. F.; Cash, D. W. & Butters, J. W. (1983). "Mirror, mirror, on the wall...?": Contrast effects and self–evaluations of physical attractiveness. *Personality & Social Psychology Bulletin, 9*, 351–358; Kenrick, D. T. & Gutierres, S. E. (1980). Contrast effects and judgments of physical attractiveness: When beauty becomes a social problem. *Journal of Personality & Social Psychology, 38*, 131–140.

130.   Weaver, J. B.; Masland, J. L. & Zillman, D. (1984). Effect of erotica on young men's aesthetic perception of their female sexual partners. *Perceptual & Motor Skills, 58*, 929–930.

131.   Polivy, J. & Herman, C. P. (2002). Causes of eating disorders. *Annual Review of Psychology, 53*, 187–213.

132.   Maharaj, S. I.; Rodin, G. M., et al. (2003). Eating disturbances in girls with diabetes: The contribution of adolescent self–concept, maternal weight and shape concerns and mother–daughter relationships. *Psychological Medicine, 33*, 525–539; Pike, K. M.; Rodin, J. (1991). Mothers, daughters, and disordered eating. *Journal of Abnormal Psychology, 100*, 198–204; Hill, A. J. & Franklin, J. A. (1998). Mothers, daughters and dieting: Investigating the transmission of weight control. *British Journal of Clinical Psychology, 37* (Pt. 1), 3–13.

133.   Carnegie, D. (1935). *How to Win Friends and Influence People*, rev. ed. New York: Pocket Books, 1981.

134.   Ibid., p. 105.

135.   Matthew 22:37–39, *The Holy Bible* (New International Version).

136.   Philippians 2:3–4, ibid.

137.   Freeman, L. (1951). *Fight Against Fears*. New York: Crown Publishers, p. 18.

138.   Ibid., p. 23.

139.   Ibid., p. 113.

140.   Ibid.

141.   Ibid., pp. 44–45.

142.   Ibid., p. 330.

143.   Ibid., p. 332.

144.   Frankl, V. E. (1962). *Man's Search for Meaning*, trans. Losch, I.   New York: Simon & Schuster.

145.   Ibid.

146.   Maslow, A. H. (1970). *Religions, Values and Peak Experiences*. New York: The Viking Press.

147.   The only text I used which mentioned purpose in life was Rathus, S. A. (1984). *Psychology*, 2nd ed. New York: CBS College Publishing. Rathus provided a discussion of Salvatore Maddi's term "existential neurosis" which was caused by a lack of purpose and led to anxiety and depression. For Maddi's article, see Maddi, S. R. (1967). The existential neurosis. *Journal of Abnormal Psychology, 72*, 311–325.

148.   Clarke, D. M. & Kissane, D. W. (2002). Demoralization: Its phenomenology and importance. *Australian & New Zealand Journal of Psychiatry, 36*, 733–742. Demoralization is a broad term which quite literally would mean "removing morals." However, in psychology and psychiatry it refers to a state of hopelessness, meaninglessness and despair.

149.   Cherry, L. (Mar. 1978). On the real benefits of eustress. *Psychology Today, 12*, 60–70. Selye's life illustrates how believing one's work is very important brings joy and

believing one's own work is meaningless can bring depression. Selye searched for a new hormone, injecting rats with ovary tissue extracts. The results were dramatic—an enlarged adrenal cortex, a reduced thymus gland, and bleeding ulcers. He later described his emotional reaction to his discovery. "You may well imagine my happiness! At the age of 28, I already seemed to be on the track of a new hormone" (Selye, H. [1976]. *The Stress of Life* [rev. ed.]. New York: McGraw–Hill, p. 25). He then had a "horrible thought . . . this entire syndrome might be due merely to the toxicity of my extracts" (ibid., p. 26). He decided to inject toxic fluids into the rats hoping the same reaction would not occur, but it did. "I do not think I had ever been more profoundly disappointed! Suddenly all my dreams of discovering a new hormone were shattered . . . . I tried to tell myself over and over again that such disappointments are inevitable in a scientist's life . . . . But all this gave me little solace and, indeed, I became so depressed that for a few days I could not do any work at all" (ibid., p. 28).

150. Warren, R. (2002). *The Purpose Driven Life.* Grand Rapids, MI: Zondervan.

151. Van Biema, D.; Booth–Thomas, C., et al. (Feb. 7, 2005). The 25 most influential evangelicals in America. *Time,* 34–43, p. 45.

152. Astin, A. W.; Oseguera, L., et al. (2002). *The American Freshman: Fifty–Five Year Trends.* Los Angeles: Higher Education Research Institute, UCLA, p. 16. The one year in which there was no increase was 1985.

153. Myers, D. (1993). *The Pursuit of Happiness.* New York: Avon Books. Myers' book made a real contribution to this subject. His analysis is excellent and his conclusions, well documented.

154. Those who consume more alcohol and drugs have been found in literally thousands of studies to have less joy—more depression. See for example Cottler, L. B. & Campbell, W. (2005). Predictors of high rates of suicidal ideation among drug users. *Journal of Nervous & Mental Disease, 193,* 431–437.

155. There are hundreds of studies on the inferior mental health of those who engage in premarital sex, cohabitation or extramarital sex. Occasionally a study is designed that seems to want to hide this fact. One example of this is the following study that controlled for "premarital levels of mental health" and then compared cohabitors and others. (Depression *is* a part of mental health, and comorbidity is widely reported for depression and other mental health problems.) Horwitz, A. V. & White, H. R. (1998). The relationship of cohabitation and mental health: A study of a young adult cohort. *Journal of Marriage & the Family, 60,* 505–514. Of course, this study, in effect, concludes that those who are more mentally unstable are more likely to cohabit.

156. Durkheim, E. (1951). *Suicide, A Study in Sociology,* trans. Spaulding, J. A. & Simpson, G. Glencoe, IL: Free Press. Originally published in French, 1897.

157. James, W. (1902/1985). *The Varieties of Religious Experience.* Cambridge, MA: Harvard University Press, p. 71.

158. This analogy is made in most of the antidepressant literature found in doctors' offices and in "education" literature produced by various organizations supported by the drug companies.

159. Effexor XR website available at http://www.effexorxr.com/depression.asp.

160. Ibid.

161. Ibid.

162. In the following study the rejected students knew who they were as did their peers and their teachers. Some students, however, saw themselves as "victims" though they were not rated so by peers (Graham, S.; Bellmore, A. & Juvonen, J. [2003]. Peer harassment in

middle school: When self–views and peer views diverge. *Journal of Applied School Psychology 19*, 117–137).

163. The quote is from NARSAD's (National Alliance for Research on Schizophrenia and Depression) "Depression. A flaw in chemistry, not character" ad campaign. The ad can still be found in some psychology textbooks. Their brochure on depression, "Conquering Depression," (available free by request) shares the same message. The brochure "was funded by an educational grant from Wyeth–Ayerst Laboratories" (noted inside the next to last page).

164. Minirth, F. B. & Meier, P. D. (1978). *Happiness Is A Choice.* Grand Rapids, MI: Baker Book House, p. 195.

Epilogue

1. Avorn, J. (2005). FDA standards—good enough for government work? *New England Journal of Medicine, 353*, 969–972.

2. Barnes, D. E. & Bero, L. A. (1998). Why review articles on the health effects of passive smoking reach different conclusions. *JAMA, 279*, 1566–1570.

3. Barnes, D. E. & Bero, L. A. (1996). Industry–funded research and conflict of interest: An analysis of research sponsored by the tobacco industry through the Center for Indoor Air Research. *Journal of Health Politics, Policy & Law, 21*, 515–542; Cho, M. K. & Bero, L. A. (1996). The quality of drug studies published in symposium proceedings. *Annals of Internal Medicine, 124*, 485–489; Rochon, P. A.; Gurwitz, J. H., et al. (1994). A study of manufacturer–supported trials of nonsteroidal anti–inflammatory drugs in the treatment of arthritis. *Archives of Internal Medicine, 154*, 157–163; Gotzsche, P. C. (1989). Methodology and overt and hidden bias in reports of 196 double–blind trials of non–steroidal antiinflammatory drugs in rheumatoid arthritis. *Controlled Clinical Trials, 10*, 31–56; Davidson, R. A. (1986). Source of funding and outcomes of clinical trials. *Journal of General Internal Medicine, 1*, 155–158; Swaen, G. M. H. & Meijers, J. M. M. (1988). Influence of design characteristics on the outcome of retrospective cohort studies. *British Journal of Industrial Medicine, 45*, 624–629.

4. Chapter 8 discusses the minimal or placebo–only effectiveness of antidepressants. Thorazine was again reviewed by The Cochrane Collaboration in 2003. The review concluded chlorpromazine (Thorazine) is "effective compared with placebo," but notes "the placebo response is also considerable" (Thornley, B.; Rathbone, J., et al. [2003]. Chlorpromazine versus placebo for schizophrenia. *Cochrane Database of Systematic Reviews* (*2*):CD000284). This review also stated, "Chlorpromazine is clearly sedating" (and, they noted, causes movement disorders, parkinsonism, lowered blood pressure, dizziness, and weight gain). Chapter 12 discusses the sedating (chemical lobotomy effect of this drug. If a more controlled patient is the goal, Thorazine is undoubtedly better than placebo. If recovery is the goal, using a placebo rather than Thorazine will increase the chances of having that outcome.

5. This fact is widely known but is discussed by Item 8 under the first question "What are generic drugs?" of the FDA's website available at http://www.fda.gov/cder/consumer info/generics_q&a.htm#whatare.

6. Matthew, A. W. (Aug. 24, 2005). Detective work: Reading fine print, insurers question studies of drugs. *Wall Street Journal*, A.1.

7. Ibid.

8. Medicare is scheduled to become the nation's largest purchaser of drugs in 2006. As of this writing, the legislation has not become law, and budgetary concerns could derail this development.

Endnotes, Appendices

Appendix 1 — Getting Off Antidepressants

1. van Geffen, E. C.; Hugtenburg, J. C., et al. (2005). Discontinuation symptoms in users of selective serotonin reuptake inhibitors in clinical practice: Tapering versus abrupt discontinuation. *European Journal of Clinical Pharmacology, 61*, 303–307. This study used a small number of subjects (66), and most of these tapered off the antidepressants. Of the 14 who ended their antidepressant abruptly, 12 experienced discontinuation symptoms, slightly more than twice the number who tapered off these drugs. Particularly prone to cause discontinuation problems were the antidepressants with short half–lives. Antidepressants with longer half–lives stay in the body longer. Thus, abruptly ending the drug is not as strong a shock to the body.
2. Examples include Ditto, K. E. (2003). SSRI discontinuation syndrome: Awareness as an approach to prevention. *Postgraduate Medicine, 114*, 79–84; Margetic, B. & Aukst–Margetic, B. (2005). Neuroleptic malignant syndrome and clozapine withdrawal at the same time? *Progress in Neuro–psychopharmacology & Biological Psychiatry, 29*, 145–147; Kim, D. R. & Staab, J. P. (2005). Quetiapine discontinuation syndrome. *American Journal of Psychiatry, 162*, 1020.
3. Yerevanian, B. I.; Koek, R. J., et al. (2004). Antidepressants and suicidal behaviour in unipolar depression. *Acta Psychiatrica Scandinavica, 110*, 452–458.
4. Glenmullen, J. (2005). The 5–step antidepressant tapering program: How to avoid uncomfortable or dangerous withdrawal reactions (Ch. 6) in *The Antidepressant Solution*. New York: Free Press, pp. 90–100.

Appendix 2 — The *British Medical Journal* Controversy

1. Lenzer, J. (2005). FDA to review "missing" drug company documents. *British Medical Journal, 330*, 7.
2. The stock dropped 75¢ per share, the equivalent of $814 million.
3. Meier, B. (Jan. 17, 2005). Dispute puts a medical journal under fire. *NY Times*, C.1.
4. *British Medical Journal* (2005). Eli Lilly: Correction and apology. *330*, 211.
5. Associated Press, January 27, 2005.
6. Available on the web at http://www.msnbc.msn.com/id/6875515/Jan27,2005.
7. Swiatek, J. (Jan. 27, 2005). *BMJ* recants, says Lilly disclosed Prozac research. *Knight–Ridder/Tribune Business News* reported in the *Indianapolis Star*, C.1.

Appendix 3 — The Real Reasons for the Decline in Mental Hospital Population

1. The population in 1850 (June 1) was 23,191,876. It was 152,271,000 (July 1) in 1950. (U.S. Bureau of Census [1990]. *Statistical Abstract of the U.S.*, 110th ed. Washington, D. C.: U.S. Government Printing Office, p. 7). The 1850 mental hospital total was 4,730 (Torrey, E. F. & Miller, J. [2001]. *The Invisible Plague*. New Brunswick, NJ: Rutgers University Press, Appendix C, Table 4). The 1950 mental hospital total was 512,501 (U.S. Bureau of Census [1965]. *Statistical Abstract of the U.S.*, 85th ed. Washington, D. C.: U.S. Government Printing Office, Table 96, p. 77).
2. Torrey and Miller's *The Invisible Plague* argues that there were measurable increases for over two hundred years in both Great Britain and in the U.S. The authors offer a fairly compelling argument supported by a host of statistics which point to an actual rise in mental illnesses. Though they are unsure as to how the rise can best be explained, they point to

urbanization as one predictor of mental instability increases, though this is not always predictive (Torrey, E. F. & Miller J. [2001]. *The Invisible Plague*. New Brunswick, NJ: Rutgers University Press).

3.   The number of insane as reported by the Census Bureau was underestimated, an admission made by the Census Bureau according to a report produced by The Council of State Governments (The Council of State Governments [1950]. *The Mental Health Programs of the Forty–Eight States*. Chicago: The Council of State Governments, p. 30).

4.   Ibid.

5.   Johnson, A. B. (1990). *Out of Bedlam*. New York: Basic Books, p. 17.

6.   Grob, G. N. (1983). *Mental Illness and American Society, 1875–1940*. Princeton, NJ: Princeton University Press, p. 92 in ibid.

7.   The Council of State Governments (1950). *The Mental Health Programs of the Forty–Eight States*, p. 4. Also see p. 42f.

8.   Solomon, H. (1958). The American Psychiatric Association in relation to American psychiatry. *American Journal of Psychiatry, 115*, 8.

9.   An exception was the attention the issue received in Ohio even in the midst of WWII. Conscientious objectors to the war were allowed to serve in other roles. Some were sent to mental hospitals where they helped care for the patients. In 1943 a group of these conscientious objectors approached the head of the Cleveland Baptist Association and a reporter for the Cleveland Press. The conscientious objectors reported that patients were put in chains, starved, beaten and abused in other ways. Their stories seemed too extreme to be fully credible, but, sadly, when investigated, they were found to be all too true. The end result was a state investigation, a number of firings and resignations, and a commitment by the Ohio legislature to construct additional hospitals to reduce crowding. However, the whole affair remained an essentially Ohio matter—until 1946 when it was discussed in a *Life* magazine article.

10.   *Encyclopaedia Britannica*, Vol. 26 (2002). Publishing: News and photo magazines. Chicago: Encyclopaedia Britannica, Inc., p. 445.

11.   Swanberg. W. A. (1972). *Luce and His Empire*. New York: Charles Scribner's Sons, p. 144.

12.   Baughman, J. L. (1987). *Henry R. Luce and the Rise of the American News Media*. Boston: Twayne Publishers, p. 93.

13.   Ibid., p. 94. Baughman notes that *Life*'s circulation was less than *Collier*'s and the *Saturday Evening Post*. However, *Life* was passed from one person to another so often that it was read more than any other magazine. The quotation "more readers every week than any other magazine in history" is from *Life* magazine itself. This is the boast that commonly appeared within the pages of the magazine in the form of a small ad. See, for example, p. 112 of the May 6, 1946, edition.

14.   W. Rich to Frank Norris, July 5, 1940, Daniel Longwell Papers, Box 29, Columbia University, New York City, as quoted in Baughman, J. L. (1987). *Henry R. Luce and the Rise of the American News Media*. Boston: Twayne Publishers, p. 2.

15.   Ibid., p. 94.

16.   Ibid., p. 170.

17.   Baughman reports that in 1955 38.8% of *Life*'s subscribers were professionals or proprietors though only 7% of the nation's residents could claim these titles at that time (ibid., p. 170).

18.   Maisel, A. Q. (May 6, 1946). Bedlam 1946. *Life, 20*(18), pp. 102–110, 112, 115, 116, 118.

19. Ward, M. J. (1946). *The Snake Pit.* New York: Random House, p. 217.

20. Before WWII began, Albert Deutsch, a social historian, published *The Mentally Ill in America* (1937). Because it was a scholarly work, it is not likely the publisher or Deutsch expected to sell many copies, yet it underwent several reprintings. It was not a book widely read by the public, but it was undoubtedly shaping the opinions of those Americans who had a particular interest in the mentally ill. Deutsch had studied the care and treatment of the mentally ill from colonial times up until the time in which he wrote and concluded that mental institutions were growing progressively worse. He clearly desired to change the status quo, but once WWII began, being heard on this issue was almost impossible. *The Shame of the States,* the *Life* exposé, and *The Snake Pit* opened doors for Deutsch to push even harder for reform. Deutsch wrote articles for magazines, gave interviews to newspapers and testified before government bodies who could no longer ignore their mental hospitals. The Great Depression and WWII had distracted America and harmed both national and state finances. The mental hospitals suffered, but now the entire nation was aware of this national embarrassment.

21. The Council of State Governments, Frank Bane, executive director (1950). *The Mental Health Programs of the Forty–Eight States: A Report to the Governors' Conference.* Chicago: The Council of State Governments, p. 1.

22. Solomon, H. (1958). The American Psychiatry Association in relation to American psychiatry. *American Journal of Psychiatry, 115,* 1–9, p. 7.

23. That admission also added momentum to the community mental health movement. When Congress passed the Community Mental Health Centers Act in 1963, even more of those who had lived in state mental hospitals for years were moved out to community housing or back into their families' homes. No, it wasn't Thorazine that was responsible for the declines. In his speech published in 1958 in the APA's *American Journal of Psychiatry* (ibid.) the APA President Dr. Harry Solomon noted that ever since the middle of the 1800s the superintendents of the nation's mental hospitals stressed that the best environment for those who had lost their minds required small hospitals with populations never exceeding 250 patients. Dr. Solomon did not indicate any awareness that the patient population was already dropping, but he did observe that "several states are experimenting with new types of facilities" and then suggested that these developments "have the potential for reducing the number of chronic patients and to lessen the need for beds." He was right, and the numbers were dropping as he spoke.

24. The Department of Health and Human Services has a website that provides an overview of "Medicaid Financing of State and County Psychiatric Hospitals." It is available at http://www.mentalhealth.org/publications/allpubs/SMA03–3830/content02.asp#1.

25. The decline was not more than 15,000 for any year prior to 1965. Between 1965 and 1966 the decline was approximately 23,000 (475,000 down to 452,000) (U.S. Bureau of Census [1970]. *Statistical Abstract of the U.S.* Washington, D. C.: U.S. Government Printing Office, Table 98, p. 73).

26. The decline was from 452,000 down to 426,000 (ibid.).

27. The decline was from 426,000 down to 399,000 (ibid.).

28. Kiesler, C. A. (1982). Mental hospitals and alternative care: Noninstitutionalization as potential public policy for mental patients. *American Psychologist, 37,* 349–360.

INDEX